Praise for
GET OFF YOUR ACID

"*Get Off Your Acid* is a must read in today's toxic world. My mission in life is spreading the truth about cancer so people can live healthy, cancer-free lives. And this is personal. Both Dr. Daryl and I lost our fathers to cancer. Everyone today suffers from this epidemic in one way or another. So knowing what causes cancer, and what prevents it, could save you or someone you love. This book empowers you to live your best life and truly prevent all chronic disease, including cancer, with smart choices."

—Ty Bollinger, *The Truth About Cancer*

"Food can either be a destructive force that leads to epidemic illness and degradation, or it can be a powerful tool that will vastly lower rates of chronic illness and improve the lives of people everywhere. *Get Off Your Acid* will help you to make wise choices, so that the food you eat can help propel you toward the health you deserve. Read it and put it into action. You'll be reaping the benefits for the rest of your life."

—Ocean Robbins, CEO, Food Revolution Network

"I'm so in love with the *Get Off Your Acid* program and the Alkamind Daily Greens and Daily Minerals. The alkaline supplements are my secret weapon for staying healthy, whether I'm at home or traveling. They are convenient, delicious, and effective!"

—Petra Nemcova, founder, All Hands and Hearts Foundation

"Dr. Daryl Gioffre is brilliant—no one like him. I work long days on the set of TV shows and would not be without my alkaline green drinks. Forget coffee, sugar, carbs—*Get Off Your Acid* is what gets me through a tough day. It gives me pure clean energy and great clarity of mind."

—Tracey Ullman, actress, comedian, singer, dancer, screenwriter, and author

"Dr. Daryl Gioffre's desire to help others comes from a very deep, special place rooted in years of commitment to his craft combined with the emotional, personal experience of dealing with his father's tryst with stage IV esophageal cancer. I understand this at a visceral level because a few decades ago, as a young 'alternative' cancer physician, I was able to help my own father successfully navigate away from advanced prostate cancer in what became a pivotal milestone in my career. It was an honor that Dr. Gioffre included me in his father's journey—a remarkable one that defied all odds, extending his survival from months to years with a high quality of life. I passionately share Dr. Gioffre's belief that taking the right steps today can help anyone, regardless of their genetic predisposition, to prevent cancer and other chronic diseases. To that end, I believe this book holds significant knowledge to unlock your potential well-being—it is a must read!"

—Antonio Jiminez, MD, ND, founder and Chief Medical Officer, Hope4Cancer Institute

"Traveling the world, searching for the biggest waves Mother Nature can offer, has led to me needing to be in peak physical, mental, and spiritual health at all times. The *Get Off Your Acid* way of life and alkaline supplements are highly effective and everything I need to keep me at the top of my game. Big thanks to Dr. Daryl Gioffre and Alkamind—I can come home to my family in one piece."

—Garrett McNamara, Guinness World Record Big Wave Champion

"There is a crisis of epidemic proportions within the blood and cells of virtually every American—and it is unleashing tragic consequences on millions of lives each year by rapidly accelerating diseases and dysfunction. Heart attacks, dementia, and diabetes will cripple the US economy, and these are increasing each year because of the fundamental nutritional imbalances that health visionary Dr. Daryl Gioffre has uncovered through arduous self-study and clinical experience. But just as careful and comprehensive in his approach to learning the root causes of most all major diseases, Gioffre brings a highly efficient, effective, and refreshing approach that drives true lifelong change. His tactics against the acid battle we all find ourselves in as a result of the plethora of toxic options around us result in lives that flourish—chemically, structurally, and functionally."

—Daniel T. Johnston, MD, MPH, CEO, and founder of BrainSpan, LLC

"With obesity rates being what they are, eating clean is a big deal in our house. As parents, it's important to model healthy eating for our kids and show them what a sensible plate looks like. We feel our best when we're taking care of ourselves physically, and that's what Dr. Daryl's book, *Get Off Your Acid*, has done for us. We're able to eat delicious food and be the healthiest versions of ourselves. Thank you, Dr. Daryl!"

—Mario and Courtney Lopez

GET OFF YOUR ACID

7 STEPS IN 7 DAYS
to Lose Weight, Fight Inflammation, and Reclaim Your Health and Energy

DR. DARYL GIOFFRE

Foreword by Kelly Ripa

Da Capo
LIFE
LONG

Da Capo Press
Hachette Book Group
1290 Avenue of the Americas, New York, NY 10104
www.dacapopress.com
@DaCapoPress

Printed in the United States of America
First Edition: January 2018

Published by Da Capo Press, an imprint of Perseus Books, LLC,
a subsidiary of Hachette Book Group, Inc.
The Da Capo name and logo is a trademark of the Hachette Book Group.

The Hachette Speakers Bureau provides a wide range of authors for speaking events.
To find out more, go to www.hachettespeakersbureau.com or call (866) 376-6591.

The publisher is not responsible for websites (or their content)
that are not owned by the publisher.

Note: The information in this book is true and complete to the best of our knowledge. This book is intended only as an informative guide for those wishing to know more about health issues. In no way is this book intended to replace, countermand, or conflict with the advice given to you by your own physician. The ultimate decision concerning care should be made between you and your doctor. We strongly recommend you follow his or her advice. Information in this book is general and is offered with no guarantees on the part of the authors or Da Capo Press. The authors and publisher disclaim all liability in connection with the use of this book.

Editorial production by Lori Hobkirk at the Book Factory
Print book interior design by Sagecraft Book Design
Cover design by Kerry Rubenstein
Interior graphics by Chris Cook

Library of Congress Cataloging-in-Publication Data has been applied for.
ISBNs: 978-0-7382-1992-9 (paperback); 978-0-7382-1993-6 (ebook)

LSC-C

10   9   8   7   6   5   4   3

For my father, and for every soul battling cancer.
Your bravery is beyond measure.
My work, and this book, is for you.

CONTENTS

PART III

ALKALINE RECIPES TO GET OFF YOUR ACID, 187

FOREWORD
by Kelly Ripa

Dr. Daryl and his plan are incredible. Our family pediatrician introduced me to him after my daughter came home sick from camp. Right around the same time, I had been experiencing unusual aches and pains at night. It was a general achiness in my elbows and knees. Overall, we both weren't feeling our best.

When Dr. Daryl recommended that we try his 7-Day Alkaline Cleanse, I wasn't sure what to expect but agreed to do it in solidarity with my daughter. The one sacrifice I would not make, though, was giving up my morning coffee each day. He assured me that the program was so effective that, even if I only followed 80 percent of guidelines, we would still see significant results.

By day three of the cleanse, my aches were surprisingly gone. My energy had skyrocketed, I was sleeping more deeply, and I even felt stronger during workouts. It was clear my body was in an overall healthier state. Dr. Daryl explained that any pain and lack of energy we experience is normally due to inflammation—a direct result of too much acid in the body. I was surprised by how much I still had to learn about acidity and its effects on our overall well being. One example

that was completely transformative during this cleanse was learning that while I drink water all day, everyday, I was drinking *sparkling* water—a carbonated beverage—which is incredibly acidic.

At the same time, my daughter was also experiencing amazing results of her own. Her symptoms disappeared, her energy increased, and her hair and skin were glowing. An already youthful young lady with a natural glow, she was even more radiant during the cleanse.

What I like most about Dr. Daryl's method is that it's not a "diet" but more of a lifestyle change. There's no counting calories or limiting portion sizes, only a new awareness of "alkaline eating." Once you learn the difference between alkaline and acidic ingredients, you will know what to eat and will be able to benefit from keeping this balance in your bodies.

This is now part of my daily routine. Whether I'm adding Dr. Daryl's Organic Daily Protein Powder to my morning smoothies or having one of his avocado recipes for lunch, I know that what I'm eating is providing me with the fuel I need to juggle my busy schedule and continue to intensify my workouts. At the end of the day, I feel healthy, balanced, and strong, *and* I'm still able to end the days with Dr. Daryl's chocolate mousse and chia pudding recipes. They're to die for!

Whether your goal is to lose weight, sleep deeper, feel more rested, think more clearly, or boost your energy, this plan will get you there. It provides a wealth of information about the importance of alkaline and offers the results you need while allowing you to truly enjoy the food you're eating!

INTRODUCTION

The Text Message
That Changed My Life

It was one week before one of the most anticipated days in New York City: Marathon Sunday. The weather was 70 degrees, sunny, and there was not a cloud in the sky. It couldn't have been a more perfect day for my final 10-mile practice run in Central Park before the big race.

Although I had run other marathons and even competed in triathlons before, something felt extra special about this race. New York City is my hometown, it would be my first time running the NYC Marathon, and I was running to raise money for charity. In addition, my wife and newly arrived six-month-old son, Brayden, would be cheering me on, along with my parents who were coming down for the big event. I had a lot to be grateful for.

I was feeling great on mile 8 when the call came in. In an instant, my life and the lives of my family would be turned upside down.

I felt the vibration in my pocket and pulled out my phone to see a missed call from one of my brothers. I decided to call him back after the run, but being the goofball brother I am, I snapped a crazy selfie midstride and texted it to him, then put the phone back in my pocket.

I continued running, but in a matter of seconds, I felt my phone vibrate a few more times. I took my phone out again and saw another missed call and two text messages: "ANSWER!!!!—EMERGENCY!" My heart sank. Without speaking to anyone, I knew it was about my father.

I called my brother immediately, and he proceeded to tell me that there had been an accident. My parents were driving in the HOV lane of a highway, going 70 mph, when my mom noticed their car was veering off the road toward the concrete divider. She looked over to see my father passed out at the steering wheel. His head was against the window, his foot still on the accelerator.

Her instincts took over, and she quickly leaned down and tried to pull his leg off the gas pedal, but couldn't. The car drove up onto the concrete divider, then back down. As the car began to ride back up the divider for a second time, she pulled the keys out of the ignition. Miraculously, the car came to a slow, grinding halt. She looked over at my dad, who looked lifeless.

I will never forget hearing this story from my mom a little later that day. She thought Dad had had a heart attack or stroke. I could not imagine what that moment must have been like for her, thinking he was gone. He was unconscious for an entire two minutes (which seemed like an eternity), but then he came to, started sweating profusely, and then passed out again. He woke again and over a few minutes gained full consciousness by the time the ambulance arrived.

At the hospital, he had an EKG and all the other heart tests. A heart attack and stroke were immediately ruled out and a CT scan of his brain was normal. The doctors then learned he'd had some dark blood in his stool for quite some time and wanted to do an endoscopy to look down his esophagus where it meets the stomach. I mentally put the pieces together: *internal bleeding, digested blood . . . something's not right in the upper digestive tract.* Afterward they dropped the bombshell. The word that everyone fears: cancer.

The next few days were excruciating, as uncertainty took over and every thought became consumed by my worst fears. Hard as you try to block negative thoughts, reality brings them right back. And it was impossible to keep focused on the things I needed to attend to: being present with my patients, my son, and my family. Those were the longest days of my life. But as with any challenge, you step up, find your strength, and come up with a game plan.

My brothers and I immediately sprang into action. Between the three of us, we were able to arrange a meeting with one of New York City's top oncologists at Sloan Kettering. We had the very first appointment at 8 a.m. After our appointment, I would head straight to the first annual NYC Holistic Chamber of Commerce Health and Wellness Expo, an event I was spearheading with a keynote speech. It was going to be a big day in many ways—and in retrospect, those two events became inextricably intertwined.

Most esophageal cancers, growing into an empty space, are not discovered until a very late stage, when you cannot swallow or eat anymore. By then, the cancer is much more advanced, harder to treat, and far more likely to have spread into the lymph and other parts of the body. Looking back, the horrific experience my mom and dad had endured turned out to be a blessing.

Because of the accident, as terrifying as it was, the cancer had been caught early. It became apparent that the cancer inside my dad's body was localized and had not metastasized or spread. With that knowledge, we all experienced a palpable relief. Though the road ahead still looked daunting, the prognosis gave us hope.

An amazing thing to happen during this trying time was the doctor's pronouncement of the cause of my father's cancer. No one could believe it when we learned the root cause of the condition, verbatim from the doctor's mouth, was "too much acid!"

When he said it, my jaw dropped, and everyone in the room looked directly at me. I was wearing a black shirt that proclaimed in bold lettering, "GET OFF YOUR ACID"—the tagline of my new company.

My research into excess acidity in the body and the alkaline diet had begun many years earlier at my Chiropractic Wellness Center in New York City. At the time, I had a very small group of patients who were fit and energetic, had perfect skin, and were really the ideal picture of health. They came to my practice for an occasional chiropractic adjustment to maintain that good health. But, on the flipside, we also had patients who were tired all the time, even after a good night's sleep; patients who were overweight, with pain in their muscles and joints; patients who were riddled with skin conditions, acid reflux, or had digestive problems and even chronic disease. This was the majority.

I kept thinking there had to be a reason that so many patients had so many ailments. I committed myself to following the clues around these basic, frequent complaints and became a sort of health detective, looking for answers to all this pain and suffering in my client audience. I followed the evidence to see where it would lead and discovered that the common denominator was always the same. The smoking gun, in every case, was too much acid. Everyone in the unhealthy group was in an acidic state.

However, I didn't yet have a comprehensive picture of what that meant. I didn't yet know that acid was a central culprit in almost every health condition, common and chronic, that I was seeing come through my practice. But in the subsequent years, as my research deepened, I started to see trends and behaviors that all pointed to something at the root of many health issues.

After 115,000 patient visits and seventeen years in practice, I'm now considered an expert on the subject of acidity and health. I'm a wellness consultant and longevity expert who specializes in the benefits of an alkaline lifestyle. From someone who battled my own health issues for a good portion of my life, becoming a chiropractor and a certified raw food chef made me understand what it means to be truly healthy. Ultimately, this journey has transformed my life. With this book, my job today is to help you with the health issues and problems *you're* having. If you picked up this book and you have pain, trouble losing weight, migraine headaches, problems with sleep, low energy, digestive issues, or skin issues, or if you find yourself uncontrollably craving sugar—whatever the problems you are having—I want you to know there is *always* a specific cause. Usually the hidden factor is acid, and you'll soon understand what that means. I'll share tools to help you determine what *kind* of acid you're suffering from and how to transform your body into a more alkaline environment, which will, in turn, address your specific health issues without pills that cover pain and treat only the symptoms.

If you have a recurrent ailment that just won't quit and you think it's "just the way it is," I can help. If you're taking medication, I can help. If you can't sleep and have low energy, I can help.

My job is to find what everyone might have missed regarding the cause of problems. To do this I investigate the three most overlooked causes of health problems: stress, lack of proper nutrition, and toxicity.

I wrote this book to empower you to make the lifestyle changes you know you need to make. The premise of this book is that an acidic state is the underlying cause of most, if not all, diseases, and ailments. But the *power* of this book is the structure designed to help you identify the *specific* type of acid that is the root of your particular health issues. And the reality is, we all have them.

In all my years, I've never met someone who didn't have some level of acid-related health issues. Sure, some people are better off than others, depending on lifestyle choices and environmental factors, but there is *not one* among us who is free from the scourge of acid in our modern lifestyle.

No one ever told me the information I am going to share with you in these pages, and looking back, I really could have benefitted from what I know today.

COMING CLEAN: MY OWN HEALTH CONDITION

I opened the book with my father's story—that terrifying episode that alerted us to his cancer. But that wasn't what led me to become an expert on acid as a foundation of disease in the body. The truth is I was already many years into my research and practice because, long ago, my personal story had led me to investigate the causes of ill health.

There's an old story of the shoemaker with no shoes; he's always too busy making shoes for other people to make a pair for himself. There's also a saying, "The plumber's faucet always leaks." Often, we are so tied up in work that we forget to take care of ourselves. Well, for years, I was that doctor. I was busy caring for others, and my own health was a mess. I was a living contradiction.

Do you know anyone with a bad sugar addiction? Well, take that and multiply it by a thousand: that was me. Growing up, one of my nicknames was Candyman. Before soccer or hockey games, I was the kid on the bus with the huge bag of candy (which made me quite popular). When I would have cereal for breakfast, every spoonful of Honey Nut Cheerios had a big spoonful of sugar on top. Yes, I added sugar to *every* spoonful, one for one!

Later on, I would drink a Coke for breakfast, one for lunch, and one for dinner. Talk about acid! Soda is ten thousand times more acidic than tap water, and it takes about twenty glasses of water to neutralize the acid in one soda.

As I grew older, my nickname became Sugar Blues. I had begun to understand the problem I was having, I was trying to kick my habit, and I was reading the book *Sugar Blues*. Some people swear by that book to help beat any sugar addiction. But at the time, it didn't work for me. My brother snapped a picture of me reading with the book in one hand and a box of Lucky Charms in the other. From time to time, he still calls me that nickname. I can only laugh about it now.

The problem persisted through my young adult years right up until I was engaged to my now-wife. I used to keep little jars of M&M's throughout my apartment. Of course, there was a jar next to my bed. One morning my wife told me that in the middle of the night in my sleep, I took a huge handful of M&M's and shoved the entire thing in my mouth, jamming them down with my palm (her imitation of the scene is hilarious). What was funnier (or sadder) was that I didn't even remember it.

It wasn't an isolated incident, either. On another occasion, when the bedside bowl was filled with gummy bears, evidence the next morning attested to my ongoing behavior. Two gummy bears must have escaped my mouth, as I sleep-fed myself, because they were stuck to my shirt.

The final straw happened in my Chiropractic Wellness Center—I will never forget it, as it was one of my most embarrassing moments, and I am happy to report that it could have been way worse had any of my patients in the office known what happened. I managed to hide my shame, but unfortunately, I couldn't hide it from my staff.

At the time, I weighed 190 pounds, with 40 extra pounds on my body. This was the most I have ever weighed. At 5-foot-9, that put my body mass index (BMI) in the overweight category. This weight gain had happened slowly over time, and it was something I barely acknowledged was going on, even though it was right there in front of me. The crazy thing was, I was doing much of what we consider "healthy" things at the time. I exercised regularly, participated in triathlons, did Pilates, took supplements, and more. But none of that was enough to offset my sugar (read: acid) addiction.

So there I was at one of the chiropractic tables when I leaned down to adjust a patient, and my pants split right down the middle of my backside. This wasn't a small tear; I'm talking the entire seat ripped open. To this day, I have no idea how I hid it from the patient. I must have just scooted out of the office backward. Thank goodness, I had a backup pair of slacks in the office. Emotionally, it was a painful experience, and pain is a mighty big motivator!

At that moment, I vowed to make a change. I knew sugar was the problem, and this time I got serious about understanding sugar, its dangerous effects on my body, and figuring out why I craved it so badly. This was the beginning of my personal journey to better health, which resulted in my breaking the sugar/acid addiction, losing those 40 pounds in less than six months, and ramping up my energy to previously unknown levels.

From that point, I alkalized and energized my body, using the concepts I'll describe in this book, adding alkaline juices and smoothies, healthy fats, and mineral salts, and adopting alkaline exercise routines (yes, that's a thing—more on this subject later). There were certain things that I would soon eat less of and eventually fully cut out of my diet. It changed everything—from what I weighed to how I breathed.

Today, my diet is typically 80/20—80 percent alkaline, 20 percent acidic—in favor of nutrient-dense foods, and I continue to keep my weight down 40 pounds from where I was then. I am 42 and running ultra-marathons, and I feel younger, leaner, and more energized than I did in my twenties. What an incredible gift!

Best of all, I didn't get to this point through an extreme diet. I simply made a commitment to my health and changed my strategy. I still remember my first green juice: it tasted like swamp water to me. It wasn't that the juice was bad; it was that my taste buds were so used to three sodas a day, my brain couldn't process what something healthy tasted like. But something interesting happened. Literally, within days, my palate changed. I started craving these green drinks because my body wanted them. The body is smart that way. It translated what it needed to what I wanted.

By gradually adding better choices to my lifestyle, it wasn't overwhelming. It didn't feel as though I was depriving myself, and to be honest it was easy and fun trying these new things. Eventually, my 20/80 diet (80 percent in favor of acidic foods) turned into 40/40, then 50/50, then 60/40, and then 80/20. This approach is not only a program I tried once—it's become my way of life. So, although I refer to it as the alkaline diet, it is more than that—it is a lifestyle. It can offer you the best health you can help yourself achieve.

IF YOU WANT TO TAKE THE ISLAND, BURN THE BOATS

How many times have you tried a diet, lost some weight, and felt great about how you looked, only to let it all go by the wayside? Those days are over, folks. It's time to step up and stand up for what your true potential can be—and make it last once and for all. What have you been tolerating in your life that you are ready to strip away? Make your commitment, and then remove the obstacles.

There is a story I once heard Tony Robbins tell about a sixteenth-century Spanish conquistador named Hernàn Cortés who conquered Cuba and Mexico. Upon arrival at the shore, Cortés would say to his army, "Burn the boats!" In other words, there is no going back. In Cortés's day, either he had to fight or he died. And really, in some ways the battle for health is no different. But unlike Cortés, your battle will be fought and won at the grocery store and on your plate.

When I talk about burning the boats, what I really mean is, remove any temptation that will set you back in your quest. Look at what is currently in the pantry and the fridge. Just as you want to detox your body and rid it of acid, you also need to detox the kitchen, getting rid of sugars and grains. Don't kid yourself about willpower. Just know that, if it's there, you will go for it. (And if it's there, your kids will go for it too!)

The first step in your journey toward a more alkaline body is to stop poisoning yourself with acidic foods. Once you do that, I will give you the proper lists and guides of healthy snacks, foods, and drinks to replace those acidic foods. And I promise, I will make it fun, easy, convenient, and most of all, delicious.

Know this: I am not here to turn you into a full-time vegetarian or ask you to completely give up your favorite foods. I'm hoping you'll find out what works for you. As you add alkaline foods into your life, follow the 7 Ways to GET OFF YOUR ACID and commit to change. All I ask is that you try this plan for seven days, give it your all, and then see how you feel. If you're like most of my patients, at the end of seven days your experience will speak for itself. I promise, you're not going to want to go back to the way you were. Chapter 5 will be your guide for beginning this seven-day plan and your new life!

• • •

I grew up addicted to sugar, suffering from chronic ear infections, chronic migraines, and IBS (Irritable Bowel Syndrome) that wouldn't go way no matter how many doctors I visited. And I can remember my parents handing me these little yellow and blue amoxicillin antibiotics all the time. That was a terrible health decision that annihilated my gut bacteria (more on that on page 8), but it *wasn't* their fault; they were doing what the doctors told them to do. And when I would get these ear infections, or migraines, or horrific acne as a teenager, the doctors said it was very normal to get ear infections because "all kids get them." They also said headaches and skin breakouts were normal. But the truth is, there is no such thing as "normal" symptoms. A symptom is your body's mechanism for alerting you that something is wrong! Symptoms that may be common are anything but *normal.*

Normal is to feel energetic, alive, and full of vitality. Symptoms are warning signs that something is out of balance. So the question is, "Are you listening?"

If you are having a health problem, we can work to find the true cause of it and do something to actually eliminate it. When patients come to me, they often tell me that traditional doctors haven't been able to help them. I see it as my job to find what everyone else has missed. After twenty years of research and thousands of clients, I have consolidated all my learning and observation into a powerful approach, which you can easily implement into your life.

Maybe you've tried several remedies; maybe you've seen many different doctors. My job is to get you on a path to truly being well. And once we get you well, we are going to stop the dreaded yo-yo syndrome and *keep* you well!

Because my methods are unique, I often get results that other doctors do not. Even people who have battled certain ailments for years can find success by adopting the methods I share in this book.

As we dive in, I'm going share a lot of detailed information that may seem overwhelming at first, but the good news is, with this knowledge, there are clear, actionable steps you can implement right away to turn your health around and achieve a greater state of wellness. The steps I share here have changed my life and the lives of my family and thousands of clients. Now I want to share that same knowledge with you. All you have to do is decide to act on it.

IS THIS BOOK RIGHT FOR YOU?

Here are the first questions to ask yourself:

How is my energy? Do I feel sluggish, heavy, exhausted, foggy, and bleary regularly, even when I get good sleep and eat mindfully? Do I often experience the 3 p.m. slump?

If you answered yes, this book is for you. As you will soon discover, these are the initial and easiest indicators of an acidic state in the body.

It's always been interesting to me to learn why some people feel weak and worn down for no good reason. Much of this is attributable to the "Law of Familiarity," or the idea that, once a condition has been present long enough, you start to think it's normal. As a society, we are used to living in extremes. An acidic state leads us to wake up feeling drained. So we grab some coffee—adding more acid to the body. Later in the day, we caffeinate again, diving deeper down the rabbit hole. When we feel sluggish, we indulge in a sugary treat, which later causes a crash. At the end of the day, we are so wired, we can't sleep, so we take sleeping pills. All of these things make the body more acidic, and it becomes a vicious cycle.

IMAGINE THE FLIPSIDE

Would you love to wake up refreshed and instantly jump out of bed?

Would you love to feel energized and ready to rock your day the second your alarm goes off—or better yet, you rise with the sun with limitless energy, without needing the actual alarm in the first place?

Would you love to be as productive at work as possible, while still having that extra energy at the end of the day to spend with your children?

As you will learn in the pages ahead, chronic, low-grade acidosis or too much acid in your system predominantly caused by stress and eating the standard American diet, has devastating health consequences.

Research shows that risk for seven of the top ten deadly diseases in this country can be significantly reduced by changes in diet.

The World Health Report 2000, Health Systems: Improving Performance, ranked the US health care system 37th in the world. Our nation ranks just above Iraq in terms of money spent on health care, but in fact, it's not health care, it's sick care. In 2012, we spent $2.6 trillion on health care, and in 2018, that number will double to a staggering $4.4 trillion. That's $15,000 per person. Could you imagine if you were given $15,000 every year and were told to use this for your health care—your organic groceries, gym, supplements, and wellness doctors? I can guarantee, there would be *a lot* less disease to treat!

I believe that if we invested as much time, money, and energy in studying the habits and behaviors of healthy people—instead of just medicating sick people—we would all be better off. So many of us think we are making healthy choices when, in fact, we are being misled about what is best for our well being. There are so many myths about what constitutes healthy food, and so many foods fool us, such as yogurt, whole grain bread, brown rice, milk, and more. I've devoted a chapter to foods that don't serve us, including the ones we thought were good choices (see page 67).

In this book, I will give you simple strategies to GET OFF YOUR ACID and discover energy all day long. Despite what you may think now, or what others may tell you, it's attainable, and it's much easier than you may think!

Increasing your energy is not about trying to be perfect or cutting out everything you enjoy for the rest of your life! It's about balance—doing the small things that make the biggest difference on a daily basis. This will help you increase your longevity and add life to your years. Studies show that we may have the genetic potential to live to 120, but we haven't yet unlocked the key to optimal health. I'd like to believe that with more education and understanding, we're going to get there.

All I ask is that you try out my 80/20 alkaline diet and my 7 Ways to GET OFF YOUR ACID over seven days, giving it 100 percent of your effort, and let the experience speak for itself. If you are like most of my patients, you are going to feel so good that you won't ever want to go back.

If you are an overachiever, you can dive right in and implement the diet and all seven lifestyle changes immediately. If you are one who likes to take it slowly, that's great too: you could implement one step per week and fully commit to it. Then, the following week, stack the new step onto the previous one. You can go in the order I've proposed, or feel free to choose your own order based on what you feel may be most suitable for you. Either way, always remember that lasting change takes time. As long as your goal is "progress, not perfection," you will be on your way!

Remember, I can tell you how to do it, but it is up to you to decide what to do with this information. And know this: the quality of your choices will ultimately determine the quality of your health, your energy, and the path of your life. Just because your parents or grandparents suffered a debilitating disease or died at an early age doesn't mean you have to. The exciting science of epigenetics shows that, even if you have a genetic predisposition to something that your family has, you have the ability to turn that gene on or off via your lifestyle choices. Knowing the right foods to put in your body, and more importantly, the foods *not* to put in your body, will make all the difference in your lifespan. And it's never too late to start—that's how amazing (and forgiving) the human body is.

I want your journey to optimal health to be enjoyable, and I want it to last. So don't worry about having to cut out all the things you love to eat. This never works. I will show you the simple strategies that finally allowed me to beat a lifetime of one of the worst sugar addictions you have ever seen and turn into the health machine that I am today. I don't say that to impress you but to impress upon you that change is possible and it's easy—it's *thinking* about change that's hard.

When it comes to making changes in health, my motto has always been moderation, not deprivation. For years, I tried to quit sugar and failed. What I didn't understand is that relying solely on willpower for long-term results isn't sustainable. When you ease into health slowly, and you gradually add back the nutrients your body is actually craving, you'll start to feel better, and you'll keep going. As long as you keep moving in the right direction, you will reach your goals . . . and surpass them.

Are you ready to GET OFF YOUR ACID? Let's go!

PART I
What's Eating You?

Do something today that your future self will thank you for.

—SEAN PATRICK FLANERY

01

What Is Acidosis?

Think for a moment about an acid chemical. What does it do? One of the strongest acids, sulfuric acid, for example, is so corrosive it will quickly burn through skin, exposing the underlayers. It is among the most powerful and potentially harmful acids known. If you were to get even the smallest amount in your eyes, you would suffer from serious burns and could possibly lose your eyesight.

Did you know that animal proteins and wheat both have sulfur-containing amino acids that are metabolized into sulfuric acid? If it can do that to your skin and eyes, consider what an excess of acid may be doing inside your body—to your digestive system, to your cardiovascular system. Many of us are walking around with too much chronic acid, inflammation, and oxidation in the body, which is really the same as slowly rusting and rotting from within.

Disease is caused by the accumulation of toxins in the body, also known as acidosis. If you suffer from low energy, muscle aches and pains, acid reflux, digestive issues, immune system issues, inflammation, or skin problems, or if you have trouble losing those last few pounds, you'll want to pay close attention, as we uncover the root cause of chronic disease: over-acidity due to poor choices in the way we eat, think, and move. There are many ways that the body undergoes this form of trauma: consuming sugar, grains, dairy, excess animal proteins, artificial sweeteners, GMO foods, and alcohol; too much stress; and exposure to chemicals and pesticides, to name but a few.

I'll go over the reasons why doing all the "right things" for your health may not be working for you, and I will give you the simple set of strategies that will turn your health around and take it to your next level.

FROM ACID TO ALKALINE

While many of us have heard of the term *pH* from other contexts, such as the pH of a swimming pool, most people have no idea what it means when it comes to our bodies. pH stands for "potential of hydrogen," and it represents the concentration of hydrogen ions in a substance or solution, which indicates how acidic or basic (alkaline) that substance is. The pH balance of the human bloodstream is recognized by all medical physiology texts as one of the most important biochemical balances in all of human body chemistry. As *Guyton's Textbook of Medical Physiology* puts it, "The regulation of hydrogen ion concentration is one of the most important aspects of homeostasis."

The pH scale ranges from 0 to 14, where 0 is pure acid (think of burning a hole through metal) and 14 is pure base— or purely alkaline (lime, for example, has a pH of 12.3 and is used to balance soil when it's too acidic). A pH of 7 is neutral. Higher numbers mean a substance is more alkaline in nature, and there is a greater potential for absorbing more hydrogen ions. Lower numbers indicate more acidity and less potential for absorbing hydrogen ions. The human body thrives when its internal environment is slightly alkaline. Likewise, the body begins to experience health problems when its terrain becomes toxic and acidic.

In fact, everything in nature depends on a proper pH balance. For example, oceans should have a pH of 8.2, but increasing levels of acidic carbon dioxide gas in the atmosphere has lowered it to 8.1. As a result, coral reefs such as the Great Barrier Reef off the coast of Australia are dying at unprecedented rates. And consider our soil. Due to unnatural agricultural methods, such as pesticide use and the genetic alteration of our crops (GMOs), the minerals, nutrients, and alkalinity in our food have been compromised. Similarly, the use of synthetic fertilizers and increasing levels of acid rain has changed our soil structure, making its pH more acidic. When a

soil's pH range is outside 6–7, plants die. Researchers feel the human body is reacting similarly to these adverse conditions: we are becoming more toxic and acidic, resulting in a staggering rise in chronic disease levels. That just goes to show how important pH is, yet how many doctors are talking with you about this?

pH is measured on a logarithmic scale, meaning it is exponential. For example, a substance with a pH of 6 (carbonated water), although only a difference of 1.0 on the pH scale from 7 (neutral), is actually ten times more acidic. A pH value of 5 (black coffee) is ten times more acidic than 6, but a hundred times more acidic than 7 (neutral). And a pH of 4 (soda) is not three times more acidic, but one thousand times more acidic!

Our body pH is very important because it controls the speed of our body's biochemical reactions. The pH affects the speed of enzyme activity as well as the speed that electricity moves through our bodies. Ultimately, the quality of your choices will determine the quality of your pH.

The various parts of your body require certain pH levels to function properly. For example, stomach pH should fall between 1 and 3, skin should be around 5.5, the large intestines at 8, saliva between 6.5 and 7.4, and pancreatic chemicals should be in the range of 7.5 to 8.8. These numbers exist on a spectrum, though, and modern dietary and lifestyle factors can make pH levels more acidic than they should be, which means the body's natural systems have to work much harder to maintain their ideal pH levels.

pH SCALE

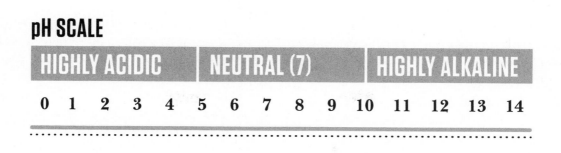

HIGHLY ACIDIC	NEUTRAL (7)	HIGHLY ALKALINE

0   1   2   3   4   5   6   7   8   9   10   11   12   13   14

You can imagine your pH is like a thermostat. If you happen to be hanging out on an iceberg, your body is going to have to work hard to maintain a temperature of 98.6°F, right? Your body would shiver and expend massive amounts of energy to create heat, and your blood would leave your hands and feet and rush to your organs. Why? To keep you alive! But eventually, your body simply wouldn't be able to sustain this temperature regulation, so you would have to get off the iceberg to survive. The same is true with your body's pH.

Think of it this way: when you measure the pH in a pool, and you see that it's not in the optimal zone, you simply add chemicals to the pool water to shift its pH to a more balanced state. Otherwise, it becomes a bacteria-ridden cesspool. Likewise, diseases thrive in a too-acidic body environment. If you want to get rid of all the bad stuff in your system, you have to restore balance.

Here's another example: What happens when you have a stagnant pond with still water? Mosquitoes. You can spray insecticide to kill off all the mosquitoes, but they will come back if the pond remains stagnant. Clean out the pond, give it healthy, flowing water, and the mosquitoes will go away. The same holds true for you. If you want to reclaim your health, you must clean out the toxicity that has been building up over the years and give your body the nutrients that it has been denied. It's that simple.

HOW DOES AN ACID STATE HAPPEN?

An acidic state means the body is *toxic* and *deficient*. Increasingly we are exposed to toxins due to the impurities of modern life, be they dietary, metabolic, environmental, chemical, or stress-related. These substances lodge in our cells and poison the body. Although is impossible to escape from it completely, you can do your best to minimize toxicity. At the same time, bodies are deficient, which means they are lacking in vital resources, such as nutrients, water, minerals, and oxygen. We need to move our bodies to the other end of the spectrum to become more alkaline, the opposite of acidity. This requires a two-pronged approach: reducing the toxicity and adding vital nutrients. In other words, we need to take away the bad and add in the good. Makes sense, right?

There are five main sources of excess acid in the body. Are any of these eating you from the inside out?

The Five Sources of Acid

DIET

Many people eat what is predominantly an acidic diet. When I say "acidic," I mean an acid-forming diet—digestion of these foods produces dangerous acid salts as by-products, and the body must work hard to quickly eliminate them. In fact, 80 percent of the standard American diet is acidic, and it needs to be 80 percent alkaline. When you consume foods such as sugar, grains, dairy, animal protein, colas, carbonated water, many teas, and coffee, they metabolize as damaging acids.

For example, eating sugar will produce lactic acid. Perhaps the worst sugar of them all, fructose, will create uric acid (which contributes to gout and kidney issues, even type 2 diabetes). Consuming grains, specifically wheat, will produce sulfuric acid. Teas and coffee are high in tannic acid. Unhealthy fats will produce acetic acid and lactic acid. Colas are high in phosphoric acid, and carbonated water—a beverage I label as one of the most surprising acidic suspects—will create carbonic acid. Eating steak produces sulfuric acid, phosphoric acid, and nitric acid—dangerous acids that *must* be immediately excreted by your kidneys.

All of these acids are extremely toxic and will lower your pH. Usually, these toxins store themselves in the adipose tissue, or in the fat cells that act as buffers to protect your body from these harmful toxins. In the short run, this will protect you. But if the toxins persist over a longer period, they will begin to corrode and cause damage to your tissues. To prevent this, your body has to work to quickly eliminate them. But before your body can expel these acids, these poisons must be neutralized with the help of the alkaline minerals. This helps prevent them from doing further damage.

METABOLIC ACIDS

Your body produces acid in the course of daily living. The body is alkaline by nature, but it's always creating acid. Your health is proportionally related to how effectively your body can eliminate these acids. Your body gets rid of waste through uric acid via the kidneys. When you work out, you produce lactic acid, and when you breathe, your body expels carbonic acid. The body has an elaborate built-in buffer system to neutralize those daily metabolic acids. But because we have become so acidic from what we eat and drink, and because we suffer from stress, and metabolic and environmental toxins, we've completely overwhelmed and depleted the natural buffers we were born with—the mineral reserves in our body.

ENVIRONMENTAL ACIDS

Our environment is deeply toxic. That's true in the natural world as well as in our homes and products. Our surroundings are full of electromagnetic fields (EMF) that radiate from many of our devices, power lines, and microwaves. In addition to toxic substances emanating from human-made sources, our natural world is toxin ridden, too. Take the water supply. You probably understand, conceptually, that water has chemicals in it, but do you know water shows traces of drugs such as Prozac and birth control pills? That's right! So many people are being medicated with Prozac that it is ending up in our water supply from their urination!

Bisphenol A (BPAs) in plastic water bottles are carcinogenic and dangerous, and tap water isn't any safer. A three-year study by the Environmental Working Group (EWG) of 20 million drinking water quality tests concluded that tap water contains 316 known contaminants.

Then there's the air we breathe. Oxygen is the most important nutrient for your body, yet we are inhaling noxious fumes and carcinogens from factories and automobile exhaust, and tons of other dangerous toxins on a daily basis. Oxygen is the major component the body uses to neutralize acids and toxins and remove them from the body, yet toxic air is providing us with less than adequate levels to perform these tasks optimally.

And if you think the air is safer inside your home, think again. We spend at least one-third of our lives inside our homes, yet according to the Environmental Protection Agency (EPA), indoor air quality is typically up to seventy times more toxic than outdoor air pollution. The average home contains between 500 and 1,000 chemicals, many of which go undetected because humans are unable to see, smell, or taste them.

The off-gassing from the fire retardants in furniture, mattresses, and carpets; the varnish from cabinets; shower curtains—they all contain polyvinylchloride, or PVC plastic, which is made up of many different toxic chemicals. Together, the toxins from these and other products have a cumulative damaging effect in the body.

CHEMICAL ACIDS

Next, we have to think about the chemicals we ingest and absorb, often by choice. Antibiotics are one of the most dangerous enemies of our natural defense system, followed by cigarettes, alcohol, medications, and illegal drugs. And then there are the chemicals found in personal care products and everyday objects. Even the antiperspirants we use daily contain aluminum, which for women, in particular, is concerning due to the proximity to breast tissue and the possibility of increasing cancer risk.

It is a devastating fact that our whole world is toxic. This is why we have to be so vigilant and work so much harder to counteract the acidic substances from every element of our environment. Choosing organic not only with your foods, but with your home and personal care products needs to become a must, because your health is at stake, and it's worth it!

STRESS

I will say this repeatedly: the mental and emotional stress in our lives outweighs anything we can eat or drink in regard to the acid it creates in our bodies. Our modern lifestyle causes daily stress that mimics our prehistoric "fight or flight" response, where the adrenal gland releases cortisol, which wreaks havoc on our system. Sure, that was beneficial when we were running from saber-toothed tigers, but now we become stressed while sitting at a desk and talking on the phone. We aren't actually using that cortisol to run for our lives; we are damaging only our bodily defenses.

YOUR GUT:
THE FOUNDATION OF HEALTH

As these sources of acid conspire to weaken the system, there is destruction of the human microbiome—the entire bacterial ecosystem, most of which resides in your gut, or intestinal tract. Here's the deal: you have ten times more bacteria in your intestinal tract than you have cells in your body. Guarding your intestines are your villi—small, fingerlike projections that form tight junctions, allowing the good stuff in and keeping the bad stuff out. These tight junctions ensure that partially digested food stays inside your intestines where it belongs, not leaking into your blood where it can wreak havoc.

When you eat, the villi aid in absorption of nutrients from foods by increasing the surface area of your intestines to a size of a tennis court (seventy-two hundred square feet!), with the primary goal of transporting them into the bloodstream where they can be used by the body.

Here's the problem. Normally, the gut should have about 85 percent "good" bacteria, and no more than 15 percent "bad" bacteria. When this healthy ratio exists, the gut stays well regulated by its microbes. But when the gut is being pounded with excess acid, the bad bacteria start to move in and take over. The gut mucosa (the intestinal lining, including the villi) becomes congested with bad bacteria, mucous, yeast, and fungus, and the villi cannot do their job.

As the harmful microbes take up more space, they trigger the release of a protein called zonulin, the "gatekeeper" in control of regulating those tight junctions. When zonulin levels rise due to stress and an acidic diet, those tight junctions begin to break down.

These harmful microbes and gluten (which I talk more about later) are the two most powerful triggers that can open the zonulin door. The result? The "security guards" of the digestive system leave the gates wide open, allowing the passage of toxins, allergens, yeast, and undigested food particles to gain entry into the bloodstream. This condition is otherwise known as leaky gut syndrome, which plagues roughly 80 percent of Americans.

In order to address this chain of negative events, it's essential to bolster intestinal villi with the right foods. They are the army defending your entire system.

It all starts with what you put in your body. Let's take the example of one problematic food that's widely consumed: gluten, a protein found in grains such as wheat, rye, and barley. Gluten is a major force behind leaky gut syndrome; it is so

> ## All disease begins in the gut.
> ### —HIPPOCRATES

acidic that it creates openings, like craters, in your gut. Because of these perforations in the intestinal wall, the body's army can't stop acid from getting into the bloodstream.

Taking antibiotics can make things even worse. To put things in perspective, if gluten creates holes in your gut, an antibiotic is like a bomb—it decimates your gut flora. Obviously, for some conditions, antibiotics can be lifesaving, but some doctors prescribe them like candy. This is why antibiotics should be taken only when necessary.

As the bloodstream becomes saturated and overwhelmed with toxins, the toxins leak into surrounding tissues until they can be eliminated. In other words, in order for the pH of your blood to remain regulated at the optimal alkaline level of 7.4, your body will dump the acids and toxins into your tissues (usually the weakest ones, whether that happens to be your kidneys, prostate, brain, lungs, or your muscles and connective tissue for example). (To learn more about blood pH, see page 21.) The acids and toxins will remain in the tissues and cause damage until your body has the energy to properly eliminate them from your body once and for all.

So what happens when tissues hold acids? It's a condition called acidosis, or chronic low-grade acidosis. When acids and toxins are parked in your tissues, they begin to rot your body from the inside out. As acidic liquids are used to tenderize meat in the cooking process, this is exactly what is happening inside your body—to your muscles, connective tissues, and organs! Even when we are trying our best and taking great care of ourselves, over the year toxins accumulate in our bodies. Chronic low-grade acidosis is the gradual build-up of toxins over time. As acids build up, they literally poison you from the inside out. Being healthy is anticipating that this is the byproduct of aging in our toxic world, and making alkalizing and detoxification a part of your daily lifestyle.

WE ALL SUFFER FROM CHRONIC LOW-GRADE ACIDOSIS

At the core of so many symptoms is chronic low-grade acidosis. Many of us try to live healthily, but there's so much misinformation about what are "healthy" foods, and we often mistake acidic choices for

WHAT IS THE MICROBIOME?

Many in the medical community consider the microbiome to be an "organ" of its own. Along with the brain and blood, the intestinal microbiome is one of the most important systems in your body.

In fact, in his book *Grain Brain*, Dr. David Perlmutter says, "Amazingly, a full 99 percent of the genetic material is housed by your microbiome! It supports and nurtures every aspect of your physiology, including what goes on in the brain. Some are even calling the gut flora the brain's 'peacekeeper.'" Despite being a system we don't widely discuss or consider, the microbiome is responsible for how often we get sick, our propensity for disease, our daily mood, and our overall organ health.

Another way to think about the digestive system is to picture the roots of a tree. Your gut and its flora are the ultimate basis of your body's health. Just as a tree will show signs of stress if the roots are damaged, the body will show signs of disease when the microbiome is out of balance and when the digestive system is inflamed and acidic. So remember, if you want to bear healthy fruit—strong organs and a disease-free system—you need to keep the roots strong.

safe choices. We consume things such as kombucha and kefir, not knowing that fermented foods are filled with yeast, sugar, alcohol, carbonation, lactic acid, and the high probability of containing poisonous mycotoxins. When we exercise, we might not realize that high-intensity activity creates great amounts of lactic acid, which does more harm than good. Many of us take medications for things such as high blood pressure and cholesterol, but these medications increase acidity in our bodies. By changing our lifestyle to minimize acid in our system, we begin to address the root cause of chronic low-grade acidosis, and we'll see our health improve.

If the underlying acidic stressors in your life are not addressed, these acids will build up and have the potential to advance into something more serious. Five progressive stages of acidosis lead to disease.

1. Fatigue/Energy Loss

Feeling sluggish on the outside? You should see what's going on inside. The first way you'll know something's not right is that you will feel run down and weak.

Before major signs appear, the digestive track backs up with acid-forming foods and toxins, which is usually experienced as either constipation or diarrhea. If all the bad stuff can't be eliminated, it damages the lining of the intestines and stomach, and toxins seep into your blood and your body.

At the same time, when this happens, your body's ability to absorb nutrients from all of the alkaline foods you're eating decreases, so you have less good stuff going in and more bad stuff building up. With all that toxicity, your body goes into overdrive trying to heal, and healing your body when it is in a state of chronic low-grade acidosis requires a huge amount of energy. It all adds up to one massive energy vampire and your first warning sign of acidosis!

2. Food Sensitivities/ Allergies/Intolerances

While the first sign of acidosis can sometimes go unnoticed, experiencing food sensitivities is a more apparent sign things aren't going well internally.

Do you have a favorite food that you *must* have and can't stop eating? Do you feel tired, bloated, and drained *all* the time? These may be signs of food intolerances. Counterintuitively, the foods we think we love the most are often the foods our bodies can't tolerate well, keeping us from losing weight and making us feel tired and even depressed.

Food allergies and intolerances are much more common than most people realize. Millions of adults and children who suffer from reactions to acidic foods, but

don't know it because the symptoms—bloating, poor digestion, skin issues, headaches, lethargy, depression, and weight gain—are common and can be hard to diagnose. Most people don't connect that these may be caused by a food they've been eating their entire lives. They think, "There must be something wrong with me." Often there is a delayed reaction from eating the food. For example, you may eat gluten one day and feel fine, but then the next day you feel bloated and tired.

Common trigger foods to watch out for include

- ▸ wheat (gluten)
- ▸ dairy products
- ▸ artificial sweeteners
- ▸ soy
- ▸ sugar
- ▸ caffeine

Ideally, these foods should be removed from your diet, as they are *all* highly acidic and often end up being trigger foods. However, if you want to determine if one specific trigger food is worse than another, you would need to consume the foods on the list one at a time, paying attention to how you feel the following twenty-four hours. If you experience any abnormal symptoms, then this food should be eliminated. Once you have eliminated these reactive foods from your life, you will be amazed at how quickly your energy and health will increase.

3. Inflammation

Unfortunately, most people arrive at this stage having overlooked the prior two.

Acne/skin breakouts

Anxiety

Gas/bloating

Slow metabolism

Depression

Headaches

Lethargy

Weight gain

Digestive issues (diarrhea,
   constipation, cramping)

Cravings for food

Binge eating

The acids have become so backed up, and the system is so overloaded, you're starting to feel chronically bad. It's hard to ignore the symptoms in this stage because they can be quite painful and uncomfortable: usually, reflux or inflammation in the joints or digestive tract (Crohn's, IBS, diverticulitis, and celiac disease). The aches and pains are your body yelling, "HELP ME," and they typically get worse as the day moves on.

At this stage, alkalizing exercises are very important. The rebounder (which you will learn more about in Chapter 8) is my favorite form of lymphatic exercise because it's easy on the joints and the back, and it is one of the most powerful ways to move the acid that's causing the inflammation out of the tissues.

4. Sclerosis (Hardening of Tissue) or Ulcers

This is where things get scary. Tissues respond in two different ways to all of the acid they're holding. Some types of tissues harden, becoming leather-like, such as with cirrhosis of the liver or hardening of the arteries. Other types of tissue form ulcerations because they are no longer protected by the delicate microbiome that's been destroyed, so ulcers crop up in the stomach or in other digestive organs such as the duodenum or esophagus.

Ulcers might not seem like a big deal. After all, they are common, right? Most medical doctors still point to stress, overconsumption of trigger foods, and use of anti-inflammatory medications as the big culprits. Some of the worst offenders are NSAIDs (nonsteroidal anti-inflammatory drugs such as Advil, Aleve, and ibuprofen) given over the counter. If these drugs can be bought in a convenience store, then you probably think "They must be safe for me." But NSAIDS are the fifteenth leading cause of death in the United States.

You probably pop these most times you have a headache or a hangover without thinking twice about it. Many of us take these drugs often and don't realize their truly detrimental effects. When ulcers occur, they are a symptom of a much larger problem that's been going on for some time. Signs of ulcers include

- pain or burning in the abdomen, especially after eating;

- nausea or vomiting, possibly with blood in the vomit;

- dark stools (indicating digested blood from the upper digestive tract);

- loss of appetite; and

- unexplained weight loss.

Finally, if not treated holistically (not only treating the symptoms of ulcers but also addressing the true cause of the acid problem), the damage continues, leading to step 5.

5. Degenerative Diseases

If bad tissue degenerates enough and no lifestyle changes are made, serious diseases can emerge. Along the digestive tract, many diseases can develop: stomach cancer, pancreatic cancer, liver cancer, colon cancer, or esophageal cancer—the latter of which is what happened with my father. His cancer was a culmination of these five progressive stages of acidosis. It began as reflux, which he had never mentioned (to me at least). As the acid perpetually invaded his esophagus, inflammation soon turned into ulceration and induration. The bleeding ulcer is what made him black out in the driver's seat, as he was driving 70 mph on the highway. And upon further testing, cancer, the fifth stage of acidosis, was the result.

Many types of cancer can be traced back to the same root causes. I still think back

to that day at Memorial Sloan Kettering in New York City when the oncologist told my family the cause of my dad's cancer was "too much acid." Let's look at what that meant in the context of his diagnosis. The first two stages of acidosis—energy loss and food sensitivities—are easy to miss. Who hasn't felt one of those things and dismissed it as an off day? Those are common side effects, yet often overlooked, so if you have low energy, it may be the first warning sign there is too much acid in your system. The same is true of food sensitivities. So many people experience these symptoms but don't realize it's because they've indulged in heavily acidic foods.

Inflammation is a big telltale sign of acidosis, which can be tested for using the HS-CRP (High Sensitivity C-Reactive Protein) test on a routine blood panel, and the Omega-3 Acid Index test. I'll be telling you about that test later in the book. Inflammation in the acute phase is good, as it is the body's healing response, bringing blood and nutrients to the injured or diseased area, but chronic inflammation is terrible for the body. In terms of my father, acid went into his esophagus, which caused irritation and inflammation.

As the inflammation did its damage and the cause was never addressed, the acid began to ulcerate his stomach and esophagus, so much so that it caused him to bleed internally, which is what caused him to pass out at the steering wheel. He was bleeding so much internally that he needed a transfusion because his hemoglobin levels were exceedingly low. The ulcer was followed by sclerosis—the hardening of the wall where the acid was doing its damage. That was making the tissue diseased, which ultimately resulted in the fifth stage, cancer.

This makes me shiver every time I think about it. But at the same time, it crystallized my mission to make sure every single person I can reach knows about the devastating effects that acidosis has on the body and what to do to GET OFF YOUR ACID! If you are experiencing reflux or GERD in any magnitude, be sure to follow the tenets I outline in this book, and consult with your health care practitioner as well.

THE 80/20 IDEAL RATIO

All health begins on your plate. In order to maintain your health, you want to put at least 80 percent alkaline-forming foods and no more than 20 percent acid-forming foods into your body on any given day. This is the first step to combating the potential for disease.

We'll talk more about which foods are acidic and which are alkaline in chapters 5 and 6. If you have a specific health challenge, I recommend following an alkaline diet plan 100 percent until your body is stabilized. For example, someone with cancer should never consume alcohol or even moderately acidic fruit, as both will feed and perpetuate the cancer. In fact, *all* sugar and grains, two of the most acid-forming foods, must be eliminated from your diet.

But, if you are in good health, having one glass of wine at dinner once a week is not a huge problem, assuming that it's part of your 20 percent for that day and you don't exceed your allotted acidic intake. The problem for most Americans is this ratio is reversed. Many of us follow an 80 percent acidic lifestyle, and that's why chronic degenerative disease runs rampant. And believe me, I know something about this, as I used to follow a 10/90 diet, in favor of bad acids!

The good news is that by using an "add the good" approach rather than focusing solely on taking away the bad, it's easy to shift your diet to be 80 percent alkaline. With your body, you can alter your nutritional intake, as well as the amount of water you drink and various other variables that you will soon learn about to bring the body back—or closer—to a healthier, balanced state. Your body is always in flux, trying to achieve balance. As you become more knowledgeable about your body's pH, you'll gain more control over your well-being.

• • •

Before we can dive into specific strategies to help you detox and reclaim your energy, you need to understand your current state of wellness or imbalance. Take the following short quiz to learn where you stand on a scale of 1 to 100. This will give you a baseline to measure against before you adopt any protocols.

QUIZ: ARE YOU OVERLY ACIDIC?

▶ **To take this quiz online, go to www.getoffyouracid.com/how-acidic-are-you-quiz**

By now, you are probably wondering how acidic you are. Take this simple quiz to give you a beginning reference point and to start to understand how acidic or alkaline your lifestyle is. *Next to each answer, write the following number of points based on the corresponding letters:*

A's = 1 point each	C's = 4 points each
B's = 2 points each	D's = 5 points each

1. Do you drink coffee?

_____ a. You mean by the gallon? Yes!

_____ b. I can't start my day without a cup in the morning.

_____ c. Coffee is my guilty pleasure, but I have switched to drinking only decaf and only every now and then.

_____ d. I never drink coffee.

2. How often do you exercise each week?

_____ a. LOL, exercise! Does changing the channel count?

_____ b. I try to take a class every week, but I don't work out as much as I know I should.

_____ c. I hit the gym or go for an easy run 2 or 3 times a week.

_____ d. I work out every day in one way or another.

3. When it comes to cooking at home . . .

_____ a. A microwave pizza is all I can count as cooking.

_____ b. I cook a few times a week, but I eat out a lot too.

_____ c. I mostly cook and I try to use unprocessed ingredients.

_____ d. I do a lot of cooking using organic, whole foods.

4. How often do you drink wine, beer, or liquor?

_____ a. I have a glass of wine (or two or three) or a couple of beers every night. Happy hour!

_____ b. A few nights a week, I like to indulge a little.

_____ c. I'll have a drink on a rare special occasion.

_____ d. I never drink any alcohol.

(Continues)

5. How stressed do you feel most days?

_____ a. Super stressed, at work, in my commute, and even at home.

_____ b. My job is stressful but I can usually unwind in the evenings.

_____ c. I have stressful moments, but they're the exception, not the rule.

_____ d. I rarely get stressed out. I try to go with the flow.

6. How much gluten (i.e., pasta and bread) do you eat?

_____ a. Gluten is my favorite food group.

_____ b. I eat gluten daily, but I try to limit my portions.

_____ c. Other than Ezekiel bread, I avoid gluten as much as I can.

_____ d. I'm completely gluten-free.

7. How well do you sleep at night?

_____ a. I never go to bed on time, I toss and turn, and then I wake up exhausted.

_____ b. I try to get a good night's sleep, but I usually wake up tired anyway.

_____ c. Falling asleep is hard sometimes, but I get enough rest.

_____ d. I get plenty of sleep every night and wake up refreshed and full of energy.

8. How much water do you drink each day?

_____ a. Hardly any because I'm drinking soda, coffee, sports drinks, or juice.

_____ b. Some, but probably not enough.

_____ c. Eight glasses a day, just like the doctor says.

_____ d. I try to drink half my body weight in ounces every day.

9. Do you have a sweet tooth?

_____ a. Sugar is my weakness! I can't say no.

_____ b. I try to eat sweets only on special occasions.

_____ c. I eat lots of fruit, but very little other sugar.

_____ d. I seldom eat sugar, and when I do, I'm balancing it with green veggies and healthy fats like coconut oil.

10. How often during your day are you taking deep breaths?

_____ a. Only when I'm about to have a panic attack.

_____ b. Rarely—only when I remind myself to breathe.

_____ c. Maybe once or twice a day.

_____ d. I intentionally breathe deeply several times a day and anytime I feel stressed.

11. What's your most common source of protein?

_____ a. Red meat

_____ b. Organic chicken

_____ c. Wild-caught, organic fish

_____ d. Hemp and chia, pea protein, chickpeas . . .

12. How often do you use artificial sweeteners?

_____ a. I can't live without my Diet Cokes (or other artificially sweetened food or drink).

_____ b. I eat many foods with artificial sweeteners to avoid the sugar.

_____ c. I avoid them, other than the occasional stick of gum or sore throat lozenge.

_____ d. I never use artificial sweeteners.

13. Do you eat many processed foods?

_____ a. Isn't that the only kind to buy?

_____ b. I buy fresh fruits and veggies, but out of convenience, I still eat a fair amount of processed foods.

_____ c. I mostly shop the perimeter of the grocery store and buy natural and organic options.

_____ d. I buy only organic, unprocessed, whole foods.

14. When it comes to cleaning your home, you use . . .

_____ a. Whatever's on sale or the cheapest at the store

_____ b. A mix of name brands and natural products

_____ c. Usually vinegar, dish soap, and other products my grandmother used

_____ d. Only organic cleaning products and essential oils

15. When you eat out, you usually go for...

_____ a. A cheeseburger and fries

_____ b. A pasta dish with seafood and veggies

_____ c. An entree salad loaded with toppings

_____ d. A simple green salad or vegetarian appetizer

16. When was the last time you had a green smoothie/green juice?

_____ a. What's a green smoothie?

_____ b. Last month

_____ c. Last week

_____ d. Today— I have one just about every day.

(Continues)

17. How much dairy do you eat and drink each day?

_____ a. If it has cheese, milk, butter, or cream, I eat it.

_____ b. I usually eat some yogurt and a little cheese here and there.

_____ c. I mostly avoid dairy, but I do cook with grass-fed, organic butter sometimes.

_____ d. I'm completely dairy-free.

18. Which drink do you reach for throughout your day?

_____ a. Soda or fruit juice

_____ b. Seltzer water or club soda

_____ c. Green tea

_____ d. Water with lemon

19. Do you eat nuts and nut butter?

_____ a. No, I stick to meat and cheese for protein.

_____ b. Yes, I am a peanut butter fanatic.

_____ c. Roasted almonds and cashews are my favorites.

_____ d. I love raw almonds and make my own almond butter.

20. How tired do you feel most days?

_____ a. I'm sorry, I fell asleep. What was the question?

_____ b. I feel more tired than I'd like to most days.

_____ c. Usually, I'm plenty energetic. Every now and then, I'm tired, even if I get enough sleep.

_____ d. Energy's not a problem for me like it is for many people. I have plenty.

_____ **TOTAL POINTS**

SCORING

▶ **75–100 Points: You are an Alkaline Ace**

Congratulations! You are living the alkaline lifestyle! You've mastered the 80/20 formula, where 80 percent of your foods are alkaline and only 20 percent are acidic, you exercise regularly, and you manage stress and are sleeping well.

You must be feeling great. Keep up the good work!

▶ **50–74 Points: You are an Alkaline Novice**

You're on the right track! While you can keep improving, you know the basics of the alkaline lifestyle, and you are trying to live it all day, every day.

Focus on drinking plenty of pure, alkaline water instead of other drinks, eating greens and healthy fats at each and every meal, cutting back on sugar, even from natural sources, adding more green smoothies into your diet, and getting plenty of exercise.

▶ **25–49 Points: You're a Recovering Acid-holic**

You've got too much acid in your body and you suffer from not having enough energy. While you make some good choices, you're probably still addicted to one or more acidic foods: sugar, grains, artificial sweeteners, processed foods, meats, or dairy.

Breaking those addictions and adding in more low-sugar produce will flip the switch for you. Soon you'll be feeling better than ever with fewer cravings for acidic foods.

Start by aiming for a few more meals each week with no meat, dairy, or sugar and see how much better it makes you feel. And make sure to read My 7 Ways to GET OFF YOUR ACID! For more info, see Chapter 8.

▶ **0–24 Points: You're Addicted to Acid**

You need to GET OFF YOUR ACID now! Your lifestyle is highly acidic, especially the way you're eating. And you feel acid's effects—from not having enough energy to being plagued by aches, pains, inflammation, and health issues.

Immediately begin to implement my 7 Ways to Get Off Your Acid and kick start your new health habits with my 7-Day Challenge. Look to my quick and tasty recipes you can make at home using whole, nutrient-packed foods to kick-start an alkaline lifestyle.

As you begin to get more energy from the way you're eating, add exercise into your routine, which will help clear built-up acid out of your body and help you start to feel better. For more info, see Chapter 8.

• • •

Now that you've taken the quiz and know where you stand, you're on your way to empowering yourself to move toward change. If we met in my office, I'd ask you these same questions and give you a saliva and urine pH test. I believe once you begin to track your health, you will learn more about your body and will have the information and the motivation to change your behavior and change your life.

02

The Secret Is a Balanced pH

There are certain metrics that a human body has to adhere closely to in order to be healthy and, on a more basic level, to be alive. Our body regulates its temperature to be around 98.6°F, optimal blood pressure is 120/80 mm Hg, and there are healthy ranges for blood glucose levels (blood sugar), cholesterol levels, and more. Usually, doctors monitor those things when you go for a checkup. However, there is another number you must know that you are probably not tracking, and I'd argue it might be the most important of all—that's the pH level in your blood, which rests at 7.4.

Why? Because if a pH balance of 7.4 were to deviate by more than one point, you'd be dead. All too often, we experience telltale signs of a poor pH level, but most people aren't aware that pH is the key to good health (I like to use the acronym pH to mean perfect health)! If you're having trouble with your energy, and you're also experiencing headaches, digestive issues, joint pains, reflux, and difficulty losing weight, pH is a number you need to learn more about.

While different parts of your body have their own optimal pH levels, the pH we are going to be most focused on is the pH of your blood and body tissues (which can be monitored through the pH of saliva and urine). Of these, blood pH is especially crucial. If any of these numbers deviate from the healthy range, you'll experience common ailments that are your body's way of saying, "I'm acidic!"

TYPES OF BODY pH
Blood pH

The pH of the blood is tightly regulated in a narrow range between 7.35 and 7.45, with the ideal pH resting at 7.4. Your body will do whatever it takes to keep that number steady because if it deviates, you can't survive. So you might be asking, if my blood pH is always self-regulated at 7.4 and can't change much, why do I need to eat an alkaline diet?

The purpose of eating and drinking alkaline-forming ingredients is *not* to try to *raise* the pH of your blood, as so many are mistakenly led to believe. Eating alkaline is important because it prevents the body from *having* to do the regulating on its own. The fact is, your body will do whatever it takes to maintain a constant blood pH of 7.4, which is good news, but this is also where the problem lies!

If you're not getting essential acid-fighting minerals in via your diet, your body will find another way to get them. Your blood will "rob Peter to pay Paul" in an effort to keep blood pH at 7.4. In other words, if you consume a high acid-forming diet, your body will be forced to use the calcium from bones and the magnesium from muscles, to buffer the high acidic potential to keep your blood healthy, so you don't die. Calcium and magnesium are "acid buffers" that act within seconds to "mop up" toxins in the blood to ensure that you maintain this healthy pH level.

We are making our bodies work too hard, and it's breaking down our systems and causing chronic degenerative disease. If your body is constantly working, day and night, to balance pH, it's going to drain your energy.

If we eat more alkaline, we support our bodily functions and increase their effectiveness. We weren't built to handle such vast amounts of toxic substances that we encounter on a daily basis. On the other hand, if 80 percent of your diet is loaded with dark-green leafy vegetables and healthy fats that are rich in minerals, vitamins, and fiber, your body will have the necessary nutrients it needs to regulate itself.

Body pH
(Saliva and Urine pH)

Unlike blood pH, the pH levels of saliva and urine do not remain mostly constant. They fluctuate based on how you have been living over the past twenty-four hours: eating, drinking, thinking, and moving. These levels are a direct measure of how acidic your body's tissues are. This means you do have some control over tissue pH, and you can take steps to improve your overall health by being attentive to it. It's also why testing and regulating pH levels are so important: it gives you an immediate, accurate window into how healthy and energetic your body is at that moment.

Saliva pH looks at what your body is retaining or holding onto (mineral reserves), whereas urine pH reflects what your body is excreting (acid waste). When saliva and urine pH are in the optimal range, enzymes function better, and digestive juices work better. As a result, your body will properly break down its food, optimally absorbing and assimilating all of its nutrients. But if urine and saliva pH are off, your digestion will be off. Food will not be broken down and absorbed properly, and your energy will suffer. Malnutrition results in fatigue, and as you've learned, this is the first of the five stages of acidosis.

SALIVA pH

Saliva pH is very important because it closely correlates with blood pH. That is because saliva is the first place your body will steal minerals from to balance blood pH. If you are pumping a hyper-acidic diet into your body, your body will go to any length to ensure it gets the minerals it needs to neutralize those acids, even if that means stealing them from other areas of your body! One of the first places it will go to is saliva. Saliva produces sodium bicarbonate (baking soda), which is an alkaline buffer that neutralizes acids as they enter your mouth. (This is why there is baking soda in many types of toothpaste.)

Testing saliva pH can offer an early indication or warning sign if your body, specifically the blood, is overly acidic. When saliva veers off course, it is a sign that the blood is acidic and is pulling in minerals to neutralize any acidity.

The general range for saliva pH should be between 6.5 and 7.4, to begin the pre-digestive process. On average, the ideal range should be between 6.4 and 6.8 (closer to 6.4 for light meat eaters, and closer to 6.8 or even higher for healthy vegetarians).

When you're eating, saliva pH should rise to 7.2 to 7.4. Your body requires this pH range for the enzyme amylase to work optimally, which is responsible for the digestion of starches. If you test "eating saliva pH" (just before you begin to eat as your mouth is salivating), and it is below 7.2, it is sign that your body is lacking the necessary mineral reserves and enzymes to properly digest food. If the enzymes are off in your mouth, you can all but guarantee that they will be off further down the digestive tract in the pancreas and the gallbladder. This why the eating saliva pH test is the most important of all pH tests.

In general, if your saliva pH is below 6.5, you are highly acidic and lack the necessary mineral buffers necessary to handle acids in its system. It's time to start alkalizing. Saliva pH should *never* dip below 6.1. A saliva pH of 5.5 (with associated urine pH of 4.5) is indicative of (or the potential for) chronic disease, and it is a clear sign that the body has been wiped out of its minerals reserves. For example, nearly every cancer patient will test strongly acidic on his or her saliva pH test.

Unfortunately, saliva does not have a large amount of mineral reserves, and it can be depleted of minerals very quickly, especially if you are consuming a heavily acidic diet.

Next, your body will take whatever minerals it can from urine and soft tissues. Magnesium is a significant buffer of acid that resides largely in your muscle tissue throughout your body. Acid drains our bodies of magnesium, which then interrupts enzyme function, causing muscle cramps, spasms, and muscle pain. When magnesium levels are depleted—and 80 percent of Americans are magnesium-deficient—your body will turn to its largest alkaline mineral bank, the bones. In fact, under dietary or emotional stress, magnesium is the first mineral to leave the body, followed by potassium and calcium.

Eating the "**S**tandard **A**merican **D**iet"— high amounts of sugar, grains, dairy, meat, caffeine, and artificial sweeteners—will rob the skeleton of almost half its calcium over twenty years. No wonder pharmaceutical companies are making millions from osteoporosis drugs.

URINE pH

Urine pH is different than blood and saliva, as urine is the output from your kidneys. That means you'll often see a higher acidic reading, especially in the morning. While you've been asleep, your body's been working to detoxify and pull acids from your tissues into the waste system. When you measure urine pH first thing in the morning, it's (usually) going to be the most acidic read of the day.

Once you transition to an alkaline diet for the first time, urine tests may initially show very acidic results. You'll be thinking, "But wait, I'm eating alkaline now! What happened?" Your new diet is helping the body rid itself of all those built-up acids, so for the first days or weeks, you'll experience them leaving your body. I can't tell you how many times I see this happen when my clients do the GET OFF YOUR ACID 7-Day Alkaline Cleanse. There is a furious dumping of acids—that means the cleanse is working! One day, you'll wake up to a higher urinary pH, and you'll know you've crossed over to clean living. It's a great feeling!

Urine pH should *always* be on the acidic side, in a range of 5.5 to 7.0. Urine pH reflects the function of your adrenal glands, kidneys, and hydration (or lack thereof), as the body has to eliminate the metabolic acids that result from the digestion of fats, carbohydrates, and proteins. This is why it is so important to consume high-alkaline foods. You will notice that urine pH is a direct reflection of what you eat. If you eat some meat or grains, then urine pH will test more acidic, as it has to eliminate those acids. Likewise, if you eat a meal consisting of a dark-green leafy salad with some avocado, then the pH will be toward the top of the range. As with saliva pH, the ideal range is 6.4 to 6.8. Urine pH should never dip below 5.0, as this indicates strong digestive issues and potential chronic disease.

MEASURING pH: CAN YOU PASS THE ACID TEST?

One of the greatest tools we have is the ability to measure pH and get a snapshot of acidity in real time. Tracking pH daily is inexpensive, extremely easy, and can be measured in just fifteen seconds! All that's needed is a box of pH test strips and a place to record your progress. I've developed pH test strips that can be used with saliva or urine, and they are available at my website, **www.getoffyouracid .com**. Generic test strips are also available at your local drugstore. They are dual color test strips, which are the most sensitive and accurate.

The Three Most Critical pH Tests

Now that you understand what the numbers indicate, pH testing can be an extremely useful way to objectively measure and track how your body is progressing.

At any given time, pH reflects your diet, how you move (or don't), how you think, and how much mental and emotional stress you carry. I will say this repeatedly because it's critical: stress outweighs anything you can eat or drink a million times to one.

I recommend testing pH at the same time consistently every day. It's easy to just wake up and test your urine right away. If you're using the urine test, try testing first thing in the morning. If you're testing saliva, aim for either 11 a.m., 2 p.m., or around mealtime. Here are the three easiest ways you can test your pH.

EATING SALIVA PH TEST (BEFORE EATING)

This is perhaps the most important of all the pH tests. It should be performed as you get ready to eat and your mouth begins to salivate in response to thinking about the food in front of you. This test determines if you have the necessary alkaline mineral reserves to act as a buffer or neutralizer of acid when your body needs it.

When you're doing an eating saliva pH test, the ideal pH range result is 7.2 to 7.4. Rest assured, if you fall into this slightly alkaline range, you have enough alkaline reserves. That means your mouth has the necessary enzymes and minerals to buffer acid and help break down and digest your food. It also means that further down the line in your digestive system you will have them as well. The same is true for the opposite. If a pH test reveals a number lower than the 7.2 to 7.4 ideal range, acid problems are more severe and chronic. The 6.0 to 6.5 range indicates mild acidic problems. Below 6.0 is strongly acidic. That

means your body is in a state of chronic low-grade acidosis and is deficient in mineral reserves.

This test is significant because with a pH range of 7.2 to 7.4, the starch-digesting enzyme amylase works best. If pH is below this range, you can expect your digestion to be inefficient, which may lead to a host of problems.

If pH numbers fall below the ideal range, there are three things I want you to do:

1. Monitor this number at least once every day.

2. Chew food at least twenty-five times and put your fork down between bites. This predigests food and encourages good digestion. I even recommend you chew smoothies!

3. Closely follow my 7 Ways to GET OFF YOUR ACID in Chapter 8 to build your alkaline reserves.

Directions: Before doing this test, swallow your saliva twice, and either put the pH test strip directly on the saliva you have gathered in between your lips or spit it into a spoon and test it there (ideal method). Read the results no more than fifteen seconds after testing.

Ideal Result Range: 7.2–7.4.

A reading of less than 7.0 signifies that you are in a state of chronic low-grade acidosis, which means you are deficient in mineral reserves (magnesium, calcium, potassium, and sodium bicarbonate) and need to start alkalizing immediately.

SALIVA pH TEST
BETWEEN MEALS

The saliva pH test between meals should be taken at least two hours after eating, ideally around 11 a.m. and 2 p.m.

Directions: Before doing this test, swallow twice, and either put the pH test strip directly on the saliva that you have gathered in between your lips or spit it into a spoon and test it there (preferred). Read the results no more than fifteen seconds after testing.

Ideal Result Range: 6.5–7.4

Mildly Acidic: 6.0–6.5

Strongly Acidic: 4.5–6.0

A reading of less than 6.5 signifies you are in a state of chronic low-grade acidosis, are deficient in mineral reserves (magnesium, calcium, potassium, and sodium bicarbonate), and need to start alkalizing immediately.

URINE pH TEST
BETWEEN MEALS

The urine test between meals should be taken at least two hours after eating, ideally around 11 a.m. and 2 p.m.

Directions: Urinate into a cup and dip the pH test strip (preferred) and then remove it, or urinate on a pH test strip midstream. Read the results no more than fifteen seconds after testing.

Ideal Result Range: 6.0–7.0

Mildly Acidic: 5.5–6.0

Strongly Acidic: 4.5–5.5

Acceptable urine pH ranges should always read more acidic than saliva pH tests, as this is an indicator of the kidneys doing their job to eliminate the dietary and metabolic acids from your body.

A reading of less than 6.0 signifies that you are in a state of chronic low-grade acidosis, are deficient in mineral reserves (magnesium, calcium, potassium, and sodium bicarbonate), and need to start alkalizing immediately.

WHAT IS YOUR IDEAL URINE & SALIVA pH?

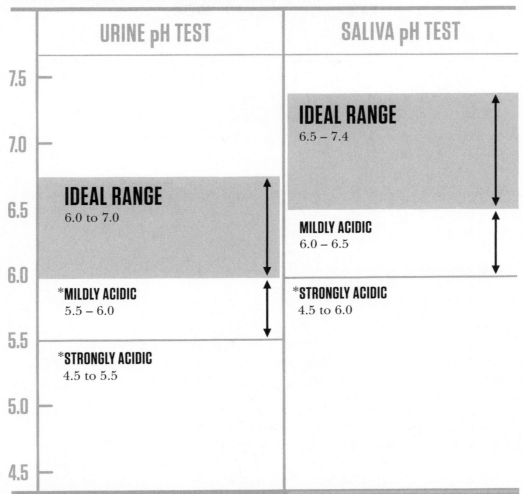

URINE pH TEST	SALIVA pH TEST

IDEAL RANGE
6.0 to 7.0

***MILDLY ACIDIC**
5.5 – 6.0

***STRONGLY ACIDIC**
4.5 to 5.5

IDEAL RANGE
6.5 – 7.4

MILDLY ACIDIC
6.0 – 6.5

***STRONGLY ACIDIC**
4.5 to 6.0

*Signifies that your body is in a state of **chronic low grade acidosis** and is deficient in mineral reserves.

- Start alkalizing immediately with dark green leafy vegetables and healthy fats
- Supplement with a dehydrated green powder high in chlorophyll
- Supplement with a mineral powder containing Magnesium Glycinate, Calcium Citrate, Potassium Bicarbonate, and Sodium Bicarbonate.

pH TESTING FOR CHILDREN

Most children's bodies are alkaline, with saliva pH in the range of 7.0 to 7.5. If their numbers are consistently lower than this range, you need to closely look at what you are giving them to eat and drink. Are they consuming common acidic foods such as orange juice, dairy, bagels and bread, pizza, cookies, chips, and soda? Test daily first thing in the morning and at least two hours after eating or chewing. Remember, give your children what they *need*, not what they *want*!

Directions: Before doing this test, have your child swallow his saliva twice, and either put the pH test strip directly on the saliva in his mouth or have him spit it into a spoon and test it there.

Children's Morning Saliva pH Test Ideal Result Range: 7.0–7.5

Monitor pH for One Month

pH testing is a science, and to avoid subjectivity you should repeatedly test yourself on a daily basis, ideally at the same times every day. In doing so, you can identify a trend after a period of four weeks. One pH test is just that—a one and done effort. It will not be highly significant.

As you test saliva and urine pH repeatedly, you will begin to get a feeling of your own body. It is the ultimate biofeedback system, and it will tell you exactly what is going on inside your body. Pay attention to the numbers, and pay attention to how you feel with your body at that specific pH level you tested at. Ask yourself, how is your energy? How is your digestion? How is your mood and your sleep? All of these help determine where in the ideal range your saliva and urine pH should reside.

In addition, monitoring pH consistently gives you excellent motivation. There is a saying, "What you inspect, you respect." Once you start examining your pH, you will have a newfound respect for your body's wondrous systems!

03

Your Body's Built-In Acid Buffers

Here's the good news: your body has a powerful defense system in the form of acid
buffers that work together to control blood
pH. It's an elaborate system comprised of
the kidneys, the lungs, the liver, your adrenal glands, the skin, cholesterol, and yes,
even fat—all beautifully designed to deal
with those daily acids. However, our bodies weren't built to withstand the onslaught
we're increasingly confronting, thanks to
all those dietary, metabolic, chemical, environmental, and stress acids.

A buffer is defined as a solution that
resists changes in pH when an acid or alkaline substance is added to it. Buffers typically involve one of the four most crucial
mineral salts: calcium, magnesium, potassium, or sodium. These alkaline buffers
keep pH balanced and resting just where
it should; without them, we would die from
acid overdose.

So if you're eating a heavily acidic diet,
your buffering system will kick into high
gear and help neutralize those acids. **But
by adopting a more alkaline lifestyle, your
buffering system can work effectively without being so heavily taxed.**

For example, when stressed by acid,
your body will deplete its store of crucial
minerals, going to your bones for calcium,
your muscles and joints for magnesium,
and your mouth for bicarbonate—finding
minerals wherever it can. There is a set
of "checks and balances" at play to keep
the most important parts of your body
healthy for as long as possible. You are pro-
grammed for survival. But over time, poor
dietary and lifestyle habits stress your body.
An acidic diet can lead to osteoporosis,
joint and muscle pain, and tooth and gum
decay—all in the ongoing effort to neutralize the acids in your blood and balance pH.

TYPES OF ACID BUFFERS
Blood Buffers

Buffers in the blood are the first to come
to your pH's defense, and they are the
most important, as they act within seconds.
One of the most powerful is an alkaline
substance called **bicarbonate**. The more alkaline you eat, the more bicarbonate your
body can make. But it doesn't work alone.

Bicarbonate ions combine with mineral salts such as calcium, magnesium, potassium, and sodium to escort the acids out of your body.

In his book *Sodium Bicarbonate,* Dr. Mark Sircus stresses the importance of having high amounts of bicarbonate in your blood at all times. Sircus wrote, "Even with healthy people, a noticeable decline of bicarbonate begins at the age of 45. . . . Loss of bicarbonates hinders the blood from effectively managing the acid the body produces. This loss, combined with mineral deficiency, triggers the onset of acid-induced degenerative diseases such as reflux, kidney stones, diabetes, hypertension, osteoporosis, heart disease, cancer, and gout."

Minerals are critical to keeping pH balanced. This is why it is so important to eat alkaline-forming foods such as dark-green leafy vegetables that are high in minerals and fiber and low in sugar. It's also why I advocate that my patients supercharge and alkalize their water. I will get into hydration more specifically in Chapter 8, but for now all you need to know is this: the most important function of drinking mineral-rich alkaline water is to increase bicarbonates in the blood because, as we age, they will naturally decrease, lowering your acid-fighting defenses.

Another important blood buffer is the protein buffering system: red blood cells and the amino acids in blood will absorb any remaining acids (H+ ions) in your blood. This is the largest and strongest buffering system in your body, accounting for 75 percent of the total buffering system.

It is responsible for fine-tuning blood pH to its healthy 7.4 level.

Lung Buffers

In addition to the acidic foods that you eat and drink, your body is constantly making metabolic acids as a byproduct of living. For example, gasoline fuels your car. As the car runs, carbon monoxide is produced as waste. Your body works the same way. It is alkaline by design with acidic byproducts.

The most important fuel for your body is oxygen. Instead of producing carbon monoxide like a car does, the body creates an acid waste called carbonic acid. Carbonic acid is either neutralized in the blood by minerals salts and bicarbonates, or it will travel to the lungs where it is converted to carbon dioxide gas and released by breathing. In fact, 70 percent of the total acid load in the body is removed via the lungs!

When acid increases, lung buffers kick in to change the way you breathe. They will increase your respiration rate (breathing faster and shallower) in an attempt to hasten the acid out of your body. While blood buffers act within seconds to neutralize acid, lung buffers can change pH in 1 to 3 minutes.

This is why it's important to watch your respiration rate (how fast or slow you breathe). Are you a shallow chest breather? Or do you breathe deeply down into your diaphragm? A respiration rate of five to six breaths per minute may indicate very good health, while a breath rate of twenty-four or higher may indicate a very serious acidic condition. As you breathe faster, your body is trying to exhale any excess carbon dioxide gas that is making your blood become more acidic.

Kidney Buffers

The kidneys will take over where blood buffers and lungs leave off. While blood buffers act in seconds, and lung buffers act within minutes, kidney buffers work within hours or days (yet they have the ability to act within minutes, if a dangerous situation arises) to help keep blood near a perfect pH of 7.4. Again, this is why the urine pH test is so important. Urine pH looks more directly at kidney function and will tend to be more acidic than saliva because it is an indicator of the toxins your kidneys are attempting to eliminate from your body.

Dietary Buffers

This is a buffer you can control more directly, which is why it is so important to eat alkaline. Not only are alkaline foods abundant in minerals, which neutralize acid, but they also release bicarbonate into the small intestines to maintain an alkaline environment and a healthy microbiome. The ideal pH of the small intestine should be alkaline at 7.5 to 8.4. When alkaline, it can absorb nutrients better.

Low Density Lipoprotein (LDL Cholesterol)

An elevated LDL level indicates your body has an acid problem. Low Density Lipoproteins (LDL, the so-called bad cholesterol) and fats bind to acids and toxins in your blood, lymph glands, and the fluid outside of the cells. Imagine a fish tank, for example. If the fish are your cells, the LDL cholesterol helps to clean up the water in the tank so the cells become less toxic. Your cells are only as healthy as the fluids they bathe in, which is why LDL and healthy fats are so crucial. Eating refined carbohydrates such as bread, pasta, and sodas increases LDL cholesterol. It will bind to these acids to help minimize their harm. Yet LDL is often considered to be a major cause of heart disease. However, LDL cholesterol does not "pull the trigger" for heart disease, but rather it is the scapegoat found at the scene of the crime. We need to understand its important role and realize it is actually beneficial.

Many doctors will prescribe statin drugs to lower elevated LDL levels, but statins just remove the self-defense mechanism that your body put in place to save your life. Acid is corrosive and can literally burn a hole, ulcerating the blood vessels and organs. LDL fats help prevent that from happening. LDL delivers cholesterol to your body, and you could not function without it. LDL levels will increase when toxins and free radical activity is present and elevated in your tissues, as it carries cholesterol to these toxic areas and serves as a primary antioxidant and buffer of acid. So, if you have increased LDL levels, heed the warning, as this is a serious sign of an underlying problem: too much acid. You will also want to test for the particle size of the LDL molecules. This is significant, and we will talk about it later.

LDL fats are acid magnets, and once they bind to the acids, ideally, they will be excreted through the four major pathways: urination, respiration, perspiration, and defecation. In other words, you pee them out, you breathe them out, you sweat them out, and you get the last one. But if your elimination methods are overwhelmed and backed up, your body will dump them into your tissues (around the organs, otherwise known as visceral fat, as well as around the belly, hips, and legs). This is exactly why obesity is an acid problem.

Acid Buffers Are Lifesavers

Your acid buffer systems are essential and are designed to keep blood pH as close to 7.4 as possible. These buffers are there to eliminate the daily acids your body is always making. But with the toxicity and stress that engulfs our lives today, our alkaline reserves quickly become depleted.

As you learned earlier, gluten, sugar, and antibiotics are destroying our micro biota, allowing toxins to bypass the intestinal wall guards, and then leaking into the bloodstream. Here it becomes a matter of supply and demand. Get too much acid, and you don't have enough buffers to neutralize them. As a result, your body is forced to deposit the acids into tissues where they are stored until the body is better equipped to eliminate them later. In the short run, this is saving your life by keeping your blood pH steady. But the longer those acids remain parked in your tissues, the more likely they will begin eating away at you from the inside out.

Next, the lymphatic system takes over. It's another very important detoxification system that your body has in place to get rid of acid. Your body will neutralize what it can, and whatever remains, the lymphatic system will suck up like a vacuum in order to remove any remaining acids from the tissues and send them back into the bloodstream to (hopefully) be eliminated. Can you see the pattern here? If you don't change your lifestyle, and the acid keeps pouring in, it becomes a vicious cycle.

This is where disease takes hold. I see it every day in my office where I do Live Blood Cell testing, which gives a real-time picture of what's going on in a patient's blood. The protocol allows me to get a detailed look at the *quality* of your blood—the internal environment or terrain that your cells are swimming in is everything. If toxins and acids are leaking into the bloodstream because of a possible leaky gut situation, a microscope at 25,000-times magnification will show it immediately.

STRENGTHENING YOUR GUT: WEED, SEED, AND FEED

Let me ask you a question. If a plant begins to wilt, what remedy comes to mind? Of course, water it! Well, why not offer drugs or surgery! You see, this is what most Western doctors would do to a "wilting" person!

It's a funny analogy, but there is some truth to it. We need to stop the approach of prescribing a pill for every ill or symptom and start addressing the true cause. Give the plant water, sunlight, and nutrients in its soil, and if it's not too far gone, the plant will heal itself. We are no different. Get rid of the toxins and give the body what it lacks, and if it's not too far gone, the body *will* heal itself. The body is a self-healing machine—give it what it needs (and more importantly, stop giving it what it doesn't need), then move aside and let it do what it was designed to do—heal! Health is as simple as that! I am very grateful for modern medicine, as it has saved both of my parents' lives. But medicine is for crisis care, not health care. The ancient physician Hippocrates wrote, "All disease begins in the gut." And I would add, "All *health* begins in the gut."

Our gut is home to 100 trillion bacteria. The healthy bacteria in our intestines produce chemicals that help us harness energy and nutrients from food. However, most people do not have a balanced intestinal environment. Instead, their microbiome is acidic, inflamed, and filled with mucous, and because of that, their health is compromised.

If you have taken antibiotics or have been on some kind of immune-suppressing drug such as Prednisone, your health is most likely compromised. If you eat sugar, grains, dairy, and meat, your health is most likely compromised. If you are dealing with a fair amount of prolonged emotional stress, your health is most likely compromised. But don't dip your head just yet. A method known as "Weed, Seed, and Feed" can help restore your gut health.

Healing is very much like growing a garden. You need to nourish the soil, give it the right seeds, water it, feed it, and if you're lucky, you might have a flourishing garden in a few months.

1. Weed: stop the poisoning; detoxify your digestive system and the blood

2. Seed: give your terrain—your digestive tract—healthy bacteria in the form of prebiotics and probiotics

3. Feed: follow an 80/20 alkaline diet that's abundant in dark-green leafy vegetables with minerals, chlorophyll, and healthy fats

This little rhyme gives you a handy way to remember the systematic approach you need to take for a more alkaline, balanced state.

Weed

You can't plant seeds if the soil is toxic. Continually eating toxic foods with a damaged gut is like walking on a sprained ankle. Your body can't begin to heal until you stop the poisoning. In this stage, you're removing all the bad stuff that crowds out your beautiful, healthy plants. In your body, that means starting by cutting out the toxic stuff: sugar, grains, white starchy foods (white flour, white potatoes, white rice), dairy, refined salt, and artificial sweeteners (see page 67). You need to weed out the pathogens while at the same time boost your immune defense.

The length of this process varies from person to person, depending on how toxic you are. This stage can take as long as one month, but it can be shortened drastically by jump-starting the detoxification process with a cleanse such as my 7-Day Alkaline Cleanse or 2-Day Detox Challenge (visit www.getoffyouracid.com for more details.) Also, the more closely you adhere to the 7 Ways to GET OFF YOUR ACID in Chapter 8, the faster you will make it through the weeding stage.

Seed

Now that you've cleaned the soil, it's time to plant all the beneficial seeds that will make your garden thrive. That means giving your body minerals, nutrients, and plenty of alkaline water. This stage also involves reviving the gut with beneficial bacteria and healing the lining of the intestinal wall. Now is a good time to start taking a probiotic supplement.

Probiotic comes from a Greek word that means "for life." Probiotics contain the helpful or friendly live bacteria that normally inhabit the digestive tract. However, not all probiotics are the same, as they all differ in species and strain. Therefore, I recommend you rotate probiotics every thirty days and opt for the refrigerated kind, as there will be less degradation (more about these and other supplements in Chapter 8).

This is also an appropriate time to eat fermented foods if you so desire, which are a source of good bacteria, vitamins, and antioxidants. The best sources are fermented cabbage, sauerkraut, kimchi, and pickles. However, there are caveats. If you are having a health challenge with cancer or candida (yeast), avoid all fermented foods. Adding yeast to a body that is already dealing with a yeast problem is like adding gasoline to a fire. In addition, if you are going to consume fermented foods, there are some you should avoid—yogurt, nutritional yeast, kombucha, and kefir grains (more about these in Chapter 5).

The seeding stage can last anywhere from a few weeks to a couple of months. During this stage, I tend to eat less fermented foods (though I do enjoy some pickles and kimchi from time to time) and rely more on a quality probiotic. With a good probiotic, I know I am getting at least 30 billion colony forming units (CFUs) every day, and as I previously mentioned, I change the probiotic monthly to be sure I am giving my body access to the different strains that my microbiome needs.

Feed

By adopting a healthy, alkaline lifestyle, you follow an ongoing regimen that keeps the body in balance, giving you plenty of energy—the telltale sign of improving health. This final stage is all about nourishment and supporting the detoxifying organs with plenty of cleansing herbs such as parsley and cilantro, salads, alkaline green juices and smoothies, raw soups, and herbal teas such as dandelion, gynostemma, or my favorite Detox Tea (see the recipe on page 153).

It's that simple. Don't think of this journey as one of deprivation but more of a gradual process to replace harmful choices with better ones. You can do this while staying satisfied, enjoying delicious food, and forgetting those warnings you've been given about calories and fats. As you read on, I'll tell you everything you need to know.

04

Acidity Is the Root of
Most Health Conditions

It may surprise you to learn just how many ailments, ranging from common complaints to acute and chronic conditions, are linked to an acid state in the body. Conditions as frequent as skin breakouts, muscle cramps, and extra weight are, in part, caused by acidity, as are more serious conditions such as heart disease, cancer, Alzheimer's, and osteoporosis.

I'm drawn to an analogy used by my colleague Dr. James Chestnut, a chiropractor, wellness expert, and author of *The Wellness Prevention Paradigm*. In his book, he talks about the notion of "rocks in the backpack" as a metaphor to explain chronic illness, and here I use it to explain pH imbalance and chronic low-grade acidosis.

I want you to visualize being born into a swimming pool, wearing water wings on your arms (to keep you afloat) and a backpack. Imagine those wings have a very slow leak, meaning that the air will run out in about 120 years (your genetically determined lifespan potential). In this analogy, any form of acid stressor that causes toxicity or deficiency—dietary, metabolic, chemical, environmental, or emotional—represents a rock in your backpack.

As the rocks accumulate, you sink a little lower in the water, and in response, you have to work harder to stay afloat. What does that do to the pressure on your water wings? It increases it. What does that do to the rate of air leakage? It increases it. What does this do to the aging process? It increases its speed. More stress is put on all of your bodily systems. Your body constantly lives in "compensation mode," draining your energy.

Now, some rocks might be little pebbles that represent small stressors, while others might be boulders. And sure, some of the rocks in life are unavoidable. In fact, the world is so toxic, the backpack may contain little rocks that were there before you were even born. The important question is, when those rocks do get into your backpack, do you have the tools to help your body eliminate them so you won't have to work so hard to stay afloat?

Remember, you're in complete control of your health.

Some of you may be lightly treading water, not having to swim very much. If so, you're in a good place and the 7 Ways to GET OFF YOUR ACID are going to elevate you to the next level, building on the healthy foundation you already have in place.

For others, your backpack may be so heavy and overloaded that you are sinking fast, in which case it is critical to begin to alkalize and detoxify your body. In this book, I will give you the strategies you need to turn this sinking ship around and get you back on track to health, energy, and vitality.

After seeing this practical analogy, many people realize why they are drained of their energy. They have more rocks than they can carry, and they are aging faster than they should. Have you ever felt older than your true chronological age? I can't tell you how many times clients come into my office and tell me they feel like they are living in a 95-year old body, and they're 30!

TELOMERES CAN PREDICT LONGEVITY— SIZE MATTERS

In a *Science & News* article from 2008, researchers from Duke University did a long-term study of New Zealanders, revealing why some people age faster than others. They discovered it's based on something called *telomeres*.

Within our cells, telomeres are the DNA protein caps at the end of chromosomes that promote chromosomal stability and protect the DNA from damage. As our cells regenerate, telomere length naturally shortens with each cell cycle, but if it falls to a critically short length, the cell is no longer able to divide and often malfunctions.

The study took a health snapshot of 954 people. All were 38 years old at the time of the study, so they all had the same chronological age. But their biological ages, based on how healthy a person is compared with the average, varied greatly. The study found ages, in effect, ranged from ages 28 to 61.

In other words, some of the 38-year-olds resembled people a couple decades older than them, while others appeared younger! The study used eighteen different markers of aging over time, and one significant marker was the length of the telomeres in their bodies. When it comes to telomeres, size does matter! The longer the telomeres are, the more longevity a person has, and the shorter they are, the more likely people will age faster and succumb to chronic disease.

And what is it that indicates having shorter telomere length? The amount of rocks in a backpack! In other words, the amount of acids and toxins in your body.

The good news is the opposite holds true as well. Just as toxicity shortens telomeres, taking positive actions toward health can lengthen them. For example, in a 2009 study from the *American Journal of Clinical Nutrition*, women who took a daily multivitamin for more than five years had a 3 percent increase in telomere length (compared to non-users), and when combined with an

HOW WE GET SICK

I'll always maintain that we don't "catch" a cold—we "ate" that cold or "thought" that cold by ingesting nutrient-deficient foods, overtaxing the body, or becoming overly stressed in a variety of ways, both mental and physical. A weakened immune system makes the body susceptible to germs it would otherwise fend off.

Why is it that when January rolls around, so many people get sick? Following all the celebrations between Halloween and New Year's, everyone winds down in January. People have become stressed, tired, and more toxic from all the acidic food and drinks consumed over this period.

Because we all share the same air, why doesn't *everyone* catch the flu? Why does one person in the office stay well while the person at the desk right next to them gets sick? Some people withstand these ailments year after year, while others continually succumb. Sick patients breathe on me all day long, yet I haven't had a cold or flu in more than twenty years. In its optimal state, the body is well equipped to fend off any germs that can cause harm. Wear your body down and weaken its defenses—now it's another story.

Germs alone don't make us sick; in fact, we are filled with bacteria. Recall microbiomes—our bodies have ten times more bacteria than they do cells! We need germs because without them we wouldn't be alive.

Illness isn't just about the germ; it's also about your internal terrain. Clean your environment, and you will make your immune system impenetrable.

antioxidant, that percentage rose to 8 percent. Conversely, a study from scientists at the University of California–San Francisco (UCSF) showed that drinking soda inhibits telomere length, even cutting years off projected longevity!

True healing is possible within us. We have the power to shift the scale either way, toward health or sickness, based on the lifestyle choices we make. As a nation, if we focus more on learning from the smaller percentage of people who are truly healthy, who are fit and full of energy, studying what they actually do to maintain their health, there would be a lot less disease to treat.

SERIOUS CONDITIONS
CAUSED BY AN ACIDIC STATE
(IN ORDER OF CAUSE OF DEATH)

- ▸ Heart disease
- ▸ Cancer
- ▸ Alzheimer's
- ▸ Type 2 diabetes

COMMON CONDITIONS
CAUSED BY AN ACIDIC STATE

- ▸ Acid Reflux/GERD (gastroesophageal reflux disease)
- ▸ Low energy
- ▸ Obesity/overweight
- ▸ Osteoporosis
- ▸ Sleep issues
- ▸ Skin issues
- ▸ ADD/ADHD

We have never been sicker as a nation, and for the first time in history, the lifespan and longevity of our children are actually lower than that of their parents. Chronic degenerative disease is skyrocketing and becoming a way of life. A November 4, 2015, article in the *San Francisco Chronicle* stated that half the people who reach age 85 over the next decade will develop Alzheimer's, the most common form of dementia. Meanwhile, so many people are dying of cancer and heart disease, they aren't even going to make it to 85! What is the common denominator between all of these degenerative diseases? It's chronic, low-grade acidosis, resulting in toxicity, deficiency, oxidation, and inflammation.

HEART DISEASE

Do you know what one of the most common symptoms of heart disease is? Death! It sounds harsh, but some diseases appear without warning and with no chance to fight them. Every ninety seconds, someone suffers a heart attack. In that same time, two people will have strokes, and one will die of cardiovascular disease.

Heart disease is the leading cause of death in the United States, and growing numbers of us have become ticking time bombs. Forty-seven percent of adults have at least one of three risk factors for cardiovascular disease: uncontrolled high blood pressure, uncontrolled high levels of LDL cholesterol (the so-called "bad" cholesterol), or smoking.

Why has this become the number-one killer for Americans? It's certainly not because of a deficit of cholesterol-lowering pills such as statin drugs, as these drugs are being prescribed at unprecedented rates. And yet, the heart disease numbers keep increasing.

The Great Cholesterol Myth

Cholesterol has been widely blamed for the heart disease epidemic we have been experiencing the 1970s. This is because most doctors have observed higher risks of heart disease with the following:

▸ **higher levels of total cholesterol in the blood;**

▸ **higher levels of LDL cholesterol ("bad" cholesterol); and**

▸ **lower levels of HDL cholesterol ("good" cholesterol).**

Consequently, the pharmaceutical industry has built a multibillion-dollar empire aimed at eliminating excess cholesterol. Roughly, 25 percent of Americans over the age of 40 and 50 percent of all people over the age of 75 are on a cholesterol-lowering statin drug. Unfortunately, not only do these drugs mask the real problem, but also many people are irresponsibly put on these drugs with no knowledge of the side effects or what I prefer to call the "non-desired" effects.

One of the major reasons why statin drugs are so dangerous is that they interfere with your body's ability to synthesize coenzyme Q_{10} (known as CoQ_{10}). CoQ_{10} is a substance similar to a vitamin that is found in every cell of your body. Your body makes CoQ_{10}, and your cells use it to produce adenosine triphosphate (ATP), the energy your body needs for cell growth and maintenance. CoQ_{10} also functions as a powerful antioxidant, which protects your body from oxidative damage caused by harmful molecules. When you take a statin drug, your body (specifically your heart) reduces its production of ATP, thus increasing the risk for congestive heart failure.

Statin drugs also interfere with your body's ability to convert vitamin K_1 (which your body gets from eating green leafy vegetables) to K_2, which plays a crucial role in where the calcium is deposit after it's absorbed. Vitamin K_2 prevents it from going to all the wrong places, such as your joints or arteries, where it would increase the incidence of arthritis and atherosclerosis.

In addition, statins massively deplete magnesium levels, one of the most important alkaline minerals and buffers of acid in the body. Unfortunately, statins do not address the true cause of cardiovascular health issues and are actually making us sicker while making the drug companies richer!

Here is what you need to know about high cholesterol: it is not a *cause* of heart disease, as so many doctors have led you to believe, but a *symptom*. In fact, you need cholesterol and cannot live without it, as it is one of the most important components of cells and the brain. When there is an increase in cholesterol production, it's a reparative response by your body to save your life from the effects of chronic low-grade acidosis. That's right: heart disease in all forms is an acid problem!

The Real Culprit

Chronic acidity in the blood causes degeneration and ulceration of arterial walls, which, over time, creates inflammation as a healing response. In addition, your body will deposit fibrin, collagen, and phospholipids to repair the acidic damage of the arterial wall. Acid is corrosive, and your body, specifically your liver, generates cholesterol as a self-defense mechanism to save you from an acid-damaged artery.

As you can see, increased cholesterol production is your body's attempt to heal itself.

When blood vessels become injured from acid, in addition to the cholesterol response, an inflammatory cascade is initiated as well. The inflammation results in plaque formation, which is akin to a scab on a blood vessel's wall. Ultimately, this inflammatory plaque build-up becomes the most dangerous effect of the underlying acid damage. The plaque has the ability to rupture, dumping all of its toxic inflammatory components into your bloodstream and general circulation.

The reality is that cholesterol is neither good nor bad. But one thing is certain: cholesterol is essential. About 25 percent of the cholesterol comes from what you eat, and the other 75 percent is made by your liver, primarily in response to toxicity and acid. Research has shown that lower cholesterol levels don't make you healthier. In fact, the evidence indicates that it actually increases your mortality risk! Nor is saturated fat the problem when it comes to cardiovascular issues.

A 2016 study in the *British Medical Journal* looked at a cholesterol-lowering diet that replaced saturated fat with linoleic acid (the harmful omega-6 fatty acids from corn oil and corn oil polyunsaturated margarine). The results showed that for every thirty-point drop in total cholesterol, there was a 22 percent higher risk of death.

Saturated fats such as coconut oil have been shown to raise HDL cholesterol, which will also raise total cholesterol. But we now know based on research that this is a *good* thing—higher total cholesterol levels are actually associated with longevity and lower cancer rates. A study published by the *International Journal of Epidemiology*, which had 47,000 participants, concluded, "The highest death rate observed was among those with the lowest cholesterol (under 160 mg/dl); lowest death rate observed was with those whose cholesterol was between 200–259 mg/dl."

Healthy saturated fats also increase large particle-sized LDL cholesterol, which are completely benign and do not contribute to heart disease. You should be more concerned about the small, dense LDL cholesterol, which oxidize easily and have a greater ability to penetrate blood vessel walls, which can contribute to plaque build-up and atherosclerosis.

The real heart disease culprit is twofold:

1. **High insulin levels** in the body, which are elevated due to a toxic and acidic diet. When you are burning sugar (carbs) as a primary fuel source, insulin levels will stay elevated, and inflammation will be the result. This results from a diet high in sugar and grains and lacking in healthy fats and dark green leafy vegetables.

2. **High dietary omega-6 fatty acids**, which create a major risk factor for coronary heart disease, systemic inflammation, and even brain diseases such as dementia and Alzheimer's. One of the most important numbers for you to know is the omega-6 to omega-3 ratio, which can be easily tested for (more about this soon). Ideally, these fatty acids should have a 1:1 ratio and no more than 4:1. Yet studies show the average American diet has a ratio of 19:1 in favor of the pro-inflammatory omega-6 fatty acids (and it is often as much as 25:1 and 50:1). Please note, it takes about four months to change your ratio once you start your fish oil protocol and begin decreasing the sources of omega-6 fats in your diet.

THE DIET SOLUTION

There is compelling evidence that a diet rich in vegetables and low-sugar fruits can lower the risk of heart disease and stroke.

The largest and longest study to date, which was done as part of the Harvard-based Nurses' Health Study and Health Professionals Follow-up Study, included almost 110,000 men and women whose health and dietary habits were followed for fourteen years. The higher the average daily intake of fruits and vegetables, the lower the chances of developing cardiovascular disease. Compared with those in the lowest category of fruit and vegetable intake (less than one and a half servings a day), those who averaged eight or more servings a day were 30 percent less likely to have had a heart attack or stroke.

Other studies show that eating a diet rich in dark-green leafy vegetables such as kale, spinach, chard, watercress, beet greens, and mustard greens; cruciferous vegetables such as broccoli, cauliflower, cabbage, Brussels sprouts, and bok choy; and citrus fruits such as lemons, limes, and grapefruit could prevent 80 percent of heart disease, stroke, and type 2 diabetes!

Seven Heart Disease Indicators That Could Save Your Life!

These blood tests will indicate if you are at risk of cardiovascular disease:

Vertical Auto Profile (VAP) Test. It is now known that LDL itself is not a marker of heart disease. A VAP test looks at the LDL particle size, which is a more accurate risk factor. Keeping it simple: larger particles are good, and smaller particles are bad. The test also provides individuals with a

> *I started the* Get Off Your Acid *program in July 2015. At that time, I had high cholesterol, peaking at 284 mg/dl. My triglycerides and LDL were dangerously through the roof. And if that wasn't bad enough, I had diabetes. I would go to the doctors every three months and they would say, 'You need to get on a diet' but could never give me any further advice on what to do. I so badly wanted to be healthy and had no idea how to get it, and at the time, this feeling caused so much stress in my life. That is when my search began, and when I found the* Get Off Your Acid *program.*
>
> Get Off Your Acid *has changed my life! I'm now off all medications for my cholesterol and diabetes. The* Alkamind Daily Greens *and* Daily Minerals *are amazing. I have lost weight and did so eating as much as I wanted, not once worrying about counting my calories. The recipes are so wonderful and very filling. My sugar cravings are completely gone! The program has such amazing support, and I can't say enough about it! Thank you!*
>
> —*Leslie J.*

better idea of their vulnerability to the metabolic syndrome, a combination of factors that significantly elevate the risk an individual has in developing diabetes or cardiovascular disease.

High Sensitivity C-Reactive Protein (HS CRP). This is a primary marker of inflammation in arteries. The following are CRP results and risk factors:

Less than 1 mg/l of blood = low risk

1–3 mg/l = moderate risk

More than 3 mg/l = high risk

Homocysteine. This is an amino acid found in blood that is a marker of inflammation and heart disease, acquired mostly from eating too much meat. Meat is acidic and should be eaten in moderation. Homocysteine is considered elevated when it's greater than 8 umol/L. Ideal homocysteine levels should fall below 6 umol/L.

A1C. Typically a blood test for diabetes, this is a primary marker for sugar oxidation of LDL cholesterol. If this number is high, it means you are eating too many acidic foods that are high in simple carbohydrates and burning sugar as a primary fuel source instead of fat (see Chapter 7). Ideally, the A1C level should be less than 5.

Total cholesterol. The optimal range is 200 to 240 mg/dl. Many doctors would be quick

> The prime cause of cancer is the replacement of respiration of oxygen in normal body cells by the fermentation of sugar.
>
> —DR. OTTO WARBURG, 1931 NOBEL LAUREATE

to prescribe statin drugs when cholesterol levels are higher than 200. However, research from the *World Review of Nutrition and Dietetics, Prevention of Coronary Heart Disease From the Cholesterol Hypothesis to O6/O3 Balance* states that there is "no reason for the majority of people to lower their total cholesterol because high total cholesterol is actually associated with longevity."

Triglycerides. These should be below 100 mg/dl.

Omega-6 to omega-3 fatty acid ratio. Next to blood pH, this ratio is perhaps the most important number in the body. In fact, some scientists have dubbed the ratio the "new cholesterol," as it offers the most accurate measure of systemic inflammation. An over abundance of omega-6s (soy, corn, meat, and eggs) and a deficiency of omega-3s (fish) causes a significant inflammatory imbalance in cells. The ratio is also known as the AA/EPA ratio, and it should ideally be 1:1 and no more than 4:1, yet the average American has nineteen times more of the pro-inflammatory omega-6 fats. The

Alkamind Omega-3 Acid Index assessment measures the amount of omega-3 fatty acids in cells and provides the specific dose of fish oil you need for optimal health. It can also reveal your specific risk factors for stroke and dementia.

CANCER

Cancer is not a disease that you happen to just get; like many diseases, it's a process that occurs over time. Think of it this way: you don't get cancer, you eat cancer, you drink cancer, and you think cancer (that's accumulated chemical and emotional stress!).

In 1971, President Nixon and the US Congress declared war on cancer and promised that Americans would have a cure by the bicentennial. Yet, in 2017, almost half a century later, cancer has become a growing epidemic. In fact, cancer has overtaken heart disease as the number-one killer in twenty-one states. In 2017, there were 1.6 million new cancer diagnoses (one every 3 minutes), and almost 600,000 Americans will die from it. That's a fatality rate of about 36 percent. Statistically, one

WANT TO LEARN MORE
ABOUT THE OMEGA 6:3 RATIO?

I'm now offering a simple, at-home test called the Alkamind Omega-3 Acid Index that measures the critical omega-6/omega-3 fatty acid ratio and can give an early indication of predisposition to certain kinds of diseases. A painless prick of the finger and a single blood droplet allows me to analyze three blood biomarkers and brain health indicators:

▸ **The Omega-3 Index** measures the percentage of EPA and DHA found in cell membranes and is a direct measure of systemic inflammation and how deficient you may be in these critical anti-inflammatory fatty acids. Fatty acids are as important to your brain and body as calcium and protein are to your muscles. Research has associated higher omega-3 index scores (optimal is above 8 percent) with up to a 47 percent lower risk of dementia, improved short-term memory, better focus and learning at school, and improved mood and lower anxiety.

▸ **The Cell Inflammation Index** checks the ratio of omega-6 to omega-3 fatty acids, which can indicate inflammation damaging to brain health, and is also a true quantifier of the inflammatory state of the cells in your body. Research has associated a lower ratio (the ideal is 1:1) with lower inflammation levels, reduced chronic pain, hormone and immune regulation, and lower risk of cancer and heart disease.

▸ **The Cell Toxicity Index** watches for cellular destruction and hormone production, which can adversely affect memory and increase inflammation. This specific index measures the amount of palmitic acid in cell membranes—toxins derived from unhealthy carbohydrate consumption that displace omega-3 fatty acids. Research has associated lower cell membrane palmitic acid with increased energy levels, optimized metabolism and fat-burning, and normalization of glucose, insulin, and leptin, which creates proper sensitivity to feeling full.

In addition to these three important blood biomarkers, a fifteen-minute online assessment will also provide you with information on how your brain is functioning, such as memory capacity, sustained attention, processing speed, and overall cognitive flexibility. To obtain an Alkamind Omega-3 Acid Index at-home testing kit, go to **www.getoffyouracid.com** or call **844-200-ALKA (2552)**.

in two men and one in three women will get cancer in their lifetime. That's 40 percent of all people, but it doesn't have to be you. The quality of the choices you make today not only can improve your energy but also can make you far less susceptible to cancer.

The typical Western diet has become fertilizer for cancer, as an acidic body creates a welcoming environment for disease to present itself and advance. **In fact, a University of Texas study stated 95 percent of all cancers are due to diet and accumulation of toxins, which leads to less oxygen going to your cells.**

Research shows that cancer thrives in an anaerobic (or oxygen-deprived) environment, and most cancers (with a few exceptions), as well as many other health conditions, happen in an acidic environment. When faced with less oxygen, the cells get their energy by switching to a more primitive mode of respiration called anaerobic metabolism, which happens through the fermentation of sugar. What's the waste product of that form of energy? Lactic acid!

So not only does acid help create a cancer-friendly environment, but there is also a vicious cycle of imbalance where cancer generates acid.

Here's the good news. If 95 percent of cancer happens due to lifestyle factors, this means we can prevent it from ever occurring in the first place!

Cancer and Toxins

Cancer is a metabolic disease of the mitochrondria that is manifested by long-term toxicity at the cellular level. There are five primary sources of these toxins:

▸ **dietary (sugar, grains, artificial sweeteners, dairy, and processed foods)**

▸ **metabolic (lactic acid, carbonic acid, and uric acid)**

▸ **chemical (antibiotics, smoking, and alcohol)**

▸ **environmental (water pollution, air pollution, and electromagnetic pollution)**

▸ **stress**

Who is susceptible to toxicity? Everyone. The average person is exposed to 167 chemicals per day, often via use of personal care products. Even our children are at risk; in fact, the leading cause of death for children over the age of 1 is cancer. How is it possible that cancer can develop at such an early age? A 2005 study from the Environmental Working Group Study (EWG) might shed some light.

This study revealed 287 chemicals in the umbilical cords from a group of babies born in 2004 in US hospitals. Of the chemicals detected, 180 are known to cause cancer in humans or animals, 217 are toxic to the brain and nervous system (including but not limited to mercury and polychlorinated biphenyls, otherwise known as PCBs), and 208 cause birth defects or abnormal development in animal tests. The dangers of pre- or postnatal exposure to this complex mixture of carcinogens, developmental toxins, and neurotoxins have never been studied.

We are surrounded by toxicity everywhere, and as cells accumulate toxins, there becomes a deficiency in the most important nutrient in your body, oxygen.

In a healthy body, cells function by burning glucose (sugar) in oxygen to create energy—what is known as adenosine triphosphate (ATP). This process of creating ATP is called aerobic respiration, which takes place inside the mitochondria, the powerhouse of your cells, and is essential to life.

When you are eating a plant-based alkaline diet, have minimal stress levels, minimize toxin exposure, move regularly, and breathe well, you are aerobically oxygenating your cells and creating a healthy, balanced blood and tissue pH. When you have a healthy pH, the oxygen-carrying capacity of the hemoglobin in red blood cells is high, allowing more total oxygen to be carried within your body, and oxygen is life. Your immune system will function optimally, and any rogue cancer cells that your body makes will be destroyed by a healthy process called apoptosis. (The average person makes roughly 10,000 cancer cells every day, but the immune system is always on the job to keep them in check.)

Likewise, when you're consuming an inflammatory diet high in processed foods, sugar, grains, omega-6 fats, alcohol, soft drinks, dairy, and meat, and have high levels of mental and emotional stress, blood is prone to becoming more acidic. At that point, the ability of your red blood cells to carry oxygen decreases. To keep blood pH balanced and to prevent this from happening, your body will dump these acids from the blood into the body's tissues to keep the blood pH slightly alkaline at 7.4.

As the acid builds, your cells and tissues will literally begin to rot (causing cancer) and rust (causing heart disease). Many of these cells will die because of the toxicity, but others will find another way to survive.

In 1931, Otto Warburg won the Nobel Laureate for discovering how cells metabolize because of increased toxicity, thus uncovering the true mechanism of cancer. In his research, he discovered the following: if a cell is deprived of 35 percent of its oxygen for forty-eight hours, it *may* become cancerous. If a cell is deprived of 60 percent of its oxygen, it *will* turn cancerous.

The Cancer-Sugar Connection

You may have heard the saying, "Cancer loves sugar." But do you know where this originated? Cancer cells rely on sugar as a primary source for energy. Cancer requires sugar to stay alive!

If cells are deprived of oxygen and ferment sugar, more lactic acid is created. Lactic acid will then push itself into adjacent cells, slowly poisoning them as well, decreasing their oxygen supply. And there you have it, the metastasis of cancer.

When healthy cells use oxygen for energy, one glucose (sugar) molecule can create as many as thirty-six ATP molecules (energy); likewise, the process of anaerobic respiration creates only two ATPs! That is an 18:1 difference in terms of the energy that a healthy cell can create compared to that of a cancer cell. In other words, in order for a cancer cell to create the same amount of energy as one normal cell, it must metabolize eighteen times more glucose (sugar). *That* is why cancer loves sugar. It requires sugar to compete and stay alive.

Here is the takeaway: sugar is not your friend; sugar is cancer's friend. Sugar, and everything that it is disguised as, is one of the most acidic substances you can put into your body. Whether you have cancer or not, you should avoid sugar like the plague. At the same time, it's necessary to increase consumption of healthy fats and minerals. Minerals neutralize the lactic acid made by high-intensity anaerobic-style exercise and cancer cells alike. If you don't neutralize the acid that's produced, your body will have to work overtime and deplete its resources to get rid it! That drains energy and leads to more illness and symptoms.

When the Doctor Says "Cancer"

I lost a piece of my heart the day my dad was diagnosed with cancer. But my family needed positivity, and we needed an immediate plan of action. If you or a loved one has developed cancer, stay positive! All healing begins with your mind, and it is more powerful than you can ever imagine. Become educated, decide right now to fight and to live, and take action to detoxify and alkalize your body.

The power to heal is yours. Cancer doesn't have to be a death sentence. It can be your journey to a better life. But you must believe that you can get well, as the most powerful medicine on this planet is *belief*!

The same incredible power that created your body keeps working for you throughout your life. In fact, in 120 days, your body can completely regenerate all new cells. It's one of the wonders of this life. Of course, no two conditions, no matter how similar they appear, ever respond the same. Everyone is different genetically; we all have a unique health history, and we all have different types of physical, mental, and emotional stresses. But the point is, your body has this miraculous power to heal and steer itself back on course, even in the most trying predicaments.

Imagine taking 120 days to give your body the best possible environment: eating a clean, plant-based alkaline diet and eliminating all alcohol, sugar, gluten, and caffeine, while exercising a bit and minimizing stress.

When my dad was diagnosed with cancer, the first thing I did was watch *The Truth About Cancer*—an empowering and educational cancer docu-series by Ty Bollinger. He traveled the world and interviewed more than 130 doctors who have been getting phenomenal results with their patients who have all kinds of cancer, even later stage, using treatment protocols other than the traditional big three used in the United States: poison it (chemotherapy), burn it (radiation), or cut it (surgery).

His interviews with these doctors revealed how cancer develops through toxicity deficiency and a lack of oxygen. We know what we must do to have our best shot in its prevention.

Detoxification must become a lifestyle. It is something that we must do every day. Did you know that increasing your vegetable intake could decrease your risk of cancer by 60 to 70 percent? Eating foods rich in healthy, alkaline, omega-3 fats and reducing the intake of inflammatory omega-6 fats can change your risk factors not only for cancer but also for heart disease and overall longevity.

In the later chapters, we dive into more ways to detox, including breathing exercises, lymphatic drainage, and consuming chlorophyll, which will build healthier cells and cleanse the toxins from your blood and your tissues.

ALZHEIMER'S DISEASE

Alzheimer's is now the third leading cause of death in the United States, right behind heart disease and cancer. A form of dementia, it is not only a horrific disease to see a friend or loved one go through, but it also shortens one's lifespan. The progressive and irreversible brain disorder slowly destroys memory and thinking skills. The buildup of beta-amyloid protein and plaque in the brain is considered one of the hallmarks of Alzheimer's disease.

When diagnosed with Alzheimer's, the average life expectancy is eight to ten years, Among people age 70, 61 percent of those with Alzheimer's are expected to die before the age of 80, compared with 30 percent of people without Alzheimer's—a rate twice as high.

Unfortunately, there is not yet a cure for Alzheimer's. Therefore, it must be prevented from ever happening in the first place. Among other factors, two processes—glycation and inflammation—are implicated in Alzheimer's disease.

Advanced Glycation

Cutting back on carbohydrates is rule number one for preventing this dreadful disease. There is an association between sugar and grain consumption and the risk of developing dementia. When you are insulin resistant and you continue to pump these acidic carbohydrates into your body, your risk factor for dementia increases by 400 percent.

Sugar and grains push your body into a downward spiral of burning glucose (sugar) as a primary fuel source, and, in turn, you end up craving and eating more sugar. The more glucose that hangs around in your blood, the greater tendency it has to attach itself to proteins in a dangerous process known as *glycation*. This breaks down the blood-brain barrier, resulting in dementia.

Inflammation

In his book *Inflammation Nation*, Dr. Sunil Pai wrote that Alzheimer's disease equals chronic inflammation of the brain. Inflammation is the body's healing mechanism to injury, so do your best to avoid any traumas to the head. When inflammation appears in sensitive brain tissue, brain function can be impaired, sometimes irreparably. Inflammation is a process that is induced by acidosis.

Elevated homocysteine (14 umol/L or higher), a direct marker of inflammation, is also associated with an increase of Alzheimer's risk. If you are a meat eater, which is a huge contributor to elevated homocysteine, limit consumption to no more than two times per week. If you closely follow the strategies laid out in my 7 Ways to GET OFF YOUR ACID, you will not only have a healthy alkaline body with a balanced pH, but you will also avoid many or all of the triggers that can increase your potential risk of developing Alzheimer's disease or any other form of dementia.

Prevention Is Everything: Ten Steps to Reduce Alzheimer's Risk

There is an old saying: an ounce of prevention is worth a pound of cure. When it comes to treating or preventing Alzheimer's, there are some specific things to focus on.

1. **Remove all sugar and grains** from your diet, including moderate- to high-sugar fruits.

2. **Balance the omega-6/omega-3 fatty acid ratio.** The brain is roughly 60 percent fat, and the fats, especially in your brain, are always in fierce competition for enzymes. An overload of omega-6 acids relative to omega-3s can lead to increased inflammation in your brain. This is why it is crucial to increase omega-3 fatty acids (taking a good quality fish oil supplement can help) and decrease the pro-inflammatory omega-6 fatty acids. Ideally, you are aiming for a 1:1 ratio, and no more than 4:1.

Tufts University researchers studied the relationship between blood DHA (a type of omega-3 fat) levels and the development of dementia and/or Alzheimer's disease in about 900 healthy men and women from the Framingham Heart study. The group averaged 76 years of age at the beginning of the nine-year study. Those people who had the highest DHA levels had a 47 percent lower risk of developing dementia than those with lower levels.

3. **Take antioxidants.** These include turmeric, vitamins C and E, glutathione, alpha lipoic acid, and molecular hydrogen.

4. **Put coconut oil in everything!** Cook with it and consume 1 to 2 tablespoons daily. The *Journal of Alzheimer's* conducted a study on the effects of coconut oil supplementation directly on cortical neurons treated with the amyloid-B peptide in vitro, which are the amino acids that make up the main component of the amyloid plaques found in the brains of Alzheimer's patients. The study found that daily consumption of coconut oil created neuron survival and helped improve the deficits associated with neurodegeneration.

5. **Take a vitamin D supplement.** Adequate vitamin D levels are above 50 ng/ml. Aim to be in the sun 20 minutes every day, with 40 percent skin exposure. Avoid toxic sunscreens, as moderate sun exposure is so important for our health and healthy vitamin D levels.

6. **Perform daily detoxification.** Ideally, focus on doing at least one detox protocol every day from the list provided in the 7 Ways to GET OFF YOUR ACID (page 151).

7. **Exercise daily.** Research shows that doing this can cut your risk of Alzheimer's by 50 percent.

8. **Burn fat, not sugar!** Insulin sensitivity is a factor in Alzheimer's risk. In Chapter 7, you will learn how to reset your body's metabolism to move away from sugar and become a fat burning machine!

9. **Reduce copper levels.** Free blood copper has been shown to be elevated in Alzheimer's patients. Never consume a copper supplement, and have your water checked, as 80 percent of the copper in our bodies comes from the pipes.

10. **Try stress relief for your brain.** Stress is like poison for your hippocampus, the part of the brain that deals with memory. Stress also activates the hormone cortisol, which can cause brain cell dysfunction and atrophy (shrinking of the brain). Follow my protocols to de-stress in Chapter 9.

TYPE 2 DIABETES

Once relatively rare, type 2 diabetes has surged to frightening new levels. More than 25 million Americans have been diagnosed with diabetes and another 80 million with prediabetes, the precursor condition. If this trend continues and with no sign of stopping, one in three adults will have diabetes by 2050.

Type 2 diabetes is a chronic condition that affects the body's ability to process blood sugar (or glucose). The pancreas produces a hormone called insulin, whose job is to move glucose from the blood into the cells, where it can then be stored as fat and used for energy later on. But when high amounts of sugar, carbs, and grains are regularly consumed, insulin levels spike, and, over time, the body's ability to produce or effectively utilize insulin becomes impaired (known as "insulin resistance"). This results in altered metabolism of carbohydrates and too much glucose in the blood and urine, putting your health at risk.

Incidence of diabetes has increased a staggering 700 percent over the last fifty years, and we can't always blame it on our genes. Our genes haven't changed over the last fifty years—but the acidity and toxicity in our lives has! Sugar and grain consumption is at an all-time high. In fact, the average American consumes an astounding 170 pounds of sugar every year, causing elevated blood glucose levels.

The pancreas and liver are two of the most important organs in charge of maintaining alkaline balance because of their abilities to produce buffering salts that neutralize acids in the intestines and blood. Chronic, low-grade acidosis increases body toxicity over time and exhausts these organs, making you more vulnerable to diabetes. It also results in a massive increase in acidic waste, which is one of the primary reasons why diabetes is the leading cause of kidney failure, amputation, and blindness. It's also a major cause of heart disease and stroke.

The average American consumes three to five times more protein than they require, which will be converted to sugar when metabolized. If you are going to eat animal-based proteins, I recommend limiting it to twice per week, and make sure it is organically grass fed. If it's not, you can almost guarantee the animal was fed with grains, and you will indirectly increase not only your insulin levels but also the unhealthy omega-6 fatty acid levels, which is mega-inflammatory.

Uric acid is also a product of fructose metabolism (more sugar!). For this reason, you need to completely remove any so-called foods that contain high fructose corn syrup, which is the sugar most commonly found in sodas. In a study by the New Harvard School of Public Health (HSPH), drinking sugar-sweetened beverages is shown to be linked to 133,000 diabetes deaths worldwide!

Yeast, which is often a result of high sugar, fructose, and protein consumption, also releases mycotoxins into the blood, leading to uric acid waste. Uric acid crystals are a common finding I see when I test patients' live blood at my wellness center. Uric acid is also associated with cardiovascular and kidney issues, including heart disease and kidney stones.

In addition to uric acid, it's important to limit consumption of moderate- to high-sugar acidic fruits such as bananas and berries, which contain fructose. Sugar is sugar in all forms.

Fructose moves directly to the liver where it does two harmful things:

1. The liver stops whatever it is doing to metabolize the fructose, so as a result, toxins build up.

2. It indirectly spikes insulin levels, turning the sugar directly into fat (and not just any fat—visceral fat, which is the worst kind). The liver immediately converts fructose to fructose-1-phosphate (F1P), and this will result in the formation of uric acid. Almost all of the F1P is turned into VLDL, triglycerides, and free fatty acids. These free fatty acids will result in insulin resistance in muscles, as well as in the liver. The resulting insulin resistance will put undue stress on the pancreas, which will pump out more insulin in response to rising blood sugar, as cells are unable to get the sugar out of the bloodstream. This is how consuming fructose in any form, including fruit, can progress to type 2 diabetes.

If you are going to consume any moderate to high-sugar fruits, add a healthy fat with it. For example, adding raw almond butter or coconut butter to apple slices not only tastes great, but also the metabolization of the sugar will slow down (keep this in mind for smoothies!). While some mild gut dysbiosis from the fermentation of the fruit may occur, this is a much better option than having insulin levels spike.

Type 2 diabetes is an acid problem. To prevent it, you need to stay away from sugar, grains, excess proteins, and starchy carbs. If you have sugar cravings, yeast issues, obesity, prediabetes, or diabetes, these foods must be removed from your diet and replaced with the highly alkalizing foods you will learn about in Chapter 6.

ACID REFLUX AND GERD

One in two Americans suffers from acid reflux. Can you believe that half of us are suffering from that burning feeling in our chests on a regular basis? What's even more unacceptable is that there is a huge misconception, even by medical doctors, about what causes and treats acid reflux—also known as gastroesophageal reflux disease (GERD) or peptic ulcer disease.

Most of us think too much acid in the stomach causes reflux. It's easy to assume that's the case because acid creeps up the esophagus. You can literally feel it. On the contrary, reflux is actually caused by too *little* acid in the stomach. Now, I'm going to make a clarification here because, usually, I'm telling you acid is bad. Usually I am talking about acidification of the blood and tissues, which is bad, but here I'm referring to the stomach acid we should naturally be producing, which is vital for proper digestion.

As we get older, our bodies, in general, tend to become weaker instead of stronger and slower instead of faster, and when it comes to our stomachs, we tend to produce less stomach acid instead of more. This lack of adequate stomach acid is commonly misunderstood and can have devastating consequences on our health.

It's compounded by the acidic lifestyle most of us are already living. When pH balance is off because of poor food choices such as fast foods, processed foods, and sugar, stomach cells produce less gastrin, which is responsible for stimulating the production of stomach acid. This sets off a chain reaction. When less stomach acid is produced, food isn't broken down and digested as well. With foods not being digested properly, blood doesn't receive as many essential vitamins (especially B vitamins), minerals, and amino acids.

Next, food moves to the small intestine for continued digestion, but because food wasn't properly broken down in the stomach, it doesn't properly break down here as well, so there is an even greater

COMMON SYMPTOMS OF REFLUX INCLUDE

▸ burning in the upper abdomen, known as heartburn;

▸ hoarseness;

▸ a feeling that food is stuck in your throat;

▸ tightness in your throat;

▸ excessive burping;

▸ wheezing;

▸ asthma;

▸ dental problems; and

▸ bad breath

deficiency of vitamins and minerals. At this point, you're more prone to infections because stomach acid is responsible for killing bacteria that enter the digestive system. However, since the stomach acid didn't kill everything, you've become more at risk for illness.

As a result, the vital microbiome—the trillions of cells in your intestines—shift from healthier bacteria to an unhealthy balance of bad bacteria. This unhealthy bacteria overgrowth produces gas that can literally raise the pressure on the small intestine and stomach, driving the contents of the stomach, including hydrochloric acid, enzymes, and bacteria, up into the esophagus. This is what you feel when you experience the burn, otherwise known as heartburn.

Heartburn, reflux, and GERD are specific problems of the lower esophageal sphincter (LES), where it becomes irritated or is not functioning properly. The LES is a flap of muscle that separates the esophagus from the stomach, and opens and closes to let food into the stomach for digestion. Reflux and GERD occurs when the LES relaxes inappropriately, allowing acid from your stomach to flow (reflux) backward into the esophagus.

Another complicating factor of reflux is a condition known as a hiatal hernia, where the top part of the stomach herniates, or protrudes, through the diaphragm into the upper chest cavity. Ultimately, this weakens the LES valve, often trapping in pockets of acid that easily reflux back into the esophagus.

Why the Current "Solution" Doesn't Work

The standard treatment for reflux is a class of drugs called proton pump inhibitors (PPIs) such as Prevacid, Zantac, or Prilosec. And by common, I mean really common.

Hundreds of millions of Americans take these drugs every year, and it's become a multibillion-dollar industry. The problem with PPI's is not only that they don't work, but they are also making the underlying problem even worse while introducing a slew of new health problems at the same time.

These drugs treat only the symptoms. Meanwhile, you're setting up a vicious cycle of imbalance in your stomach. PPIs fully inhibit acid production in the stomach and make you feel better temporarily in the process. Yet, in the end, suppressing stomach acid production is one of the worst things you can do for your health.

As we age, acid production in the stomach tends to decrease, not increase, and usually begins to decline at the age of 45 for females, and after age 30 for males. Stomach acid is essential to proper digestion, and the last thing we want to do is deplete what little levels of acid you may have, and that is exactly what PPIs do. Every pill you swallow takes any acid you currently have and brings it down to very low lever for about a twenty-four-hour period.

Other treatments used are H2 blockers such as Tagamet, Zantac, and Pepcid AC have bad digestive side effects (nausea, diarrhea, constipation, and even heartburn). They also interfere with the metabolism of certain hormones, including estradiol and testosterone.

Taking these pills every day may expose you to a host of health issues, as you get older, from poor digestion to increased bacterial infection from H Pylori, to

heartburn, GERD, ulcers, and even cancer. On pages 10–13, we discussed the five stages of acidosis. Something that may seem as insignificant as heartburn, if left to its own devices, is a perfect example of how that acidic progression can take place. This is exactly what happened with my father.

Here is my plea to you. If you have any underlying symptoms of heartburn or reflux, please don't take it lightly. Your body is telling you that there is a problem. Trust me, I don't say this to scare you. I say this because I care about you and don't ever want to see you go down the path that my father had to go down. Crush it while it's small and you still can.

All of that said, if you are taking PPIs for your reflux, it's imperative that you don't stop taking them cold turkey. If you do, you will experience severe withdrawal symptoms, as your stomach begins generating more acid. Instead, decrease your PPI dose gradually over several weeks in conjunction with your general practitioner's advice.

Use my approach to "add, don't take away." Follow the 7 Ways to GET OFF YOUR ACID in Chapter 8, and you can stop this problem in its tracks before it can cause significant damage. Once you've addressed the true cause and moved your body into a healthier and more balanced state, then you can begin the weaning process in conjunction with your doctor.

At-Home Test for Low Stomach Acid

Approximately 90 percent of those over age 40 who see their doctor will, in fact, have low acid. Wondering if this is the case with your acid reflux? Try this simple test. Take 1 tablespoon of lemon juice or apple cider vinegar with a little water at the beginning of a meal. If it alleviates your symptoms during and after eating, you should investigate further and have your stomach acid levels tested. You likely have a deficient amount of stomach acid, which could be the contributing factor to your reflux or GERD. Once confirmed, follow these steps to increase stomach acid production and sooth any potential inflammation or "burn" from the corrosive effects of the acid reflux.

Eliminate high-acid food triggers. Caffeine and alcohol are two of the biggest sources of reflux symptoms, and not so coincidentally, they are highly acidic.

Increase your body's natural production of stomach acid. Since reflux is usually a problem of too little stomach acid, encourage your body to make sufficient amounts of hydrochloric acid (stomach acid). You can easily increase the acid content of your stomach by drinking 1 tablespoon of raw, unfiltered apple cider vinegar in a large glass of water. The acetic acid found in the ACV fights against

66 *After being diagnosed with severe GERD more than four years ago, I thought I would be on PPIs forever. I originally went to the doctor because very quickly I went from having what I perceive as 'regular' heartburn to feeling a constant burning in my chest that went through to my back. I also frequently experienced acid coming up into my throat. It was debilitating, and I never felt good. I had an endoscopy done, and they found some small, healing ulcers but nothing that could tell them why I felt awful every day.*

When they couldn't give me any answers, I started searching and reading, and I found Alkamind *and the* Get Off Your Acid *program. It was the start of my journey back to being me. It has now been just about one year since I took my last pill! The* Get Off Your Acid *program works, period. It has changed my life by giving me back my quality of life. Now, instead of packing my medications when I travel, I pack my* Alkamind Daily Minerals *and* Daily Greens *instead, and the knowledge I have gained from this program is truly invaluable.* 99

—*Kelley O.*

bacteria and other foreign bodies in the intestinal tract. Drink 1 teaspoon daily to start and, if necessary, increase to 1 tablespoon in 8 ounces of water. In addition, a good, healthy alkaline sea salt provides the body with the chloride it needs to produce HCL, in addition to the minerals.

Take a good alkaline mineral supplement in a powder form. The sodium bicarbonate in Alkamind Daily Minerals will soothe the esophagus and stimulate HCL production. It is important to choose a supplement in a liquid form (from powder) that can have a direct effect on the irritated tissue of the esophagus and stomach.

Supplement with probiotics. Because reflux stems in part from an imbalance of bacteria in your gut, add a good probiotic supplement.

Digestive enzymes. These help break down food that is not broken down efficiently because of the decrease in stomach acid as we age. Try this first, then after some time you can always graduate to a digestive enzyme with betaine HCL (if needed).

Supplement with molecular hydrogen. (See page 140.)

Low Energy

If I were to ask you right now to rate your energy level on a scale of 0 to 10, 0 being *rigor mortis* is about to set in and 10 being the Energizer bunny, where would you *honestly* be? Now that we are being truthful with ourselves, are you okay with that?

Your health comes down to this in one word: *energy!* You will hear me talk a lot about it because when your energy increases, your health improves, and vice versa. When your energy is high, everything in your life is better. But the reality is that most people are tired 24/7, even after a good night's sleep.

Are you the kind of person who rolls out of bed and heads straight to the kitchen first thing in the morning to start the coffee brewing? Coffee is a drug, so much so that many people can't start their day without it. They are caffeinating with coffee or drugging with sugar to counter the effects of the energy crash, and all they're doing is becoming more acidic. A vicious cycle's hard to break.

Acid Is an Energy Vampire, Sucking the Life Right Out of You

Being drained of energy is a sign that something more significant and concerning is happening. Just like when the air-conditioner filter gets clogged with dust, so much more energy is required to maintain the desired room temperature you want, and the air-conditioner needs so much more output just to keep up. Sometimes it has to work so hard, it can blow a fuse. Your body is no different.

When you are stressed and eating an acidic diet filled with sugar, grains, caffeine, alcohol, energy drinks, and carbonated water, you are making your body work

> If the body is an engine, then food is its fuel. Food gives the body the energy it needs to function. If we don't make sure the fuel we pump through our system is the right quality and quantity, we're going to run ourselves right onto the scrap heap.
>
> —KRIS CARR, HUNGRY FOR CHANGE

that much harder to neutralize all that acid, just like that air-conditioner.

Stress and acidic foods are energy vampires! If you don't change your lifestyle *now*, eventually something has to give. You can always buy another filter for your air-conditioner, but you can't buy yourself another body. Take care of the body you have now, and I promise it will take care of you. When you're healthy and fit and eating alkaline, your body will work the way that it's supposed to. You will have energy all day long, and you can consider your energy crisis solved!

And here is the amazing thing: your body is resilient, and when you alkalize your life, your energy can return quickly. When you GET OFF YOUR ACID, you can reclaim energy levels that you haven't experienced since your teens and early twenties, and that feeling and what it gives you back in your life is priceless.

Now, if you are chronically acidic and toxic, you may experience a couple days of fatigue at first as your body heals. Listen to what your body is telling you to do. Get extra rest and continue to pound the water—**the solution to pollution is dilution!** A small drop in hydration levels can zap your energy for days. Stay ahead of it by giving your body the things it needs to help the detoxification process (see Chapter 8).

OBESITY

Obesity is a bigger health crisis globally than hunger, and it's the leading cause of disabilities around the world, according to a report published in the British medical journal *The Lancet.*

After remaining relatively stable in the 1960s and 1970s, the prevalence of obesity among adults in the United States increased by approximately 50 percent per decade throughout the 1980s and 1990s. Today, the United States has the highest incidence of obesity in the world, with

64 percent of all adults being considered overweight or obese.

Someone who is overweight weighs more than what is considered normal for their height, age, and sex, and their body mass index (BMI) falls in the range of 25 to 29.9. Obesity, on the other hand, is a disease marked by excessive generalized deposition and storage of fat, with a BMI over 30. Obesity has been shown to have a substantial negative effect on longevity, reducing the length of life of people who are severely obese by an estimated five to twenty years.

To make matters worse, we are seeing the same rise in numbers among children, and the massive amounts of money being spent to try and combat this issue isn't working. In 2012, $40 billion was spent to combat obesity. Still, one in three children are overweight. Kids are consuming a steady diet of acidosis-friendly foods: candy, processed food, pizza, chips, and sodas. In fact, 25 percent of the "vegetables" consumed by Americans are French fries. Between grains and processed foods, the sugar consumption in children has skyrocketed and is at an all-time high.

The American Heart Association recommends no more than 9.5 teaspoons of refined sugar per day, yet the average child consumes a whopping 32 teaspoons of sugar every day. To make matters worse, a significant portion of this sugar comes in the most acidic and dangerous form— high fructose corn syrup (HFCS)—a sweetener commonly found in soda and baked goods. In fact, sugar from soft drinks, desserts, and fruit juices accounted for half of kids' overall added sugar intake. One study found school-age children in Oklahoma on average drink four 12-ounce soft drinks every day—that's scary!

Aside from soda and baked goods, many more foods contain high-fructose corn syrup. Fruits canned in heavy syrup—peaches and pears—condiments, such as ketchup, jelly, syrup, barbecue sauce, and many salad dressings contain the sweetener. Many types of commercially manufactured bread, buns, rolls, and bagels also contain high fructose corn syrup. And the sweetener could be lurking as well in certain kinds of breakfast cereal, crackers, muffins, granola bars, juice, and spaghetti sauce.

High fructose corn syrup has been found to have similar addictive qualities to heroin and cocaine and has been linked to weight gain and the obesity epidemic. Here is why fructose is more dangerous than any other form of sugar. While glucose can be metabolized anywhere in the body, fructose cannot. When consumed, fructose is shuttled directly to the liver, where it acts more as a fat (instead of a carbohydrate) and is converted to triglycerides. Once converted to triglycerides, fructose alters the function of insulin receptors on cell membranes, causing insulin resistance. With elevated triglyceride levels from fructose and elevated insulin levels in the blood as a result of insulin resistance, the body will store these triglycerides as fat rather than being burned by the body for energy.

To make matters worse, the consumption of fructose also causes leptin resistance, which many researchers say is the key hormone linked to obesity. Leptin is the "satiety hormone" made by your adipose (fat) cells that helps you regulate energy balance by inhibiting hunger. Here is how it works: the more fat you accumulate, the more those cells tell your body to produce leptin. The more leptin you produce, the more your body tells you you're full and the less food you eat. Likewise, the less fat you have, the more leptin is inhibited, and hunger feelings kick in. It is an important survival mechanism.

Here's where the problem occurs that could be a primary cause for developing obesity. When you are consuming high amounts of sugar, specifically fructose, leptin resistance develops. As a result, you will always be hungry and crave food (and it's usually not the green foods!). This is an alteration in your body's chemistry. I don't care how much willpower you have, fructose is a powerful addiction that is difficult to overcome.

Here is what scares me the most about parenting. A *New York Times* article stated, "For the first time in two centuries, the current generation of children in America may have shorter life expectancies than their parents . . . [and] the rapid rise in childhood obesity, if left unchecked, could shorten lifespans by as much as five years."

This is scary but preventable. Being obese or overweight is fundamentally an acid problem. When your body has too much acid, it uses fat as an additional way to store it in the tissues, so that it won't be of any harm in the blood. In the short run, fat is saving your life from the damaging effects of an acidic lifestyle. In the long run, it's making you more toxic and acidic. This

is why all those fad diets fail—because they haven't addressed the true cause, which is the acid. If you are looking to lose some weight, GET OFF YOUR ACID so that your body can heal and melt the pounds.

OSTEOPOROSIS

Osteoporosis a medical condition in which the bones become brittle and fragile from loss of tissue. In America, in 2017, 10 million men and women have been diagnosed with osteoporosis, and another 34 million are at risk for low bone mass, or osteopenia, a precursor to osteoporosis.

Many people believe they can prevent brittle bones by increasing the consumption of milk and dairy products. However, this is a myth but one that has really caught on thanks to the dairy industry. I know this may be a shock to many reading this. It was a shock to me as well when I first read the research.

Growing up, I had to drink milk every night at dinner. Our parents were doing what they thought was the right thing. They didn't know milk is acidic, and it drains calcium from your bones. This is not my opinion, but rather what the research shows. After twelve years of study, Harvard researchers noted a correlation between increased dairy consumption and increased hip fractures in women. It is true that milk has a high calcium content, but the problem is the human body is able to utilize very little of that.

In the book, *Lessons from the Miracle Doctors*, Jon Barron wrote, "The problem with milk is that because of its high sulfur and phosphorous content, your body needs to buffer it with even more internal calcium (from your body) than you get from the milk itself. Besides, even if the absorption issue was not enough by itself, the 10 to 1 ratio of calcium to magnesium found in milk is too high and devastating to the human body." Thus, the high incidence of osteoporosis in countries that consume a lot of dairy such as the United States is incredibly high because of these reasons. The ratio of calcium-to-magnesium is crucial for its absorption and should ideally be 1:1 for the calcium to be absorbed into the body.

In addition to the ratio of calcium to magnesium, the form of calcium is critical. The most bioavailable form of calcium is calcium citrate; the most detrimental form is calcium carbonate, which primarily composes coral calcium. So if you are taking a calcium supplement, always look at the ratio of calcium to magnesium, as most people think more is better; however, it is not.

It may also surprise you to learn that you can take an optimal calcium supplement every day and still develop osteoporosis. That's because osteoporosis is not only linked to a calcium deficiency, it's also an excess acid problem! When you're overly acidic, your body goes on a scavenger hunt for minerals to neutralize the acid to maintain a healthy balanced blood pH. If you're not getting minerals from your diet, your body will find another way. It will grab some minerals from your mouth, which can lead to tooth decay. It will also rob your bones of precious calcium, and your muscles of magnesium, causing cramps, muscle pain, and energy depletion. The pH of

your blood is so important that it will let your body fall apart before it allows its pH to veer off course.

The more dairy, meat, sugar, and grains we eat, the more calcium gets leached from our bones, and the more prone we become to osteoporosis. The purpose of eating alkaline foods, drinking alkaline water, and avoiding acidic foods is not to try to raise the pH of your blood outright. It's to prevent your body from having to do the regulating on its own by depleting its own resources, such as calcium in the bones, to neutralize all that acid.

I had a 34-year-old client named Andrea, who discovered from a DEXA scan (a bone-density scan) that she had lost 25 percent of her total bone mass. Would it surprise you that she also had a massive addiction to sugar and never exercised? She was ready to raise her standards and change her life. We jump-started her healing with the 7-Day Alkaline Cleanse, removed all the acidic triggers, and modified her diet by adding plenty of dark-green leafy vegetables, healthy alkaline fats, green juices, and green smoothies. She used the rebounder every day for lymphatic drainage to detoxify her body (see page 151). Twelve months later, on a follow-up scan, her bone density was perfect. Hers is a true testimonial to the power of the body to heal and to what a phytonutrient- and mineral-rich alkaline diet can do.

SLEEP ISSUES

A great day starts with a good breakfast, but even before that, it starts with a full night's sleep. Do you think stress is to blame for an untamed mind at bedtime? Your busy schedule probably isn't much help, but tossing and turning throughout the night could be a result of acid from the foods you ate that day.

Maybe it was the 12-ounce steak you had for dinner (or the sweet treat afterward) that was to blame for your restless night. Consuming too much animal protein or sugar in the evening is a surefire way to lose sleep. A gradual buildup of acid throughout the day will also cause nighttime discomfort and insomnia.

Your body is most acidic in the middle of the night, peaking at 5 a.m. If you have a habit of waking up between 1 a.m. and 3 a.m. to use the bathroom, you're acidic and your liver and kidneys are asking for help!

Every acid and toxin you ingest must be filtered through your liver, and waking up around this time can signal that the liver and the body are exhibiting acidity and need some cleansing. When we get up to urinate during the night, the body is doing whatever it can to get rid of the acid that it's having trouble handling. Kidneys are some of the most powerful acid buffers, and urination is one way of keeping pH balanced. I have a saying, "Pee your way to better health!" This is also why if you test your urine pH first thing in the morning, it will be acidic, as it is a sign that the kidneys are doing their job. As you eat more alkaline, upon further testing, this pH reading should go up the pH scale and become more alkaline.

Ultimately, the more alkaline you eat, the better you'll sleep. Try to limit your consumption of sugar, dairy, caffeine, carbonated beverages, meats (even most fish!), yeast, alcohol, grains (especially white bread and pasta), vinegary foods, margarine, and MSG, as these are the most acidic foods that will contribute to a poor night's sleep.

You should be eating dark greens (bonus points if they're raw) and getting plenty of fiber and probiotics to help keep your colon clean. Allow food to digest for at least three hours before you go to bed, and keep in mind that dinner should not be your biggest meal of the day.

Before slipping into your pajamas, do some breathing exercises and take a detox bath to relieve your mind from a chaotic day. I share instructions for baths and the powerful 3:6:5 breathing—another detoxification protocol—on page 138. Not only is a clear mind conducive to a good night's sleep, but taking a few minutes to breathe deeply can change your pH within one to three minutes!

Finally, give your body a dose of alkaline minerals thirty minutes before you go to sleep. Taking minerals such as magnesium, calcium, potassium, and sodium bicarbonate is a fast way to neutralize acid so that your body doesn't need to do it all on its own. Alkaline minerals are also very calming to the nervous system and will put your body into a deeper REM sleep when it needs it most. You'll find that when you wake up with an alkaline body, you'll be full of energy and ready to take on the day, rather than allowing stress to keep you up at night.

Now, go get some sleep!

SKIN ISSUES

If, like millions of Americans, you've ever struggled with acne, eczema, dry skin, psoriasis, rosacea or skin redness, dermatitis, or even just the effects of aging on skin and hair, you know that the conventional treatments out there just don't work very well. You can slather on all of the chemical treatments you want, but stubborn skin and hair problems just won't go away.

Why? As with so many health conditions, these products never address the true cause, which are the toxicities and deficiencies that are at the heart of these issues in the first place. Fortunately, there is a better way, and that's to take care of your skin, nails, and hair from the inside out.

When best-selling author and world-famous makeup artist Bobbi Brown launched her book *Beauty from the Inside Out*—a gorgeous guide in which she reveals the secrets of radiance—I was grateful to be one of her chosen wellness experts. And when I was asked what all beauty and skin issues had in common, my answer, of course, was acid.

You can trace all skin issues back to the gut. Acidic foods such as gluten and sugar, or chemical stress in the form of antibiotics, wipe out the healthy bacteria in your gut microbiome, allowing toxins, undigested food particles, yeast, and bacteria to leak into your blood through your intestinal barrier where they don't belong. From there, it's all hands on deck, as your body uses any means necessary to get the acid out.

Skin is the largest organ—sometimes referred to as the "third kidney" for its ability to assist with the detoxification process. When your body becomes overly acidic, it turns to the skin to reduce the toxins via perspiration. Roughly 20 percent of the total acid load in your body is eliminated via the skin. No matter what the skin condition may be, it is a sign that you're acidic, your liver is stressed, and your lymphatic system is backed up. You are most likely dehydrated, and need to start hydrating, rebounding (more on this later), and focusing on eating alkalizing foods to help cleanse and detoxify your blood and body. Soon, your skin will look younger and will begin to glow.

ADHD

Poor diet is also linked to concentration and behavior problems such as attention-deficit/hyperactivity disorder (ADHD). In the United States, an astonishing 8 million children are taking medication daily for hyperactivity. In my opinion, for the majority of these children, drug treatments such as Ritalin and Adderall are not the answer. The Controlled Substances Act (CSA) classifies this medication as a schedule II controlled substance, which is in the same class of highly addictive substances as cocaine, morphine, oxycontin, and opium.

In some cases, a child's diet has been neglected, and doctors have not performed a micronutrient depletion test to look for any possible deficiencies that could be contributing to the ADHD in the first place.

America's children are more deficient and overweight than ever, and it's directly related to how they move (or lack thereof) and eat. Instead of running around outside, most kids come home and are glued to their devices. In addition, the average American child consumes a whopping 32 teaspoons of sugar daily. Soft drinks, in particular, are loaded with high fructose corn syrup and caffeine, both highly acidifying to the body. Excessive sugar and caffeine intake cause symptoms of hyperactivity and distraction in children.

Researchers have also observed signs of essential fatty acid deficiency in hyperactive children. Deficiencies in long-chain omega-3 fatty acids are known to affect behavior and cognition. The human brain is 60 percent fat, and when your child is consuming a diet that heavily favors omega-6s over omega-3s, the structural integrity of the brain will be altered.

Did you know that the level of DHA in children's blood cells significantly predicts their ability to concentrate and learn at school? An Oxford University study involving nearly five hundred school children found that blood levels of omega-3 fatty acids significantly predicted a child's behavior and ability to learn. Higher levels of omega-3, DHA in particular, were associated with better reading and memory, as well as with fewer behavioral problems, as rated by parents and teachers.

This is why every child, whether dealing with ADD/ADHD or not, should have an Alkamind Omega-3 Acid Index assessment (with cognitive function tests), to determine if these omega-3 deficiencies could be contributing to the problem. This test will confirm this and let you know exactly what your child needs to become sufficient in omega-3 fatty acids. I mentioned these tests in the Heart Disease section on page 41, and you can purchase them at www.getoffyouracid.com.

This is why it is so important to be dietary role models for our children and stress the importance of consuming more dark-green leafy vegetables and healthy, alkaline fats to help rebalance their bodies.

PART II
The GET OFF YOUR ACID Program

Success is nothing more than a few simple disciplines, practiced every day.

—JIM ROHN

05

Out with the Bad:
Acidic Foods

How do you know if a food is acidic? Remember, it doesn't matter to us what the food does outside your body, but rather what happens once it is metabolized. Digestion of some foods produces dangerous acids in the body (see page 6).

How "acidic" or "alkaline" a food is depends on three factors: mineral content, sugar content, and fiber content. Take four citrus fruits, for example—lemons, limes, grapefruit, and oranges. You may think all of these are acidic because they contain citric acid, but this is not the case. Three of these are alkaline forming, and one is acid forming—which one out of the four would you say creates an acid state *inside* your body? Lemons, limes, and grapefruit are very high in minerals and fiber, but low in sugar, so their effect is alkaline forming. Oranges are high in minerals and fiber but also high in sugar, so they're acid forming.

In this chapter, we'll look at some of the worst offenders of acidic foods in our diets.

SUGAR AND ARTIFICIAL SWEETENERS: THE BIGGEST BAD GUY OF ALL

I'm very passionate about sweeteners, and I don't think there is one single person reading this who is not affected by sugar. Skin issues, allergies, digestive problems, arthritis pain, and sleeping issues or fatigue are all underlying symptoms of too much acid in your diet. Sugar is easily at the top of the list about why most people have a pH problem. In fact, sugar is one of the most acidic substances you can put inside your body.

Here are some facts about the history of sugar consumption that might surprise you:

▸ In 1700, the average person consumed about 4 pounds of sugar per year.

▸ In 1800, the average person consumed about 18 pounds of sugar per year.

- In 1900, individual consumption had risen to 90 pounds of sugar per year.

- In 2012, more than 50 percent of all Americans consumed ½ pound of sugar *per day*—and a whopping 170 pounds of sugar per year!

As good as sugar may taste, it is not your friend; it is, however, the friend of cancer and type 2 diabetes and every other chronic degenerative disease. Here's another set of alarming statistics:

- In 1890, only 3 in 100,000 people were diagnosed with diabetes.

- In 2012, almost 8,000 in 100,000 people were diagnosed with diabetes.

It's not only a coincidence that our appetite for sugar has risen so dramatically in the last three hundred years. A peer-reviewed study from the journal *Public Library of Science* (*PLOS one*) showed that sugar is eight times more addictive than cocaine!

Sugar is big business that wants you to be addicted. A September 2016 article in the *New York Times* exposed the sugar industry's efforts to purposely shift the blame for heart disease and other chronic illnesses away from sugar to fat by funding biased studies since 1965. According to the article, "Marion Nestle, a professor of nutrition, food studies, and public health at New York University . . . said the documents provided 'compelling evidence' that the sugar industry had initiated research 'expressly to exonerate sugar as a major risk factor for coronary heart disease.' . . . 'I think it's appalling,' she said. 'You just never see examples that are this blatant.'"

Sugar Is Everywhere

Most of the sugar in our diets doesn't come from those packets of sugar on the table at the restaurant or in those 5-pound bags at the supermarket. Even as consumer purchases of refined sugar have actually been declining since 1970, actual sugar consumption is skyrocketing. Research has found that most Americans consume up to 40 teaspoons of sugar per day, when the maximum should be 4 to 5 teaspoons per day. Sugar is hidden in almost every food you buy, one way or another.

Check the labels—sugar lurks in so many common foods! Besides the places you'd expect, such as doughnuts, ice cream, candy, and chocolate, sugar is often hiding in seemingly wholesome foods—bread, cereals, pasta sauces, salad dressings, and yogurt. One bagel has 45 grams of carbs and 11 teaspoons of sugar. That's the same sugar content as a can of soda! These insidious sugars add up and cause all the problems.

How Sugar Makes Us Sick

You may be consuming carbs and sugar in many different forms, and whether you realize it or not, you're most likely burning sugar instead of fat as your primary fuel source. Sugar is a dirty fuel and a dirty burn. In Dr. Joseph Mercola's book,

HOW TO READ A NUTRITION LABEL

You should read labels for three things: sugar, total carbs, and fiber. High fiber content is always a good thing. High sugar is not. Avoiding sugar as much as possible, so look for low numbers there. To determine net carbs, subtract the grams of fiber from the total carbs, which are the unhealthy carbs (see Appendix II, page 243).

Fat for Fuel, he states, "Using sugar for energy produces 30 to 40 percent more ROS (reactive oxygen species) than burning fat," which massively increases inflammation and oxidative damage on your body. Oxygen is the most important alkalizing nutrient, bar none. When sugar is metabolized, it burns up oxygen, ferments, and turns to lactic acid and alcohol.

When you eat sugar, blood glucose levels spike and in order to maintain healthy blood glucose levels, the pancreas needs to release more and more insulin. This can become a chronic inflammatory issue, leading to diabetes, heart disease, cancer, and more. A sugar-laden diet also leads to weight gain—when insulin levels spike, your body stores the sugar as fat!

Additionally, sugar consumption, paradoxically, keeps you feeling hungry. It alters hormone function, especially when it comes to two hunger hormones—leptin and ghrelin. These are the hormones responsible for letting you know when you are hungry and when you're full. When insulin levels spike from eating sugar, the effects of these two hormones are negated,

so you continue to feel hungry, and you never feel satisfied.

If that isn't bad enough, sugar consumption makes your body highly acidic and causes massive depletions in one of the most important minerals, magnesium. Research shows that 80 percent of Americans, and probably even more, are lacking in this vital mineral. Magnesium is critical for more than six hundred metabolic reactions that involve enzymes, and every cell needs it. It helps regulate glucose, insulin, and the neurotransmitter dopamine. If you crave sugar, your body is really craving and deficient in magnesium and other mineral salts.

Having been a former sugar addict, I know firsthand how hard it can be to overcome those cravings. Here is my suggestion to you: **add, don't take away.** And as you add more of the good to your diet, it will soon crowd out the bad. Begin eating some alkaline foods rich in good, healthy fats: avocados, coconut oil, flax seeds (ground right before consuming to avoid oxidation), chia seeds, hemp seeds, raw nut butters, and wild-caught salmon. Also, opt for foods high in natural fiber and minerals: dark leafy greens, watercress, kale, spinach, romaine, and chard. Start taking an alkaline mineral supplement such as Alkamind Daily Minerals. You'll see the cravings will soon disappear.

Zero-Calorie Artificial Sweeteners

You might be saying to yourself, okay, I understand sugar is bad, but what's wrong with sugar substitutes? Let's take a closer look.

You know the saying: if it sounds too good to be true, it probably is. As a society, we keep using artificial sweeteners because they seem so great, right? They have all the sweetness of sugar with none of the calories. However, zero-calorie artificial sweeteners are a big problem. They are highly acidic and may be carcinogenic—many studies have linked artificial sweeteners to cancer. And, unfortunately, the health claims about these sweeteners when it comes to weight loss and diabetes prevention don't hold up. Artificially sweetened foods, often marketed as "reduced calorie," "sugar-free," and "diet," can actually sabotage your weight-control efforts.

One study found drinking diet soda, often sweetened with aspartame, was linked to increased belly fat. Another study concluded that with each can of diet soda consumed daily, there was a corresponding 41 percent increase in obesity risk. Eating or drinking something sweet-flavored triggers a release of the body chemicals dopamine and leptin. You feel good from the dopamine, first, and then the leptin kicks in and give you the sensation of feeling full once you've consumed a certain number of calories. With calorie-free sweet things, however, that full feeling never kicks in. So what does your body do? It craves more sweets. As a result, people who consume diet drinks regularly experience more weight gain and worsened insulin sensitivity—a precursor for diabetes.

In 2010, the *Journal of Clinical Nutrition* studied 59,334 pregnant Danish women and associated artificially sweetened sodas with increased risk of preterm birth.

Let's break down what's so bad about a few of the most popular artificial sweeteners.

ASPARTAME (NUTRASWEET, EQUAL)

Calorie-free and 180 times sweeter than sugar, aspartame comes in those little packets usually in restaurants. But even if you don't use these products, aspartame can be found in more than six thousand food products and five hundred prescription drugs. It hides in very unsuspecting places, including the following:

> breakfast cereals
> diet sodas
> carbonated beverages
> chewing gum
> chewable vitamins
> dessert mixes
> diet foods and diabetic foods
> jam
> all sugar-free foods
> yogurt

This means that there's a good chance that you and your family are among the two-thirds of the adult population and 40 percent of children who regularly ingest this artificial sweetener. Aspartame is perhaps the most controversial food additive in history. At one time, the Pentagon listed aspartame as a biochemical warfare agent. Yet, it's become integral part of the modern American diet for its sweetening properties.

For years, studies have linked aspartame to cancer, and now there is evidence that links it to leukemia and lymphoma. Additionally, one of the ingredients in aspartame is methanol (wood alcohol). Once consumed, methanol breaks down to form formaldehyde—the same stuff used in paint remover and embalming fluid! Formaldehyde is a poison that is several thousand times more potent than ethyl alcohol. In fact, the Environmental Protection Agency (EPA) has concluded that formaldehyde causes cancer in humans, specifically breast and prostate cancer. It shouldn't come as a shock that formaldehyde is also heavily acidic. Its end waste product inside your body is something called formate, which can cause metabolic acidosis, or acidity in your blood. Metabolic acidosis can result in massive nutrient depletion, blindness, fatal kidney damage, multiple organ system failure, and even death.

Additionally, 90 percent of aspartame is comprised of two amino acids—phenylalanine and aspartic acid—which are known to stimulate the rapid release of insulin and leptin, two hormones that are responsible for regulating metabolism, hunger, and weight management. The more diet soda or sugarless products you consume, the more prone you will become to insulin and leptin sensitivity, triggering more fat storage and less satiety. I don't care how strong-willed a person may be, when he or she becomes leptin resistant, the hunger signal becomes too powerful and will always prevail.

Dr. Sharon P. G. Fowler of the University of Texas Health Science Center at San Antonio, conducted a nine-year study on people over the age of 65 and told Reuters the following about consuming diet sodas: "Diet sodas are very acidic, more so even than acid rain, and the acidity of the artificial sweeteners may have a direct impact on things like gut microbes, which influence how we absorb nutrients."

SACCHARIN
(SWEET'N LOW)

If I were to dare you to eat coal tar, would you do it? What if I told you it was 350 times sweeter than sugar, would you do it then? Probably not, because the vision of coal tar inside your body would not be too appetizing. Well, that is exactly what saccharin is—a coal-derived, calorie-free sweetener that just so happens to be in practically every restaurant across the country.

In March 1977, a Canadian study with rodents linked saccharin to an excess of bladder tumors. Despite once being labeled as a human carcinogen by the Department of Health National Toxicology Program at the National Institutes of Health, the Food and Drug Administration (FDA) now declares saccharin safe for human consumption.

SUCRALOSE (SPLENDA)

Since about 2000, people have turned to Splenda as a supposedly safer alternative to other artificial sweeteners that have been linked to cancer. Unfortunately, sucralose is no better than aspartame or saccharin. Sucralose, the chemical compound in the brand name Splenda, has been ringing more and more alarms. The Center for Science in the Public Interest, a nonprofit watchdog group, graded sucralose as "caution," claiming the additive could pose a risk to public health and warranted further study and testing.

The *International Journal of Occupational and Environmental Health* conducted a study in which mice were fed sucralose daily throughout their lives, similar to the way many humans consume the chemical daily. These mice developed leukemia and other blood cancers. Even if there were no links to cancer or other health risks ranging from headaches to seizures, because it is six hundred times sweeter than sugar, it poses the same threat as aspartame of causing body chemistry to crave more sweet foods. Studies have found that sucralose creates peaks and valleys for blood sugar and insulin levels that could lead to cravings, headaches, and mood swings. Again, more sugar cravings lead to more weight gain, not weight loss.

High Fructose Corn Syrup

I am blown away at how many products contain this genetically modified food (GMO) sweetener. High fructose corn syrup (HFCS) is found in everything from crackers to bread, chips, yogurt, and sauces. And it has been shown to damage immune function, speed up the aging process, and contribute to weight gain,

Glucose and fructose are two forms of sugar. Unlike glucose, which can be metabolized in any part of your body, fructose must be shuttled straight to the liver to be broken down. And herein lies the problem: during this breakdown process, uric acid—a dangerous waste product—is produced. The liver must stop whatever it's doing to handle this highly damaging acid. These uric acid crystals can lead to hypertension and gout.

Fructose activates the switch that turns the food we eat into fat—the visceral fat (the most dangerous fat!) that surrounds your vital organs. And many people are living with chronic insulin sensitivity because of so much sugar in their diets. It's an awful cycle: consuming sugar, burning sugar, and then craving more sugar!

Also, high fructose corn syrup is often loaded with alarmingly high levels of mercury. One study by *Environmental Health* found mercury in more than 50 percent of samples tested. Mercury exposure can result in irreversible brain and nervous system damage—especially in young, growing bodies.

Agave Nectar

One day I was sitting in Pittsburgh at this great farm-to-table breakfast restaurant, and I listened to the host explain one of the menu items. He was talking about a fresh green drink, juiced in the kitchen, with all

SWEETENERS

NEVER	BETTER	BEST
Artificial Sweeteners	**Coconut Sugar/Nectar** *(40% Fructose)* **Honey** *(52% Fructose)* **Molasses / Maple Syrup**	**Stevia & Lo Han** *(Monk Fruit)*

the "good stuff," including kale, spinach, cucumber, celery, apple, and *agave nectar*. I love that you can go out and actually now get fresh juices like this with your breakfast. But he was talking about how healthy all of these ingredients were. Well, he was right about all of them, except one—the agave.

Agave is one of the most acidic foods you can put into your body, which is a surprise to most people. Although agave is a natural sweetener, it is perhaps worse than high fructose corn syrup since it has an even higher fructose content. HFCS has a fructose content of 55 percent, which is bad, but agave nectar has a fructose content of 70 to 97 percent, which is dangerous!

High fructose levels are heavily acidic and cause conditions such as insulin resistance, type 2 diabetes, increased weight, and increased triglyceride levels, heart disease, and even cancer!

Truvia/PureVia

Truvia and PureVia are the new "all-natural" sweeteners created from the stevia plant. Thanks to claims of being natural, many health-conscious shoppers have been swayed into believing these products are a good alternative to sugar.

They should not be an alternative, and they are far from healthy! While liquid organic stevia is okay, Truvia and PureVia are processed, altered, and mixed with chemicals in a laboratory. Don't eat them. Truvia contains erythritol, which, according to the manufacturer, is produced by a natural process. It's a sugar alcohol made from a food-grade starch—genetically modified corn—and is broken down by fermentation (the process of decay becomes acid!). Is it still "natural" if it's coming from fermented genetically modified corn?

So What Can You Do Instead?

First, if you're regularly consuming artificial sweeteners, don't stop cold turkey. These chemicals are highly addictive, perhaps as addictive as any drugs. You'll want to wean yourself off in order to prevent side effects that will just make you crave the additives even more.

That said, *do* cut back on sweets. Because of the biochemical reaction of dopamine and leptin, the more sweets you eat (especially with artificial sweeteners), the more sweets you'll want to eat. Fortunately, the opposite is also true. The more you cut back, the less you'll want them.

In addition, when you find yourself craving sweets, there's usually a mineral deficiency. Load up on dark-green leafy vegetables and healthy fats, and start taking an alkaline mineral supplement every night. This will help you begin to feel good, so it'll be easier to cut out more and more of the sweet stuff.

What About Fruit?

Sugar in all its forms, even in most fruit, creates acid. Fruit contains the type of sugar known as fructose (sound familiar?). Does this mean you shouldn't eat any fruit? No, because fruit also provides a lot of good stuff, too, such as vitamins, minerals, antioxidants, and fiber. Ideally you want to limit fruit consumption to once a day, in season, and not too ripe. (Exceptions include alkaline fruits, such as lemons, limes, grapefruit, avocados, tomatoes, coconut, pomegranate, watermelon—you can eat more of these.)

What about fruit juice? I recommend avoiding it because fruit juice contains no fiber and is very high in sugar (and very acidic). Fruit juice is often as acidic as a soft drink and may have more total calories! For example, orange juice has 18 grams of fructose per ounce, compared to that of a can of soda, which has 1.7 grams per ounce.

Look at the breakdown for a 12-ounce portion of Coca-Cola versus apple juice:

Coca-Cola: 140 calories and 40 grams of sugar (10 teaspoons).
Apple juice: 165 calories and 39 grams of sugar (9.8 teaspoons).

If you do drink juice, stick to homemade, cold-pressed juices made from green vegetables and low-sugar fruits. If you are transitioning to an alkaline lifestyle, it is perfectly okay to add a green apple or a pear for a slightly sweeter taste, but as your taste buds become more alkaline, you can remove them from the equation.

Ten Ways to Crush Your Sugar Cravings

1. GET PLENTY OF KEY MINERALS

If you crave sugar, the number-one deficiency in your body is alkaline minerals, specifically magnesium and potassium. The most important thing you can do is start incorporating more dark-green leafy vegetables into your diet. Foods that are high in magnesium include the following:

▸ **dark, leafy greens**
▸ **broccoli**
▸ **raw cacao**
▸ **raw nuts and seeds**
▸ **quinoa**
▸ **avocados**

Think about where you can sneak these foods into your diet. For example, my wife will add 2 cups of spinach to pasta sauce, curries, and soups. Spinach can also be added to any cooked, savory breakfast. It is great in smoothies because it has a very non-green taste. Broccoli can be grated like cheese into soups and salads.

That said, it's almost impossible to get the amount of minerals your body needs from foods alone, and here's why: our food supply just isn't as nutritious as it used to be.

- ▸ **There was a study about spinach in 2010 that showed it would take sixty servings of spinach to give you the same mineral content that spinach gave you in 1948.**

- ▸ **Since the mid 1990s, the calcium in broccoli has dropped 50 percent.**

- ▸ **Compared to vegetables grown in 1975, veggies today have 37 percent less iron and 30 percent less vitamin C.**

- ▸ **We have to eat eight oranges to get the same amount of vitamin C as our grandparents got from one orange.**

Why has the mineral content in these vegetables and fruits changed so much? It's because of things like synthetic fertilizers and acid rain, to name a few. So if you want to crush your sugar cravings, I recommend taking a mineral powder added to water that contains the four most crucial alkaline minerals: magnesium, calcium, potassium, and sodium bicarbonate.

Never take magnesium by itself, as it can deplete the other minerals in your body. Make sure the supplement you choose has both calcium and magnesium (at a ratio of 1:1) in order to prevent a deficiency in either mineral. My Alkamind Daily Minerals is a high-quality product that comes in a canister or single-serving packets you can use on the go.

2. SPICE UP YOUR MEALS

Turmeric, ginger, cinnamon, nutmeg, and cardamom will not only naturally sweeten your food but also will help balance blood sugar and reduce sugar cravings. You can add these to fresh juices, smoothies, soups, and even grate them over salads and alkaline desserts! Turmeric and ginger can be stewed in nut milks for nice, creamy drinks.

3. CONSUME HEALTHY FATS AND MCTS WITH YOUR MEALS

Healthy fats include those found in avocados, nuts and seeds, extra-virgin olive oil (EVOO), coconut, flax, hemp, chia seeds, raw nut butters, and the natural fats found in animal products such as wild salmon, sardines, anchovies, herring, and trout. These fats provide satiety and help to keep blood sugar stable. Take a fish oil supplement or eat a tablespoon of cold-pressed coconut oil one to three times per day. Add a tablespoon of coconut oil to smoothies, dressings, sauces, soups, and stir-fries. Some people like coconut oil in their morning coffee, assuming they're still drinking that (very acidic) beverage. It's a great way to fight hunger cravings, too!

Aim to consume 7 to 10 servings of healthy oils every day including EVOO and coconut oil, avocado oil, macadamia nut oil, sesame oil, MCT oil, and black cumin oil. Avoid polyunsaturated oils that have the ability to oxidize and go rancid, such as flax, chia, and hemp. The seeds are fine, and if you make the oils yourself for immediate consumption, that's fine as well. However, most manufactured polyunsaturated oils are rancid and oxidized by the time you open the bottle, so buyer beware!

Fish oil, which is a source of omega-3 fatty acids, is a powerful anti-inflammatory supplement. However, even good polyunsaturated fats such as fish oil have the potential to oxidize. When any oil oxidizes, it turns rancid and transforms into trans-fatty acids and free radicals, which are dangerous. Therefore, I recommend you always take an antioxidant along with the fish oil—alpha lipoic acid, glutathione, or the master antioxidant, molecular hydrogen (a good quality fish oil will have antioxidants in the supplement).

4. EAT MORE ALKALINE FOODS THAT ARE HIGH IN FIBER

Some foods encourage cravings, and some foods fight cravings. Incorporate high-fiber foods into your regular diet to prevent cravings from popping up in the first place. Foods high in natural fiber are dark, leafy greens (watercress, kale, and spinach), avocados, broccoli, celery, cucumber, artichokes, peas, okra, squash, Brussels sprouts, red bell peppers, cabbage, cauliflower, and quinoa.

5. EAT FOODS HIGH IN THE MINERAL CHROMIUM

Chromium regulates blood sugar and cholesterol levels and helps to reduce sugar cravings. Chow down on broccoli, sweet potatoes, green beans, raw onions, tomatoes, and romaine lettuce.

6. EAT FOODS HIGH IN ZINC

Zinc is abundant in spinach, chickpeas, pumpkin seeds, and Brazil nuts. Zinc is needed for insulin and glucose utilization, and a deficiency can lead to sugar cravings.

7. READ LABELS

I was in the natural food store one day, looking for some healthy snacks for my father that didn't include any sugar, and it was nearly impossible. And this was in a health food store! Going forward, you need to become a Nutrition Facts label reader. Once you read the sugar and carb counts, you can assess if you really want to put that food in your body (see page 69).

8. CUT BACK ON CAFFEINE, ALCOHOL, SUGAR, AND PROCESSED FOODS

Caffeine and alcohol dehydrate the body and can lead to mineral deficiencies. Processed foods have a tendency to be very high in sugar and table salt, which both lead to sugar cravings. Don't keep these in your house. Whatever your greatest weakness is, don't have those within reach when strong cravings hit. Instead, look around the kitchen and find something much better to snack on that satisfies what your cravings are really about. A smoothie, homemade alkaline trail mix, or an avocado with lime juice and hemp seeds might do the trick. But don't be too hard on yourself. It's okay to have a cup of coffee or a glass of wine occasionally. It's all about moderation.

9. STAY HYDRATED WITH FRESH WATER AND HERBAL TEAS

Dehydration is linked to food cravings. You should be drinking about half your body weight in ounces of water daily. If you weigh 150 pounds, you need to drink 75 ounces of water each day. Add a slice of lemon or lime to the water to improve the taste and alkalinity (while citric acid is acidic out of the body, a lemon's effect is alkaline once it's ingested). And water should be filtered, ideally with a pH of 8 to 9.5.

10. GET ADEQUATE SLEEP, MANAGE STRESS, AND EXERCISE REGULARLY

Do more of what nourishes your body, mind, and soul, such as reading, meditating, yoga, and other exercise, and remember that stress is not created by external factors but by the way we perceive situations in life. Get plenty of sleep. When we're tired, we have the tendency to eat sugary foods. Regular exercise will help

boost energy levels and reduce stress. Enjoy a serving of Alkamind Daily Minerals thirty minutes before sleep to get a deep REM sleep and shortly after working out to replenish the minerals you lost.

GLUTEN: THE SILENT KILLER

Gluten is a protein made up of the peptides gliadin and glutenin and is found in many grains, such as wheat, semolina, spelt, kamut, rye, and barley. Gluten (the term derives from the Latin word for "glue") is what gives elasticity to dough and often gives the final product a chewy texture. But it's not just limited to bread and dough; it is also hidden in many processed foods—salad dressings, soy sauce, cereals, pasta, beer, and even beauty products.

Many people rightly avoid wheat because they have gluten allergies or autoimmune diseases such as celiac, which gluten consumption can trigger. Actually, gluten is bad for everyone. It is literally like glue in the digestive tract that clogs everything. Next to sugar, wheat is one of the most acidic and inflammatory foods in the modern diet. I don't care whether you think you can handle gluten or not, you shouldn't be eating it.

When you eat glutinous grains, the gliadin triggers the production of another protein in your digestive tract called zonulin, which we discussed in Chapter 1. When zonulin is stimulated, it affects the gut lining and increases the perforations in the gut.

Now, the barricade that's in the gut to protect your system is compromised. We call this leaky gut syndrome. So all the bad stuff—toxins, yeast, mold, the bad bacteria, and undigested food particles—all leaks into the blood; it has bypassed the body's defense system. It's like a security breach, and once it's happened, you're looking at inflammation, autoimmune diseases, arthritis, and more. Next, the white blood cells start attacking these interlopers, creating inflammation. Your body will drive the toxins out of the blood into the tissues. Now you're looking at problems in the joints, the muscles, and the skin, as well as breakouts, arthritis, osteoporosis, and obesity . . . the list goes on. We talked about the five stages of acidosis (see pages 10–13), and here they are, showing up in all kinds of health challenges.

Gluten and Celiac Disease

Gluten is an instigator of celiac disease, which affects an estimated 1 in 100 people worldwide, with the number of diagnosed cases quadrupling over the past fifty years. There may be 2.5 million undiagnosed Americans who are at risk for long-term health complications. One of the main reasons for the huge number of misdiagnosed cases is that celiac disease symptoms are common—bloating, constipation, diarrhea, and vomiting.

Celiac disease is a severe disruption of the small intestine's health that is triggered by a severe reaction to gluten. It is an autoimmune disorder where the body mistakenly attacks its own intestinal cells. The gut mucosa is wiped out, leaving the intestines more permeable for these toxic compounds to gain entry into the bloodstream where

they don't belong. Once they gain entry, they fully activate the immune cells into attack mode. Doctors label this an autoimmune condition, but what is actually happening is your body's immune defense is kicked into full gear, trying its hardest to get rid of the toxicity that entered your blood that doesn't belong there in the first place.

Ever Feel Like You Have a Gluten Addiction?

When you eat bread, bagels, or pasta, you are eating carbohydrates, which of course means that you are eating sugar. Eating carbohydrates produces a natural, physical high caused by the release of dopamine. The human body loves that happy feeling and starts craving more of it. Gluten will cause a rapid spike in blood sugar levels, increasing insulin sensitivity, and leaving you craving more.

Wheat also has a direct effect on the opiate receptors in your brain. But different from most opiates (drugs), wheat stimulates your hunger center. When you try to eliminate anything with wheat from your diet, you can experience something I call wheat withdrawal: a feeling of fatigue, shakiness, brain fog, and depression. The symptoms can last up to one week. The truth is, wheat is something we all should cut down on and ideally remove from our diets.

Why Have Grains Suddenly Become a Problem?

Forty thousand years ago, humans were nomadic and mostly ate plants and meat.

They ate no grains and no dairy other than breast milk. They were healthy then. Now it's a different story; we are drowning in sugars and grains.

As grains such as wheat began to be cultivated, our ancestors could harvest and ingest wheat and other glutinous grains without the harmful effects we see today. However, today's wheat is not the same as what our ancestors ate. Since the 1980s, grasses have been genetically changed to meet the demands of a growing population and an unsustainable environment. They have been altered to increase yield and generate more profit, like so many other industries, harming our own health.

William Davis wrote this in a 2012 article called "Put Down That Slice of Bread: Even 'Healthy' Whole Wheat is Linked to Heart Disease, Arthritis and Dementia." "The whole wheat that we eat today has little in common with the truly natural grain. Decades of hybridization by the food industry to increase yield and confer certain baking and aesthetic characteristics of flour have created new proteins in wheat the human body isn't equipped to handle."

What Do Acid Rain and Wheat Have in Common?

In *Wheat Belly*, a phenomenal book I suggest you all read, Dr. William Davis explains the prevalence of wheat in the American diet and its responsibility in contributing to our overall acid burden. Wheat is a major source of sulfuric acid, much more so than any meat. In its natural state, sulfuric acid

burns holes in stone and metal. Imagine what it does to your intestinal lining. Of course, the amount of sulfuric acid in wheat is tiny, but if it's ingested in great amounts for a lifetime, it will be problematic. Davis says, "Grains such as wheat (gluten) account for 38 percent of the average American's acid load, more than enough to tip the balance into the acid range."

That's insane! In fact, 38 percent is enough of a shift that if you fully removed grains from your diet, it would be enough to move you from a net acid state to a fully alkaline state, which would be great.

There's Nothing Free about Gluten-Fee

Gluten-free eating is one of the hottest trends in food, and rightfully so. Here's the bad news. Unfortunately, many gluten-free, processed foods are loaded with sugars and artificial sweeteners, simply replacing one dangerous acid for another. These food manufacturers need to sell product, and to do so they need to make it taste good. There's nothing free about gluten-free. For something to be considered gluten-free, it needs to be free of only one gluten-containing protein—gliadin—but there are many others. For example, gluten-free oatmeal may not contain gliadin, but it does contain avenin, a glutinous protein in oats that's similar to the gluten in wheat.

Do you see where this is going? The only way to eat gluten-free is to eliminate glutinous foods from your diet and eat whole foods instead, not replace them with artificial foods that try to re-create the gluten versions. For example, it's better to skip bread altogether than to eat a gluten-free version that's full of sugars or sweeteners. If bread is one of those foods that you refuse to give up, then replace it with a sprouted version, such as Ezekiel bread. While this still has small amounts of gluten, it is a much better option than white or whole wheat.

As you transition off wheat and perhaps other grains, if you want to replace rice, try quinoa or cauliflower "rice." Replacing pasta? Try spaghetti squash or zucchini noodles, sometimes called zoodles. Also, you want to be sure to add in healthy alkaline fats such as avocados, coconut oil, chia, hemp, and flax seeds, raw nut butters, and plenty of dark-green leafy vegetables.

DAIRY IS SCARY

The average American typically consumes close to 630 pounds of dairy products per year (milk, yogurt, cheese, and ice cream), which makes it the single largest component of the Standard American Diet! Contrary to marketing claims, drinking cow's milk doesn't have significant health benefits. In fact, cow's milk is the number-one allergy of children. It was not designed for children and adults; it was designed for cows (think about how much an infant grows in one year, compared to that of a calf)!

Milk is filled with sugar and casein, a protein that is linked to certain cancers in humans, due to its high acid content. Cow's milk has twenty times more casein than human milk and is poorly digested and very damaging to the human immune system. Most dairy products are made from milk of cows that feed on grains and are loaded with pro-inflammatory omega-6 fatty acids and other acidic hormones and pesticide residues. Additionally, dairy products contain the sugar lactose, which like all sugars, is highly acid forming. The body converts lactose into lactic acid, which acidifies blood and tissues, ultimately *pulling* calcium from your bones and magnesium from your muscles, while your body is hard at work to neutralize the acid.

Like fruit juices, milk is pasteurized and homogenized, and although this kills the bad bacteria, making it safe to drink, it has the unfortunate effect of losing most of the nutrients right along with it. In addition, the homogenization of milk makes the fat particles so small so that they are easily absorbed, while at the same time scarring and clogging the arteries. It is a dangerous process and you flat out don't need it. Plenty of plant-based sources of calcium are much better than milk, such as broccoli, chia and sesame seeds, Chinese cabbage, raw almonds and collard greens. There is more usable calcium from these plant-based sources than there is in any type of dairy.

Humans are the only species that consumes another mammal's breast milk after weaning. Cows don't even drink cow's milk after weaning! Forget about the fact that we are consuming another mammal's breast milk for a second. Even when consuming human breast milk, a human baby will digest the milk differently once the gastric juices begin to appear, around eighteen to twenty-four months. Before the gastric juices are flowing, human breast milk is alkaline-forming in the body. Once the gastric juices appear, the milk becomes acid forming, creating mucus, allergies, sinus congestion, and potential immune issues. That is why every mammal weans their young off milk, *except* the human species. What's the takeaway? **Cow's milk was designed for baby cows, not humans, period.**

But don't just take my word. Here are a few statistics:

▸ Men who have two or more servings of dairy per day have a 60 percent greater chance of getting prostate cancer.

▸ 30 million women suffer from osteoporosis, even though Americans are among the highest consumers of dairy in the world.

▸ 18 percent of dairy cows have been injected with artificial growth hormone, which boosts milk production by 15 percent.

▸ A Harvard study tested children (ages 6–11) before and after drinking American milk for one month and noted an increase in their hormone levels.

▸ The growth hormone insulin-like growth factor (IGF-1), often found in milk that has been treated with bovine growth hormone, has been shown to cause early puberty in girls. IGF-1 is also known to mutate healthy human breast cells to cancerous cells,

contributing to breast and colon cancer.

▸ The cow's milk protein beta-lactoglobulin has been found in the blood of lung cancer patients, suggesting a link to cancer.

Cow's Milk

People believe milk makes bones strong. In fact, it's the opposite! As I mentioned earlier, drinking milk actually *leaches* calcium from bones. Furthermore, you drink milk, and you more than likely consume antibiotics, growth hormone pesticides, pus, and painkillers. Did you know that 80 percent of all the antibiotics in America are fed to livestock? Not only is this creating a terrible problem with resistant bacteria, but it is also contributing to leaky gut syndrome and the destruction of our delicate microbiome.

If you must drink milk from an animal (and I'm asking you not to), choose raw goat's milk, as it most closely resembles human breast milk. Preferable to cow's milk or raw goat's milk is hemp and coconut milk (unsweetened and carrageenan-free), or homemade almond milk from raw, non-irradiated almonds. Skip soymilk and store-bought almond milk altogether. Not only is 95 percent of all soy genetically modified (GMO), but it is also higher in phytoestrogens than just about any other food source. Phytoestrogens are plant-based estrogens that mimic the estrogen in our bodies. Soybeans also have the highest amounts of phytic acid, an antinutrient

ARE ALMONDS TOXIC?

Eighty percent of the world's almonds come from California. After a salmonella outbreak in the early 2000s, the US Department of Agriculture imposed "mandatory sterilization" of almonds. Methods of pasteurization include oil roasting, dry roasting, blanching, steam processing, irradiation, and, shockingly, the use of propylene oxide (PPO).

Dr. Jane Goldberg wrote that the first three processes could also cause a reduction of nutrients; heat also oxidizes the omega-3 fatty acids in almonds, leading to rancidity and creating free radicals. But most alarmingly, PPO is a treatment that is classified by the Environmental Protection Agency as a class B2 carcinogen that has caused tumors in rodents and is used to make polyurethane plastics.

For these reasons, I recommend avoiding store-bought almonds and almond milk, instead buying organic almonds in bulk from a roadside farm or other reputable source whenever possible.

---

that will block the uptake of your most essential alkaline minerals, such as magnesium, calcium, and zinc.

Cheese

Cheese is acidic. It takes 10 pounds of milk to make cheese, so it has even higher levels of the residues we mentioned in milk. It's essentially concentrated milk, so it's effectively ten times worse for you. It's very processed as well as high in unhealthy acidic properties. I know most people are going to keep eating cheese, and so I won't forbid it, but do cut back significantly—make sure you're keeping to that 80/20 rule. Raw and unpasteurized cheeses are slightly less detrimental overall, but I advocate for real moderation.

Remember, cheese is mold, and that's not something you want in large amounts.

Butter

Rather than cook with butter, I suggest choosing many other healthy fats first, such as coconut oil, coconut butter, and avocado oil. That said, raw butter or butter from grass-fed cows is a smart transition food. For those of you who cannot find raw butter, the Kerrygold brand is an excellent grass-fed option. I also like ghee, which is clarified butter popular in Indian cooking.

A warning: some people think they are doing the right thing by avoiding butter and using margarine or even yogurt-based spreads instead because these don't have cholesterol or saturated fat. But what might

MILK

NEVER	BETTER	BEST
Cow's Milk and Soy Milk *(Raw Goat's Milk - Best Animal Based Option)*	Almond Milk	Coconut Milk & Homemade Almond/Hemp Milk

NOTE: *When buying store-bought coconut or almond milk, be sure ingredient panel excludes the following 2 ingredients: Carrageenan & Cane Sugar/Syrup*

they have in place of saturated fats? Trans fats, which are worse than saturated fats and more likely to lead to heart disease.

Even the brands that claim to be trans-fat free can contain trans fats in up to 0.05 percent of the ingredients! Stay away from any food that includes partially hydrogenated oils on the list of ingredients. This applies to vegetable oils and canola oil as well. Instead, stick to healthy fats such as coconut oil and extra virgin olive oil. When stored below 76°F, coconut oil is solid and can be used as a great spreadable alternative to butter. Cacao butter and raw nut butters (peanut butter aside) are excellent options as well.

Yogurt

It's a common myth that yogurt is good for you. It's actually one of the most acidic foods on the planet. People consume it because they think they're getting healthy probiotics, which they may be, but at what expense? Yogurt is highly congestive and acidifying to the digestive tract and is filled with yeast from the fermentation process. You may be getting probiotics, but there are better options out there. Even when you buy fat-free yogurt, there's often sugar added, including high fructose corn syrup or agave nectar (which is 90 percent fructose). And most yogurts are loaded with artificial sweeteners.

Kefir

Traditional kefir is a fermented drink made from cow's milk and kefir grains (consisting of lactic acid bacteria, and yeast). The fermentation of the lactose sugar yields a sour, carbonated, slightly alcoholic beverage, with a consistency and taste similar to thin yogurt. Some health nuts think they're doing a great thing because they've graduated from yogurt to kefir. Guess what: The kefir grains initiating the fermentation are highly acidic, consisting of lactic acid, bacteria, yeasts, in a matrix of proteins, lipids, and sugars. You most certainly want to avoid this one.

Ice Cream

Who doesn't love ice cream on a hot summer day? Sadly, with a combination of sugar *and* dairy, and often additives as well, ice cream is one of the most highly acidic foods there is. Most ice creams today are chemical concoctions that shouldn't be allowed for human consumption, yet our children eat it on a regular basis. It takes 12 pounds of milk to make 1 pound of ice cream, and the many additives consist of high fructose corn syrup, hydrogenated oils, food coloring, and dry milk solids. According to the Hippocrates Health Institute, a typical ice cream label may include the following:

▸ **ALDEHYDE C-17, an inflammable liquid dye that is used in dyes, plastics, and rubber, which also serves as a flavor enhancer**

▸ **DIETHYL GLYCOL is an inexpensive chemical used as an egg substitute and is also used in antifreeze and paint removers**

▸ **ETHYL ACETATE, which also cleans leather and textiles, and can cause chronic lung, liver, and heart damage**

▸ **POLYSORBATE 80 is a surfactant that has been shown to have damaging effects on the reproductive and immune systems.**

Fortunately, there is a solution. If you must indulge in ice cream, there are many great alternatives, from coconut-based desserts to low-sugar fruit sorbets.

BAD FATS

There are two major problems with the standard American diet when it comes to fat. First, Americans have been trained by physicians and the media to fear fat, and therefore, we don't eat nearly enough of the right kinds. Second, with the fats that we do happen to consume, a dangerous imbalance exists that is harmful to our health.

As I've said, there are two types of essential fatty acids, omega-6 and omega-3, which we need ideally in equal amounts in order to be healthy and pH balanced. "Essential" means our bodies need it but don't manufacture it, so it needs to come from dietary sources. The ideal omega-6 ratio to omega-3 should be 1:1 and should never exceed 4:1. With that said, the average American has a ratio of 19:1, and in many cases, 25:1, and even 50:1, imbalanced toward unhealthy omega-6 fats.

Omega-6 fats are in nearly every processed food we eat. Omega-6s and omega-3s act differently. Omega-6s are pro-inflammatory, while omega-3s have an anti-inflammatory effect. Omega-3s will thin the blood, while omega-6s will thicken and clot the blood. Both are essential to our survival, but they need to be balanced.

The omega-6 fats are linoleic acid (LA) and arachidonic acid (AA), which are found in animal products. When you consume a heavily acidic diet high in omega-6 fats, chronic and excessive inflammation occurs, and chronic disease is the result. Because your brain is primarily fat, a diet that heavily favors omega-6 fats causes inflammation of your brain. In health research on murderers and people in mental institutions, researchers found an average omega-6/omega-3 ratio to be 70:1! Remember, the brain is about 60 percent fat, so behavior shifts dramatically when a healthy nutrient balance is achieved.

Omega-6 fats also generate dangerous free radicals that contribute to cancer and atherosclerosis, or narrowing and hardening of your arteries. Too much arachidonic acid can trigger blood clots. A 1993 study found, "The increased consumption of many vegetable oils particularly of the omega-6 series is . . . viewed as pro-inflammatory and is suspected as one of the possible causes for the rise in certain malignant tumors, rheumatoid arthritis and autoimmune diseases primarily due to the increased production of pro-inflammatory cytokines."

In addition, a diet that favors omega-6 fats will trigger greater fat storage. Many studies show animals fed a diet high in omega-6 fats will become fatter than animals on a non-omega-6 diet with identical calories. If you have been trying to lose some weight and have been unsuccessful, bringing your omega-6/omega-3 ratio back into balance may be the answer.

Not only do you need to increase the healthy omega-3s in your diet, but you also have to decrease the omega-6s to get back to that healthy 1:1 relationship. A typical American diet has too many acid-forming omega-6 fats in the form of corn and soy, safflower, sunflower, cottonseed, palm, margarine, and hydrogenated vegetable oils. These dangerous fats are hidden everywhere—in baked goods, pasta sauces, salad dressings, mayonnaise, and most of the meats and fish you eat. Cottonseed oil is most acidic, with the omega-6 fats outnumbering the good fats 234 to 1, which is off the charts!

Soybean oil is a major culprit, as it is added to so many processed foods. It is also fed to animals as well as farm-raised fish, which is why it's so important to eat grass-fed meat and wild-caught fish. According to a study from Dr. Joe Hibbeln, **from 1909 to 1999, the estimated per capita consumption of soybean oil increased one-thousand-fold. No wonder we are so inflamed and acidic.**

If you want to lose the toxic fat, replace it with good fat. Start eating more avocados and wild-caught salmon, and add coconut oil to everything, as these fats will satiate you, making you crave less sugar and helping you lose weight.

Now, you will never see "omega-6 fats" on an ingredient label from a product you buy in a store, so how will you be able to identify them so that you *can* remove them? You have to become a conscientious label reader. Refer to the Inflammatory/Acidic Fats list (see page 86). Ask yourself, is there soybean, sunflower, or safflower oil? Is the meat grass fed or fed with grains? Is the fish farm-raised? Once you know this information, you will know if it contains acidic omega-6s. As you change your diet, not

INFLAMMATORY/ACIDIC FATS (Including Omega-6 Fats)

OILS: Hydrogenated Vegetable Oils, Cottonseed Oil, Safflower Oil, Sunflower Oil, Wheat Germ Oil, Grapeseed Oil, Walnut Oil

Soybean Oil *(93% of margarines, 72% of salad dressings like Caesar, Italian, Thousand Island, and Mayonnaise)*

Soy *(tofu, soy milk, soybeans /edamame)*

Corn, Corn Oil, HFCS *(High Fructose Corn Syrup)*

Peanuts, Peanut Butter, Peanut Oil *(Peanuts contain 21 different kinds of aflatoxin, a fungus that is a known carcinogenic)*

Canola *(a partially hydrogenated refined oil that is 95% genetically modified)*

Trans-Fats *(cooking oils other than coconut / all roasted nuts)*

Margarine

Shortening

Flax, Hemp, and Chia Oils *(Their seeds are healthy. When manufacturers produce them as oils, they got oxidized and turn to trans-fatty acids)*

COMMON SOURCES OF OMEGA-6 FATS:

Eating Meat, Eggs, Poultry, Dairy *(Indirect Source)* — a majority of the animals are fed unhealthy grains and omega-6 fats to "beef" them up. These foods are a major contributing factor to the dangerous levels of inflammatory omega-6 fats. Many people's omega-6 fats are too high due to this source.

Farmed Fish, including Salmon *(5 times higher in omega-6 fats than wild-caught)*

Chicken Sandwich *(i.e. McDonald's Chicken Sandwich)*, Hot dogs *(vegetarian, turkey, and chicken)*

Sunflower and Safflower seeds *(These seeds are on both lists, because they are a good source of omega-3s, but they are also very high in omega-6 fats, so consume in moderation)*

Cookies, Crackers, Candy, Dairy Creamer, Frozen Pizza, Granola/Granola Bars, Mozzarella Cheese Shreds, Pie Crust, Pastries, Popcorn

A study by the Harvard School of Public Health revealed that omega-3 fatty acid deficiency is the sixth biggest killer of Americans—even more deadly than excess trans-fat intake. The study utilized 2005 data from the US National Health Center for Health Statistics and revealed there are between 72,000 and 96,000 preventable deaths each year due to omega-3 deficiency.

only will this ratio improve, but your body will begin to reset its metabolism away from sugar as its primary fuel source and transform into a fat-burning machine, as you'll learn in the next chapter.

ANIMAL PROTEINS

You might think of a lean chicken breast or a piece of fish as diet food, but meat is actually one of the biggest acidosis culprits you could consume. Though I follow a mostly plant-based diet and believe it to be the best option for maintaining an alkaline body, I won't tell you to cast off meat completely—I get it, you like your occasional steak and sushi! In fact, your body needs protein, as the amino acids are the building blocks for your bones, muscles, and hormones. But here's the problem: most people are eating way too much—consuming three times the protein they

actually need—and more times than not, the meat is poor quality.

Protein is a necessary part of your daily diet, but much less than what most people are currently eating. It's a fact that Americans eat too much, too often, and the wrong kind. In addition to quantity and eating far too much, the quality could be the damaging component to health. For example, research shows that excess animal protein is linked with osteoporosis, kidney disease, calcium stones in the urinary tract, and some cancers. Increasing red meat intake by more than half a serving per day raises the risk for type 2 diabetes by 48 percent.

According to a Harvard study, people can live up to 20 percent longer by eliminating or at least reducing how much red meat they eat. People who ate the highest levels of red meat died the youngest, most often from colon cancer and cardiovascular diseases. In addition, excess protein converts to glucose and is stored as fat, just like sugar and grains.

Now, if you enjoy meat, I'm not telling you that you can't ever have it. Quality is important, so always go for grass-fed, organic, and free-range. Meat is okay in moderation (no more than two to three times per week), but meat is acidic and requires a lot of energy to break it down. So if you are going to have meat or fish, make it the sideshow and not the main event. If you're eating red meat or processed meat every night and it's the major part of the meal, you may be on the fast track to health problems.

When you consume more than half of your calories from protein, not only do you stress your digestive system and your liver, you also increase your likelihood of chronic disease such as cancer and heart disease. The byproduct of protein metabolism is blood urea nitrogen (BUN), which is turned into ammonia and urea, both highly toxic. To make matters worse, BUN has a diuretic effect on your body, causing your kidneys to get rid of water. As a result, you become dehydrated. But water is not the only thing the kidneys dump out—they also eliminate vital alkaline buffering minerals such as calcium, magnesium, potassium, and sodium bicarbonate.

Protein is a double-edged sword. By itself, it is highly acidic and toxic because of the sulfuric acid, phosphoric acid, ammonia, and urea it produces as it's metabolized. Second, proteins use up minerals by neutralizing the above acids that they produced in the first place. Lastly, consuming too much protein can actually produce sugar! That's right, excess protein in your diet will cause the liver to convert the amino acids found in protein into sugar.

Where Should I Get Protein?

People always ask if they can get enough protein on an alkaline diet. The answer is a resounding yes!

One way to limit consumption of meat is to declare one day of vegetarianism per week, a "meatless Monday" of sorts. But be careful—vegetarians who merely replace meat with pasta and carbohydrates are some of the unhealthiest people around. So many vegetarians I come across are sugartarians and can be worse than meat-eaters, and the product of that way of eating is acid.

It doesn't take much to give your body the nutrients it needs, even after giving up meat, as long as you aren't just trading in that portion of your plate for empty carbs. With my seven favorite plant-based proteins list (see page 131), you will never have any trouble fulfilling your body's requirements!

If you are going to eat animal-based proteins, opt for proteins rich in omega-3 fatty acids such as wild caught salmon, sardines, anchovies, herring, or trout. In addition, increase plant-based proteins by consuming quinoa, dark-green leafy vegetables, chia and hemp seeds, hummus, and smaller beans that have been soaked and sprouted, such as chickpeas or adzuki beans.

A Word about Bone Broth

Bone broth has become very trendy. You wouldn't believe how many questions I get in my practice about it. Bone broth can be very nutritious and loaded with minerals and collagen. But the caveat is, it is of course, animal-based, which is why you must carefully read the label to know what is inside.

When you buy bone broth, if it doesn't say grass-fed organic, it's all but guaranteed it will contain an indirect source of antibiotics, growth hormone, and omega-6 fats that are inflammation-producing and acidic. The source must be organically raised, pastured, and grass-fed.

Many companies use vinegar in the process of extracting as many minerals as possible, and anything that has vinegar is a big no-no because of the yeast and sugar. If you are considering bone broth, make your own and use apple cider vinegar because it is a better option that is unfiltered and unpasteurized.

I prefer broth to be plant-based and alkaline. If you are looking to get some of the collagen and mineral effects from bone broth, make my high-alkaline vegetable broth instead, which I call Boneless Broth (see recipe, page 213). To replace the benefits of the collagen, take a good organic sulfur supplement or MSM (to purchase pure organic sulfur, refer to the Resource section on page 249). If you are still intent on having bone broth, I again, strongly suggest you make your own and know your source!

OTHER ACIDIC FOODS TO AVOID

When it comes to acidic foods, sugar, wheat, dairy, and animal proteins are the worst offenders, but other nefarious characters add acid as well.

Caffeine

If you're a coffee drinker, then you probably won't argue that caffeine is addictive. The more you drink, the more likely you will suffer from withdrawal symptoms once it is removed. There may be some good components to it, but the fact is this: when you consume caffeine, you crave it more, and it is an adrenal and liver suppressor.

And I'm not just talking about coffee—caffeine is also found in green tea, matcha tea, energy drinks, sodas, chocolate, and even decaffeinated coffee (8–12 mg per cup).

Coconut Oil in Your Coffee? Absolutely!

Okay, so if I can't convince all coffee drinkers out there to quit, here is the next best option: replace all dairy products (milk and cream) with cold-pressed coconut oil. It is a powerful neutralizer of acid that is rich in healthy medium-chain triglyceride fats (MCT). It will energize and fuel your day.

Directions: First, choose organic coffee. Next, carefully pour your coffee into a blender. Add 1 tablespoon of coconut oil, and if you need a sweetener, swap out the refined sugar for organic stevia or lo han (monk fruit). Place the lid on the blender and blend up your coffee. Once blended, pour it into your cup and get your drink on.

Now, there are many reasons why people crave and drink coffee. For some people it's the taste; for others, it's the morning ritual; and for some, it is the energy spike. When most people drink coffee, the nail in the coffin is not so much the coffee itself but what they add to it: milk, sugar, syrups, or heavy cream, which contribute even more acid to the body.

If you want to stop drinking coffee, drink lots of water with lemon during the detoxification process, and I always recommend supercharging it with a scoop of Alkamind

Daily Greens. The chlorophyll helps accelerate the detoxification of the liver from the toxicity the caffeine created.

I also suggest making a detox tea in its place. My recipe (see page 153) is detoxing, energizing, tastes yummy, and fulfills my morning ritual.

Soy-Based Foods

I don't eat any soy-based foods, and you shouldn't either. Soy is problematic for many reasons. Around 2000, everyone was singing the praises of soy and tofu, but since then, we've learned that 95 percent of it is genetically modified to make it resistant to herbicides. Even if you buy GMO-free, soy foods inherently have isoflavones, which resemble human estrogen, so they block natural estrogen receptor sites in your body.

Soy interferes with healthy thyroid function and includes anti-nutrients such as saponins, which are natural plant "toxins" that can create digestive issues, inhibit enzyme function, and damage your red blood cells. Soy foods also contain phytates, which can block the essential minerals, including calcium, magnesium, iron, and zinc. (One thing to note is that meat can stop the effects of mineral blocking, so if you do decide to eat soy, eating meat with it can help counteract the effects. However, both should be avoided.) Here is a list of common soy products:

- tofu
- tempeh, miso, natto
- soy sauce
- edamame
- soy formula
- soybean oil
- soymilk
- soy cheese, soy ice cream, soy yogurt
- soy "meat" (meatless products made of TVP or textured vegetable proteins)
- soy protein

SOY SAUCE SUBSTITUTIONS

Some people prefer tamari (made from soybeans, but it's wheat and gluten free, which is a plus) or Bragg's Liquid Aminos (nonfermented, gluten free, and GMO free with sixteen amino acids and sodium bicarbonate). The best choice by far is coconut aminos—made from raw coconut sap and natural sea salt and free of all soy, plus it tastes great!

Mushrooms, Peanuts, Corn, and Vinegar
MUSHROOMS

Fungi are mistakenly thought of as being healthy since they are vegetables. The truth is, any foods containing fungus are acidic and harmful. Avoid eating them, especially if you are having any health challenges with cancer, yeast, or mold.

Mushrooms are the fleshy, spore-bearing fruit of the fungus that typically grows in a damp, moldy, rotting environment. Out of the thousands of mushroom species, most are poisonous with only a few being edible.

SOY SAUCE

NEVER	BETTER	BEST
Soy Sauce	Braggs Liquid Aminos/Gluten-Free Tamari/*Shoyu Soy Sauce	Coconut Aminos

*Raw, contains wheat, but gluten levels are below detection limit <5ppm

I never recommend eating mushrooms. However, there is some research showing that medicinal mushroom supplements (different from eating the mushrooms) such as Reishi, Cordyceps, Maitake, and Turkey Tail can be very powerful for certain conditions, including cancer. If you are going to choose one of these supplements, discuss it with your healthcare provider first, and second, make sure the supplements are from a very reliable source.

PEANUTS AND CORN

You'll want to avoid peanuts and corn like the plague, as you are being exposed to poisonous fungal mycotoxins. In fact, peanuts (which are actually not a nut but a legume) have twenty-one different types of fungus that produce a dangerous mycotoxin called aflatoxin. Corn has twenty-five! Aflatoxin is not naturally found in peanuts but rather is produced by a naturally occurring fungus that lives in the soil that peanuts are grown in, organic or not.

Aflatoxin is a potent carcinogen (especially known to cause liver cancer) and is easily absorbed by soft-shelled peanuts as well as corn, which is why I dub them both as two of the most acidic and dangerous foods.

VINEGAR

Vinegar is a popular ingredient, especially for all salad lovers. But vinegar is a

PEANUT BUTTER OPTIONS

SWAP THIS FOR THAT: *Instead of peanut butter, use raw almond butter, cacao butter, or coconut butter.*

AVOID PEANUT BUTTER

Peanut butter is something all kids love. However, it is the very last food I would ever give my children. It is acidic and toxic, and because of the high amounts of aflatoxin, can contribute to certain forms of cancer. I sincerely hope this motivates you to go into the kitchen right now and throw out the peanut butter. Peanut butter is even worse than whole peanuts, as manufacturers take the prettier peanuts with fewer molds and use those as cocktail peanuts. Consequently, the peanuts with the most fungus (and aflatoxin) are mashed up and made into peanut butter.

If you still refuse to give up peanut butter, here are some tips to lessen aflatoxin exposure:

▸ **Always refrigerate peanut butter.** By placing peanut butter in the refrigerator, you are stopping any fungus that may be present from multiplying.

▸ **Eat more chlorophyll!** Research has shown chlorophyll consumption reduces the absorption of aflatoxin, which makes green vegetables and dehydrated alkaline green powders great for decreasing its carcinogenic effects.

fermented alcohol byproduct that is filled with sugar, yeast, and acetic acid. Avoid it and swap it for fresh lemon or lime juice. Apple cider vinegar is an exception (in moderation), as it does have an alkaline-forming effect inside the body. It also is a great adjunct if you are dealing with reflux: take 1 tablespoon with water every day on an empty stomach (if dealing with cancer, avoid completely).

Table Salt

Natural salts are rich in minerals. However, commonly used table salt is often packed with numerous additives such as anti-caking agents, fluoride, and bleach to name a few. Choose mineral salts instead.

People hear they should be on a no-salt diet, but that's not true. Your body requires salt to live. The most important things to neutralize acids are mineral salts: calcium,

ALCOHOL

NEVER	BETTER	BEST
Beer, vodka, and gin (made from grains)	Wine	Chopin Vodka (from potatoes only) Ciroc Vodka (from grapes)

magnesium, potassium, and sodium. This is why dark-green leafy vegetables are so important, as are low-sugar citrus fruits—lemon, lime, and grapefruit. These are all high in mineral salts.

The two types of salts you need are sea salts (Celtic Grey, or Himalayan salt which is not a sea salt, but is of equal quality) and mineral salts. Anything else is heavily processed and heavily acidic.

Carbonated Water

People seem to think carbonated water is a healthy option, but it is—you guessed it—acidic. The same waste product of breathing, carbon dioxide gas (CO_2) is what is infused to give this popular beverage the carbonated effect. If you have to drink it, add some lemon or lime to make it more alkaline. The rule of thumb is, if it's carbonated, it's acidic.

Fermented Foods

Fermentation is a metabolic process that uses yeast and bacteria to convert sugar to acids, gases, and alcohol. Avoid ALL fermented grains (in many alcohols) because of their ability to become impregnated with fungal mycotoxins. While many people tout kombucha as a health drink, avoid this one too, as it's filled with saccharomyces yeast, bacteria, carbonation, some sugar, caffeine, and alcohol—an acidic nightmare!

Alcohol

Alcohol is acidic, period. I'm not saying you should never have a drink, but I am saying, indulge in moderation. Alcohol is acidic, period. I'm not saying you should never have a drink, but indulge in moderation. Alcohol producers often use grains that are contaminated with fungal mycotoxins (poisons from fungi), so there is a good chance you are consuming more than just alcohol in your cocktail. Stay away from beer because of the fermented grains, and wine because of the yeast and sugar. The best option is grain-free vodka made from potatoes and grapes, such as Ciroc and Chopin, respectively.

06

How to Become a
Fat-Burning Machine

I've been super excited to share with you the ways I crushed my cravings and overcame my lifelong addiction to sugar. I want to show you how I turned my body into a fat-burning machine and lost 42 pounds in a safe, healthy, sustainable way over a six-month period. I didn't get there by starving myself or by doing one of the dozens of fad diets. I got there by eating as much as I wanted—the alkaline way. If you follow the strategies I'm going to share with you, not only can you lose any unwanted extra weight, but you will also turn your body into an energetic, healthy machine.

This information has changed my life, and it has the potential to change yours. When you lose weight with my method, you will lose it for one reason—because of reduced acid levels. There are many ways to lose weight, but most methods don't address the true cause of why the person gained the weight in the first place. With the same acidic habits in place, it's just a matter of time before the body returns to where it was previously.

Excess body fat is an acid problem. So to reach your ideal weight, you first have to transition to eating an 80/20 diet in favor of alkaline-forming foods. This is a minimum goal, and you can eat even more alkaline if you'd like. Then, as I'll detail in the next chapter, follow the 7 Ways to GET OFF YOUR ACID. By the end of this section, you will know exactly what I did to transform my body into a fat-burning machine in just a few months.

I have taken thousands of clients through this program with a very high success rate. People lose pounds off their bodies and inches off their waists, and more importantly, they are keeping it off. But they're losing the weight as a byproduct of health and energy. As Kelly Ripa said, "This is a lifestyle, not a diet!" (Look at the first three letters of the word "diet." What does that spell? Exactly!)

The GET OFF YOUR ACID program and the alkaline way of life is so powerful, you will enjoy pHenomenal results (pun intended!), even by following it only

80 percent of the time. We all love food, and depriving ourselves of favorite foods sets us up for failure. Deprivation drives resentment, and that is why so many diets fail. That's what I love about this program—you don't have to give up anything completely. For example, I will never tell you to stop drinking coffee, if that is something you truly love and don't want to give up.

Now, is coffee highly acidic? And will you achieve your weight loss goals faster without it? You bet! But I want you to have lasting change, and when you consistently fuel your body with high alkaline foods, including healthy fats, your body will have all the tools it needs to neutralize the acid so your body has no need to hold onto the excess weight anymore.

What I am going to show you works. At the end of the day, it is all about results! However, we need to first talk about how to reset your body so that it burns fat instead of sugar.

When it comes to healthy versus unhealthy foods, there is a lot of confusion and misinformation out there and that could be sabotaging your goal of losing weight. We talked earlier about heart disease and cancer. Most of the time, there is not a single event that creates those conditions, but a process. There's a saying, "Kill the monster while it's small." I want you to begin to recognize all the little things that may seem insignificant in the moment so that they don't build up to have a more harmful effect on your weight, your health, and your longevity.

With that said, by the next chapter you will know how often you should be eating in order to burn fat fast and exactly what your plate should look like. I've also included a short quiz so you can determine whether your body is currently primarily burning fat or storing fat. This way you will have a good baseline against which to measure progress. I always say, "What you inspect, you'll respect!" Finally, I am going to teach you one of my best tips and tricks that ultimately catapulted my body into becoming a fat-burning machine!

SECRET #1: EAT (THE RIGHT) FAT TO LOSE FAT

If you want to burn more body fat, you need to load up on more healthy fats. The more fat you want to burn, *the more fat and fewer carbs* you need to eat. Don't be afraid—as you follow this diet, 50 to 75 percent of calories may come from these healthy fats. Yes, we've been taught (by the sugar industry) to think that all fat is our enemy, and it's true that some types of fats should be avoided, but the body needs healthy fats.

Wait, you say, he wants me to eat more fat? But isn't fat what I am trying to lose? Won't eating more fat make me fatter? No!

Consuming the right fats is an essential part of being healthy. They boost your metabolism and reduce cravings for carbohydrates and sugar. The right fats fight stress and inflammation, slow down premature aging, and prevent chronic disease. In addition to helping you lose weight, they are the ideal fuel to energize your body.

Have you heard of the fifteen-minute sugar crash? This is what happens after you consume carbs, grains, and processed foods. Imagine lighting a tissue on fire . . . *poof!* It's gone. This is what happens when sugar is your primary source of fuel. It burns hot and fast, and it doesn't last. The dirty burn generates more acid. As a result, your body's minerals reserves, especially magnesium, become massively depleted. And because sugar burns so quickly, what do you think you are going to crave more of?

Fat, on the other hand, is like slow-burning coal. In the absence of carbohydrates, your body breaks down fat (dietary fat and/or stored body fat) to generate ketone bodies, or ketones, for energy. Ketones are a very clean source of energy and the ideal and preferred source of fuel for your body and your brain.

When you look at your total body calorie load for usable energy, 95 percent of those calories are stored as fat and only 5 percent as sugar. By training our bodies to burn fat rather than sugar for fuel, we can tap into this nearly endless supply of energy and at the same time melt the fat off for good. In fact, your health and longevity will ultimately be determined by the proportion of fat versus sugar you burn in the course of your lifetime. But the reality is most people are getting their energy from burning sugar.

Now, if I happen to see a saber-toothed tiger, I don't want to wait for my body to access its stores of fat to get the energy I need to run from the dangerous situation—I'd be lunch for the tiger! I need energy, and I need it fast, and that is exactly what sugar (glucose) is designed for. When you're in fight or flight mode, sugar can save your life. But here's the problem: so many of us are chronically stressed and living in a perpetual state of fight or flight, and our bodies don't know the difference! While we will always be able to make good use of both fuels, resetting your body's metabolism to use more fat for fuel is the goal. You just need to learn how to access it!

Once you tap into that boundless energy supply, you will become an alkaline Energizer bunny. This can be achieved in a relatively short period by avoiding carbs and grains, keeping protein at a moderate level, and substantially increasing levels of healthy fats and dark-green leafy vegetables. (See the Food Plate diagram on page 117). Follow this formula, and your body can reach a state of ketosis rather quickly, where it is using a slow-burning super fuel (again, known as ketones) instead of sugar for fuel.

In general, the body will burn carbs first. So guess what happens when you reduce the carb load and feed your body healthy fats instead?

This is what will lead to weight loss. This benefit even applies to you if you are slim, as some of the most dangerous fat in the body is visceral fat that parks itself around the organs. The other great thing is, eating more fat will keep you satisfied so you won't feel the need to snack between meals.

QUIZ: ARE YOU A FAT BURNER OR A SUGAR BURNER??

▶ Take this quiz to see if your body is most likely burning fat for energy, or burning sugar (while storing fat)! This quiz was developed by my good friend, colleague, and one of the leaders of the chiropractic profession, Dr. David Singer.

If you answer yes to more than 3 of these questions, chances are you're burning sugar for fuel, and you're in a fat storage mode.

_____ Have you ever done a diet, lost weight, and put it back on and then repeated losing weight and gaining it back? This roller-coaster effect causes the loss of muscle mass. Most people do not diet correctly. This causes the body to burn muscle for energy. Muscles require more energy keeping your metabolism high. When you lose muscle mass your metabolism slows down and so does your fat burning capacity.

_____ Have you ever completed a diet, yet still returned to your original weight? In order for your body to have a new normal weight it needs to maintain the new weight for approximately six months in order for it to become your new normal.

_____ Does emotional baggage overpower you? Eating for the wrong reasons, using food as an emotional comfort when you are depressed or a celebration when you are happy? That behavior puts on fat.

_____ Do you consume alcohol? Alcohol triggers insulin, which stimulates the body to store fat, thus causing weight gain.

_____ Do you skip meals or let yourself get hungry? Skipping meals, reducing calories and letting yourself get hungry makes the body think it should store fat. It goes into survival mode.

_____ Do you eat refined grains, white bread, cakes, cookies, etc? Eating refined carbohydrates, eating refined sugars and refined grains, white bread, cakes, cookies, etc. all stimulates insulin production, which stimulates fat storage.

_____ Do you have recurring or chronic pain? Cortisol is your body's anti-inflammatory hormone. It is released when you're in pain but when cortisol is elevated it controls the body to hold onto fat. This hormone causes the storage of belly fat, so getting any body pains reduced helps put you in a fat burning mode.

_____ Do you overeat? Overeating stimulates fat storage hormones. What you don't need the body stores.

_____ Do you consume caffeinated drinks like coffee or cola? Caffeine stimulates cortisol, which triggers fat storage.

_____ Do you often get stressed? Stress causes an increase in the hormone cortisol, which triggers fat storage.

_____ Do you have poor sleeping habits? If your body is not well rested; metabolism is reduced, adrenals are stimulated, and this puts you into a fat storage mode.

Becoming a Fat Burner

Did you take the quiz? Are you surprised, or did you get the result you expected? Now that you know where you stand, change can begin! Let's get you to a state where your body can flip this switch.

INCREASE HEALTHY FATS

Once you know what the bad fats are and what the good fats are, you can slowly start to add more of the healthy fats into your daily diet. Soon, more than 50 percent of your calories should come from healthy fats (see the list on page 122). If 50 percent seems crazy, based on where you are currently, don't stress about it. Start by adding a little bit at a time to what you eat normally, and remember to think progress, not perfection. Add healthy fats to your smoothies, salads, soups, snacks, and desserts. Add them to everything you eat.

REDUCE CARBS

As you increase calories in the form of healthy fat, initially you _must_ also reduce carbohydrate levels to no more than 25 to 50 grams of net carbs per day (net carbs equals total carbohydrates minus fiber). Ideally, these carbs should all come from whole food organic vegetables. This amounts to no more than 5 to 10 percent of total calories coming from vegetable carbohydrates at any given meal. Of these 50 grams of net carbs, no more than 25 grams should come from fruit. That's roughly equivalent to one banana.

Once you are in ketosis—a fat-burning state (which you can determine with a urine dipstick)—it is okay to increase daily net carb levels to between 50 to 150 grams. This is because you do not want to stay in ketosis 100 percent of the time. Our ancestors lived in feast and famine and routinely shifted in and out of fat burning. We should be no different. For the net carb counts of many common vegetables and foods, see Appendix II on page 235.

When you maintain a high alkaline diet—high in healthy fats and greens, moderate in protein, and low in vegetable carbohydrates—you can burn fat and lose weight while calming your appetite and cravings at the same time. Following this model can begin the fat-burning process rather quickly. In Nora Gedgaudas's book, *Primal Fat Burner*, in regards to producing ketones, she writes,

> The body begins to produce ketones after being without carbs for about twenty-four to seventy-two hours. Within about three days, the brain is already getting 25 percent of its energy from ketone bodies. After four days, this increases to 70 percent! Soon the body begins to generate ketones and free fatty acids from body fat. When this happens, the body has shifted from a glucocentric (sugar-focused) metabolism to an adipocentric

(fat-based) one. The basic definition of being ketogenically adapted is that you are burning your own body fat for fuel.

WATCH PROTEIN

How much protein do you really need? The average person should fall between the 30- and 70-gram zone per day. When calculating your target daily protein intake, the biggest mistake is using your current weight, which for many people, is overweight and not ideally where you want to be.

So I want you to try Gedgaudas's helpful formula, which will give you the number of grams of protein you should eat each day: first, come up with your *ideal* weight, and then convert that number into kilograms by dividing by 2.2. For example, if you weigh 200 pounds, and your ideal weight is 150, then divide 150 by 2.2, which is 68.18 kilograms. Next, round to the nearest whole number, which is 68. Finally, multiply this by 0.8, which equals 54.4, and round this number again to the nearest whole number. That means your goal throughout the day should be a target of 54 grams of daily of good quality protein, spread out throughout your meals (18 grams per meal).

A 3-ounce serving of cooked meat equals about 21 grams of protein. This is about the size of a deck of cards or bar of soap. Thin, flat slices of fish should resemble a standard checkbook for a 3-ounce (21 gram) serving size. Remember, too, that plant-based proteins are excellent sources that should contribute to the 54 grams.

HOW WILL I KNOW IF I AM IN
KETOSIS AND BURNING FAT FOR FUEL?

When you are in ketosis, blood tests will show ketone levels between 1 and 3 millimoles per liter (mmol/L). You can also purchase Ketostix, which is a test strip that you can urinate on that will let you know if you are producing ketones. Or, use a special Breathalyzer called Ketonix, which detects ketones and interprets the results by displaying a visual spectrum of the quantity of the gases in your breath.

Please note that ketosis should not be confused with diabetic *ketoacidosis*, where ketone levels are too high, between 15 and 25 mmol/L. Ketosis and ketoacidosis are two completely different terms—the first is good and the latter is dangerous. Risk of ketoacidosis is why people who were on the Atkins Diet and were consuming tons of animal-based protein were recommended to urinate on Ketostix test strips every day. They had to make sure their ketones weren't at dangerous levels (and that is why consuming too much meat is so bad—it's too much acid). When in a ketoacidosis state, it's very common to have a rapid breath rate of twenty to thirty breaths per minute, as the body is expelling massive amounts of CO_2, which results from acidic blood.

This all may sound daunting at first, but believe me, as you start to add those healthy fats, you will begin to automatically crave less sugar (see Chapter 7). As you crave less sugar, you will eat less sugar. And as you eat less sugar, what mode of calories will be available for your body to burn? Fat! You see how this works? Again, I want to stress this, if you are looking to lose weight, don't be afraid of the fat—you need to really trust me on this one. Add more healthy fats, and you'll win this battle.

SECRET #2:
THREE ALKALINE
MEALS A DAY WILL
BURN THE FAT AWAY

You have probably heard this advice time and time again: "Eat five to six smaller meals throughout the day and focus on putting something into your body every two hours or so." This is otherwise known as grazing. I can't tell you how many different sources I have heard this from. Our pre-agricultural ancestors didn't have access to food around the clock, as we do in modern times. While having food at our fingertips 24/7 can be quite convenient, the negatives can outweigh the positives.

When grazing, your body will quickly get used to this way of eating. When this happens, cravings will increase and your body will come to expect food on a more frequent basis. In addition, blood sugar and insulin levels will spike, ultimately leading you down the path to insulin sensitivity. This is why I urge you to move away from grazing, if this is what you are doing.

Ideally, stick to three meals a day, with nothing in between. Focusing on eating three alkaline meals, while avoiding sugar and grains, instead of eating every couple of hours accomplishes a few important things. Eating this way keeps blood sugar and insulin levels low. When this happens, your body moves from burning sugar as its primary fuel source to burning fat instead, which is ideal. This transition to reset your body can take anywhere from a few weeks to a few months, but once there, insulin levels will remain at bay and your body will turn into a fat-burning machine!

I always aim to have two substantial meals, with the third being a little lighter. My preference is for breakfast and lunch to be heartier. Those give me solid energy to jump-start and carry me throughout the day. If your job requires a lot of physical activity or if you are an athlete or pregnant, starting your day with a hearty alkaline breakfast is even more important (see my favorite breakfast options in the recipe section, beginning on page 187).

Dinner is always lighter. Try a Rainbow Salad, which is super simple and is just as it sounds—greens with any combination of healthy veggies from all colors of the rainbow, from bell peppers to carrots and beets to cucumbers. Zucchini noodles are also good (avoid foods at this time that take longer to digest, such as animal proteins). Be sure to finish dinner at least three hours before going to sleep (this is a must!). Now, I know sometimes with our busy lifestyles this doesn't always happen. For that reason, it is even more important to make dinner the most alkaline meal of the day. Your body requires the fewest calories when sleeping, so the last thing you want is to have a heavy dinner loaded with slow-digesting, animal-based proteins right before bed. In addition, your body is always most acidic in the middle of the night, peaking at 5 a.m., so give your body as many alkaline minerals through what you eat at dinner to help it neutralize all that acid, and so that you can get a deeper REM sleep.

Aim for alkaline meals loaded with vegetables. My greens will come from spinach, kale, chard, watercress, and/or romaine, and I always color it up with red bell peppers, cucumbers, red onions, carrots, celery, sprouts (thirty times more nutritious than their vegetable counterpart!), beetroot, and jalapeño, as well as healthy fats such as avocado, extra virgin olive oil, coconut oil, and raw nuts and seeds such as almonds, macadamia nuts, hemp, and chia, and tahini dressings.

To summarize, if you are looking to lose weight and prevent chronic disease, you need to eliminate sugar, grains, and other acidic foods and be extremely careful about the quantity and quality of the proteins you choose to eat. Your meals and your plate should consist primarily of dark-green leafy vegetables and healthy alkaline fats, moderate proteins from a plant-based or fish source, and little to no carbohydrates in the form of vegetable carbohydrates.

Perhaps my best recommendation is to simply let your hunger, not your emotions, dictate when you eat (guilty as charged!). Make it your goal to stick with three meals every day, but if you find you are hungry and it happens between meals, by no means am I telling you to starve yourself. What I am telling you to do is dial in and truly listen to what your body is telling you.

SECRET # 3: INTERMITTENT FASTING— THE ULTIMATE WEAPON

Okay, hear me out. When people hear the word *fast*, they shudder. They tend to think of going days or even weeks without eating. While there is some health benefit to giving your body and digestive system a long break, this is not what I am talking about. I am talking about intermittent fasting, and if done correctly, it can be the most preferred metabolic intervention you can do for your health, weight, energy, and, ultimately, longevity.

While intermittent fasting has been getting a lot of buzz in the health world and press, fasting has been around since the beginning of time. Fasting is one of the most ancient and widespread healing traditions in the world, having been advocated since the days of Hippocrates, the father of modern medicine. Hippocrates wrote, "Instead of using medicine, rather, fast a day."

Whether you realize it or not, you are doing some form of fasting every day—it's called sleeping. Putting it simply, if you eat dinner at 8 p.m. and then eat breakfast at 8 a.m., you have fasted for twelve hours. You "break" the "fast" with breakfast. Your body enters into a fasting state eight hours or so after a previous meal, when the digestive system is finished absorbing all of the nutrients from the food. When your body is in this state, it uses up all its glucose, first, for energy and then moves to fat. This is where the power of intermittent fasting comes in.

The minute you wake up and swallow the first bite of food, your body starts producing insulin, a fat-storage hormone I've mentioned a lot. By practicing intermittent fasting, you are simply prolonging that state for a few more hours with the goal of keeping insulin levels low, getting the most out of your body being in a fat-burning mode.

There are many ways to go about intermittent fasting, but my favorite is time-restricted feeding. The idea is to consume all of the day's calories in a narrow window, typically within eight hours, and fasting for the remaining sixteen (minimum fourteen).

Let's clear up one misconception right now: intermittent fasting is not a deprivation

EATING GUIDELINES

▶ Aim for 80/20 in favor of alkaline-forming foods (at minimum 70/30, and 90/10 for all you overachievers).

▶ Eat three meals per day and try to avoid grazing in-between unless necessary.

▶ Don't eat your last meal within three hours of going to sleep.

▶ Eat organic, homemade, or locally grown when possible.

▶ Limit or avoid artificial sweeteners, sugar, grains, omega-6 fatty acids, and processed foods.

▶ Add—don't subtract! As you begin to add these healthy foods into your diet, soon enough the good will outweigh the bad and the ratio will shift in favor of alkaline versus acid.

Rules for Combining Foods

▶ **Avoid combining starch with animal protein.** The combination of animal-based proteins and non-vegetable starch in a single meal is the worst possible food combination there is. A hamburger on a bun or spaghetti and meatballs are classic examples and a recipe for disaster in regards to digestion. So many of our favorite comfort foods are anything but comforting to our bodies. That's because proteins are digested in the stomach by acid, while starches are digested in small intestine by alkaline compounds, so they neutralize each other, and we end up with undigested food that will putrefy and rot in your small intestine.

▶ **No fruits for dessert.** Eat fruit *before* a meal or on an empty stomach. Fruits consumed during or after a big meal can interrupt the digestion of almost anything else, especially carbohydrates and proteins. Fruit digests the quickest and has a very fast transit time through the digestive tract (roughly 20 to 30 minutes). Eating fruit for dessert will cause a traffic jam in your digestive tract. The fruit will sit on top of whatever else is in your stomach and begin to rot and ferment, giving you gas and making you feel bloated! By the time it reaches your intestines where the nutrients are absorbed, there won't be anything beneficial left to absorb. Melons especially should be eaten alone.

▶ **Combine acidic fruits with fat.** If you are going to eat moderate- to high-acidic fruits (berries or bananas), combine them with a healthy fat. For example, combine berries with coconut butter or add one of these fruits (ideally frozen) to a smoothie, as they will make the smoothie taste better. It is very important to add some healthy fats as well, such chia or hemp seeds, coconut oil, and some raw nut butters, which will slow down the metabolization of the sugars in the fruit, preventing an insulin spike. Even though there will be some fermentation of the sugar in the fruit, it will be the lesser of two evils compared to that of your insulin spiking, which should always be avoided. In doing so, you will have a great-tasting smoothie that is net alkaline.

▶ **Some general rules.** If eating fruit, wait one hour for it to digest before eating something else; if eating starch, wait two hours; and protein, three hours.

diet, as many people are led to believe. It's a way of incorporating the healthy, alkaline lifestyle you are already on the road to achieving in a specific way or schedule so it will have a more beneficial impact on your body. The only difference will be eating everything within a specific time frame.

Intermittent fasting will help you lose weight by increasing enzymes that burn fat, and your body becomes far better at using stored fat as a primary fuel source, rather than relying on carbs and sugar as a quick fix for energy.

You see, when you rely on carbs and sugar as a primary fuel source, you're unable to access the large amount of stored fat fuel you already have for energy. And if you recall, your body has 95 percent of its total calories stored away as fat just waiting to be tapped into. What's the result? You burn more sugar. And if you're burning sugar, what do you think you crave? More sugar. It becomes a vicious cycle; your body becomes more acidic and more depleted of the essential minerals it needs to thrive.

There is no downside to intermittent fasting, and it will help move your body into a healthier, alkaline state.

Intermittent fasting can be more challenging for women. Why? Because women's bodies are set up to nurture a fetus, and hormones remain on high alert for interruptions in nutrition. If women have a tough time with these guidelines, I recommend starting with a twelve-hour fasting period no more than once a week for a better-regulated experience.

What Does a Day of Intermittent Fasting Look Like?

It's simple. You can fast intermittently by timing meals and allowing for regular periods of fasting. First, select an eight-hour window to eat and fast the remaining sixteen hours. *You* are in control of this, and it's not as intimidating as it sounds. You can decide if the eight-hour window is 9 a.m. to 5 p.m., 10 a.m. to 6 p.m., or 11 a.m. to 7 p.m.—it's whatever time works best for you and your schedule.

During the eight hours that you can eat, it's important to make smart and healthy food choices. You will still be eating alkaline foods ideally 80 percent of the time and acid-forming foods no more than 20 percent of the time. Your goal should be to minimize your daily intake of net carbohydrates to less than 50 grams. The more you minimize acidic foods, the better results you will get.

Some people skip breakfast, and others skip dinner. As I mentioned earlier, if you are going to have three meals during an eight-hour window, the two biggest meals should be breakfast and lunch, and dinner should consist of a nice rainbow salad with some healthy fats. Remember, this is not a calorie deprivation fast.

Here is the *most* important part and where I see people make the most mistakes: you will need to eliminate all forms of sugar and grains and substantially increase healthy alkaline fats. The healthy fats will be easily metabolized for energy and are essential to getting your body into a fat-burning state. Also, limit the net carb intake in order to produce ketone bodies for energy and fuel.

During fasting, it's important to stay well hydrated. Drink water with lemon, herbal teas, and alkaline green juices. Some people incorporate intermittent fasting every day; others fast every other day, once per week, or once per month. Whatever you decide to do, do it 100 percent and keep it consistent.

As you transition to a fat-burning machine and your metabolism begins to change, you may experience some cravings and hunger pains. At this stage, you have momentum so don't give in to cravings, as this will set you back. Instead, add 1 tablespoon of coconut oil to some herbal tea (or coffee, if you must!), or eat the 1 tablespoon straight up. This will quell hunger pains and help you control cravings.

LIMITING NET CARBS

In *The Primal Blueprint*, author Mark Sisson refers to the 0 to 50 grams of net carbs as the **Intermittent Fasting and Ketosis Zone**. He states this zone is for rapid fat loss, and is not recommended for long periods, which is why once you achieve a ketotic state, it is advisable to go in and out of the fasting state, simulating the times of "feast and famine." For example, once you confirm your body is producing ketones, you can raise the net carb intake to the next zone, which Sissen labels the **"sweet spot" for continued weight loss**. In this zone, you can eat the 50 to 100 grams of net carbs per day, which will enable 1 to 2 pounds of fat loss per week while your body continues to minimize insulin production. The next phase he terms the **Primal Maintenance Zone**, where net carbs do not exceed 100 to 150 grams per day. Once you arrive at an ideal weight, as long as you do not exceed the threshold number of 150 grams of net carbs each day, you will maintain this weight quite easily by following an alkaline diet. Once you exceed 150 net carbs, weight gain will ensue, as will increased risk for other chronic diseases such as obesity, metabolic syndrome, and type 2 diabetes.

Other benefits of intermittent fasting include

- stimulating autophagy, a process by which the body cleans out acidic and toxic debris;

- promoting healthier gut microbiota (the "good bacteria" in your digestive system);

- normalizing insulin sensitivity, which is essential for optimal health and lowering the risk of diabetes and even cancer;

- lowering triglyceride levels;

- reducing inflammation and lessening free radical damage, which comes from too much acid in your lifestyle;

- promoting memory functioning and learning;

- promoting muscle growth and improving metabolism, which in turn, helps fat loss; and

- reducing cravings.

SECRET #4:
FEEDING A SNACK ATTACK

I want to make sure you are listening to your body throughout this process, giving it what it's asking for. Most of the time, if you are eating three meals a day, loaded with healthy fats, a big green salad with tons of alkaline goodies, moderate protein, and some steamed or sautéed greens, you'll likely be satiated enough that you won't feel that urge to snack between meals. But if you're hungry, I don't want you to starve and not have a snack because of the information I just told you. However, please be sure you are truly hungry and not eating emotionally.

If you find you're hungry between meals, do the following:

1. **Drink a tall glass of room temperature water.** Supercharge that water with lemon, Alkamind Daily Greens, or Daily Minerals. Do this and then wait fifteen minutes and reassess. If you are still hungry, move to step two.

2. **Take a brisk walk for fifteen minutes.** The thing is, we are all emotional eaters to some extent. I am guilty many times over. Exercise and just moving in general (and going for a fifteen-minute brisk walk will do that) will change your mood. One of my heroes, Tony Robbins, says, "Motion is emotion," and moving your body will stimulate happy hormones (endorphins and enkephalins).

3. After that, if you are *still* hungry, then I give you permission to **eat a small, healthy alkaline snack**, preferably one with some healthy fat in it. Eat some guacamole or hummus with raw vegetable sticks or half an avocado with lime juice and hemp seeds. Eat a celery boat, which is a stalk of celery with raw almond butter and hemp seeds. Or eat 1 tablespoon of cold-pressed coconut oil, which is filling and is loaded with healthy saturated fat. Go to the recipe section of this book to see more of my favorite alkaline snacks.

Energy Boosters

Every morning, I consume 2 tablespoons of cold-pressed coconut oil with my omega-3 fish oil supplement. The healthy fats are energizing and give me so much energy to start my day. Later in the day, I have my third tablespoon of coconut oil, right out of the jar. This not only adds to my energy inventory, but it also helps keep my body in a state of ketosis where I am burning fat instead of sugar all day long!

You can also drink a smoothie loaded with dark leafy greens and healthy omega-3 fats. As a foundation, grab a huge handful of dark-green leafy vegetables like spinach, kale, Swiss chard, or romaine lettuce, and then add healthy fats such as chia, hemp, flax seeds, unsweetened coconut flakes, raw nut butters (not peanut butter), and some super foods such as ginger, turmeric, or propolis. Finally, add some coconut milk or coconut water for the liquid.

GET OFF YOUR ACID ULTIMATE SMOOTHIE FORMULATOR

CHOOSE YOUR BASE - DARK GREEN LEAFY VEGETABLES *(1 Big Handful or combination):* Spinach, Kale, Watercress, Cabbage, Swiss Chard, Collard Greens, Romaine, Dandelion Greens

CHOOSE YOUR FATS *(at least one, ideally two, three optional):* Avocado, Avocado Oil, Hemp Seeds, Chia Seeds, Flax Seeds, Coconut Oil, Unsweetened Coconut Flakes, Coconut Meat, Raw Nut Butter *(Almond, Coconut, Tahini,* or *Cacao)*, Raw Almonds, Macadamia Nuts, and Brazil Nuts

CHOOSE YOUR LIQUID *(1-1.5 Cups):* Alkaline or Spring Water, Raw Coconut Water, Coconut Milk, Almond Milk, or Hemp Milk.

ADD-ON SUPERFOOD BOOSTERS *(use 1-3):*
Alkamind Daily Greens, Alkamind Daily Minerals, Alkamind Organic Daily Protein *(Creamy Chocolate or Vanilla Coconut)*, Ginger, Turmeric, Black Pepper, Cayenne Pepper, Goji Berries, Cacao Powder, Cinnamon, Spirulina, Chlorophyll, Chlorella, Blue-green Algae, Bee Pollen, Propolis, Micro-greens, Sprouts, Maca, Camu Powder, Celtic Grey Sea Salt or Himalayan Salt.

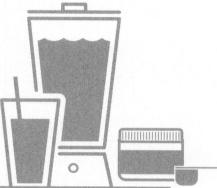

OPTIONAL:

CHOOSE A SWEETENER: Stevia, Lo Han *(Monk Fruit)*, Date

VEGETABLE BOOSTERS *(choose 1 or 2):* Parsley, Beets, Carrots, Broccoli, Cucumbers, Celery

CHOOSE YOUR FRUIT: Lemon, Lime, Grapefruit, Blueberries, Raspberries, Banana, Strawberries, Acai.

DIRECTIONS:
Place ingredients in a high power blender*(for example, Vitamix or NutriBullet)* and blend on high speed to your desired consistency.

NOTE: *If you are transitioning to an alkaline lifestyle, it is okay to add one moderate sugar fruit to your smoothie for better taste (some of the fruits in this list are acidic). Adding some healthy fats to your smoothie from this list will slow down the metabolization of the sugars, thus preventing any spikes in your insulin levels.*

Listen to Your Cravings

The more you succumb to nasty cravings (chocolate, cheese, ice cream, and salty carbs), the more your body will long for the junk you've been feeding it. A craving is your body saying something else is missing. Usually a craving is a deficiency in minerals and phytonutrients. The key to overcoming cravings is understanding what they really mean, and *then to give your body the necessary nutrients to fight them.*

For example, when you eat sugar or carbs (bread, pasta, and other grains), insulin levels spike. And what does that make your body do? You know the answer by now. If you've ever eaten pizza and then had a craving for ice cream, you know what I'm talking about. Your body is just begging for more sugar. This sets you up for insulin resistance, which over time can lead to chronic disease.

Cheat Sheet: What Cravings Mean

Craving ice cream, cheese, milk, or yogurt. If you crave sugar and unhealthy fats, increase minerals and *healthy* fat intake to 50 to 75 percent of total calories (start adding more of the following into your daily diet)—avocado, coconut oil, chia seeds, hemp seeds, flax seeds, nut butters like raw almond butter, coconut butter, and cacao butter, and omega-3 fatty acids from organic, wild-caught salmon, and be sure to take a good fish oil supplement (even if you eat fish!)

Craving pretzels. If you crave salt, increase mineral salts.

Craving vinegar. If you crave the sugar in the vinegar, increase mineral salts.

Craving red meat. Most meats have a high content of unhealthy fats. If you crave red meat, opt for healthy fats, including MCTs (medium chain triglycerides) such as coconut oil—a healthy saturated fat and a good alternative to the fats in meat. A red meat craving may be a sign of iron deficiency, especially for women during their menstrual cycles, which can lead to more intense PMS symptoms.

Aim for dark-green leafy vegetables such as watercress, kale, spinach, chard, and romaine lettuce. These vegetables are high in chlorophyll, which has the same molecular shape as red blood cells, except for the center atom, where chlorophyll has magnesium, and red blood cells have iron. If you want to build more iron, eat more chlorophyll. Also, have on hand a dehydrated alkaline green powder such as Alkamind Daily Greens, where one scoop gives you five servings of organic alkaline greens high in chlorophyll. When it comes to protein, opt for healthy, alkaline choices (lentils, chickpeas, adzuki beans, lima beans, raw almonds, hemp and chia seeds, and organic plant-based protein powder such as my Organic Daily Protein).

Craving sushi or fatty fish (tuna). If you crave fatty fish, eat more healthy fats.

Cravings happen most commonly when blood sugar is at its lowest between meals and are most likely at these times:

▶ in the morning, if you haven't eaten any breakfast;

▶ in mid-afternoon about halfway between lunch and dinner; and

▶ late at night a few hours after eating dinner.

To avoid cravings at these most common times, aim to eat three meals a day, and make it a rule never to miss a meal. In addition, make sure those meals are loaded with dark green vegetables, plenty of healthy fats, some moderate protein, and small amounts of vegetable carbohydrates (no more than 5–10 percent of the meal).

Again, the goal is not to eat between meals in order to keep insulin levels low. A consistent habit of eating this way will allow your body to shift from burning sugar as its primary fuel source to burning fat instead. Fat is a much cleaner and healthier source of fuel for your body. In addition to keeping you satiated and free of cravings between meals, fat will help melt away the excess pounds.

We need to rethink how we look at food. I'd like everyone to move away from eating for instant gratification and start looking at food as fuel. This is what I ask myself when I eat: Is this food going to cleanse or clog me? Is it going to fuel health or fuel cancer? Every time you put something into your mouth, ask yourself these things. To reclaim health and energy, make sure healthy fat is a major player in your diet. The quality of food choices will determine how healthy you are.

07

In with the Good: Alkaline Foods

Living the alkaline lifestyle is actually very simple. In order to ensure the body is balanced at its ideal, a slightly alkaline pH of 7.4, you have to eat about four times more alkalizing foods than acidifying ones. I recommend making sure that your diet is 80 percent alkaline and no more than 20 percent acidic. If you make only one change, add more greens to your daily regimen. Greens are packed densely with essential nutrients and are highly alkalizing. (In fact, if you look at many popular diets, as conflicting as they may all seem, the one constant is they all advocate eating more greens.)

The major problem, revealed in a US government survey, is that we're simply not eating enough green food. Out of twenty-one thousand people surveyed, none (yup, as in 0 percent) was consuming the recommended amount of vegetables and fruits. On an average day, only 8 percent of us eat the recommended amount of fruit, and just 6 percent eat the recommended amount of vegetables. So,

as a basic acceptable bottom line, aim for at least five servings of vegetables and low-sugar fruits every day. However, the *ideal* goal should be seven to ten servings.

Here's the problem: most nutrients have been stripped from conventionally grown produce, so even when you try to eat enough veggies, you're most likely not getting enough nutrients. For example, the nutrient levels in broccoli have shrunk by 50 percent since 1995! This is why it's important to buy organic veggies—from the local farmers market, if possible—or grow your own.

In addition, begin every morning with an alkaline supplement. Take one scoop of Alkamind Daily Greens dehydrated super food powder. One scoop is equal to five servings of organic greens. Before the day even begins, you will be sure to get the necessary nutrients your body requires. Additionally, I recommend drinking a fresh green juice or an alkaline smoothie, which will allow you to get roughly seven servings of vegetables in *one* glass! You still need to eat your greens, but drinking greens is best, as you can get the micronutrients and the fiber in a liquid, predigested form.

Now, back to that 80/20 alkaline-to-acidic food ratio. The good news about this way of eating is everything is on a spectrum; you don't have to be 100 percent strict to improve your health. If you can't quite get to an 80/20 split between recommended and less-optimal foods at first, that's okay. When I first heard about the alkaline diet, my diet was the opposite: 20/80 in favor of foods loaded with sugar. The key is to make alkaline living a priority. Set goals to steadily increase alkaline food consumption: get to 50/50, then 60/40, and then 70/30 (alkaline/acid, respectively). If you are an overachiever, go for 90/10. In any case, you'll be following a ratio superior to most people, thus moving your body to a healthier state.

I had a rocky start with my personal struggle of quitting sugar. My willpower got me only so far—a day here, a day there, the occasional weeklong boycott. My problem? Initially, I associated pain with stopping sugar. I thought I'd have to hit rock bottom to make behavioral changes, and that doesn't always work. I had to retrain my brain to make changes for a positive goal and outcome, rather than associate the change with deprivation.

By associating the change you want to make with positive outcomes, such as increased energy, you will be far more likely to see the desired results. In reality, it isn't renewed energy that invokes the change; it is what that energy will allow you to do in life that matters. Think about that: increased energy isn't only a nice thing to feel, it's also the reason you'll be able to play with your kids, go for a walk, tackle the workday, and more. Increased energy is the key to better quality of life in every possible way.

So ask yourself this: Why do I want more energy? Once you figure that out, and it's a powerful enough purpose, the change will follow.

In this chapter, we'll look at most powerful foods you can eat to turn your health around.

What really drives my passion in educating others on the benefits of living an alkaline lifestyle is opening peoples' eyes to the an abundance of natural foods that can actually make your body work better, stay healthier, and live longer. It's amazing to live in a time when we can go to a grocery store and select ingredients from all over the world that can heal us when we're sick, give us more energy when we need it, and make our overall quality of life better.

The following section lists the most alkaline foods available and discusses why they're so good for you. I will also show you how to find ways to eat more of them. Eating these foods will help you get the most vitamins and minerals, and of course, the least toxins and pollutants. I really believe everybody should always demand organic food. Yes, it's more expensive, but this is your health we're talking about. And without health, you don't have anything. So let's jump right in!

WHAT IS A SERVING?

One serving is equal to about 80 grams of vegetables or fruit. Let me give you some examples:

▸ **Salad greens:** 2 cups mesclun greens, 2 cups raw spinach, or 1 cup cooked greens

▸ **Other vegetables:** 1 cup of carrots or 12 baby carrots; 1 cup of green beans; 1 cup chopped, raw, or cooked red or yellow bell peppers or 2 small bell peppers; 1 cup of chopped tomatoes or 2 small raw tomatoes, or 15 to 20 cherry tomatoes (dependent on size); 1 cup cooked or raw broccoli or 10 broccoli florets; 1 cup of mixed vegetables; 3 celery sticks; ½ large Haas avocado; 5 spears asparagus; ½ large zucchini; 8 Brussels sprouts; 1 cup chopped cucumber; or 1 cup raw or cooked cauliflower

▸ **Legumes or starchy vegetables:** 3 to 4 tablespoons of beans, such as chickpeas, adzuki beans, or lentils; 1 cup green peas; 1 cup squash; or 1 medium baked sweet potato.

▸ **Fruit:** half of larger fruit (grapefruit), 1 medium-size fruit (green apple, pear, or banana), or 7 strawberries (½ cup)

▸ **Green juice/smoothie:** depending on what vegetables you use, you can easily get 5-9 servings of vegetables in a green juice. However, while these drinks can fulfill your daily veggie requirements, I do not count them toward the 7 to 10 daily vegetable servings I've recommended—they are a bonus.

THE GET OFF YOUR ACID FOOD PLATE

What does following the food pyramid look like on the plate? A powerfully alkaline meal primarily consists of the following:

Your goal should be to have three meals per day, consisting of seven to ten total daily servings of vegetables (with a mixture of dark-green leafy vegetables and sprouts, low- and non-starchy vegetables, cruciferous, and sulfur-based) and low-sugar fruits.

GET OFF YOUR ACID FOOD PYRAMID

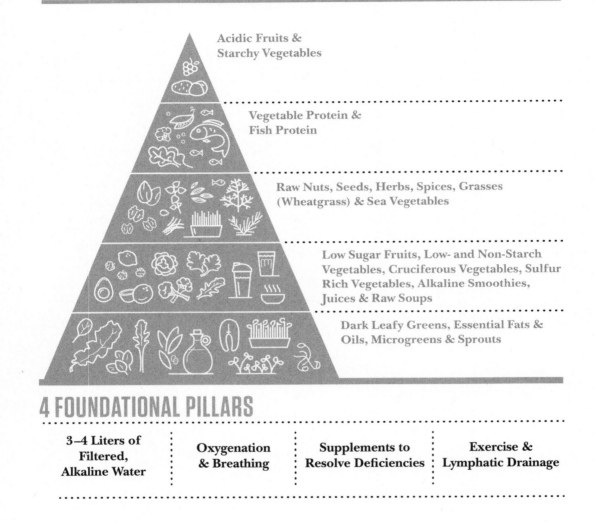

Acidic Fruits &
Starchy Vegetables

Vegetable Protein &
Fish Protein

Raw Nuts, Seeds, Herbs, Spices, Grasses
(Wheatgrass) & Sea Vegetables

Low Sugar Fruits, Low- and Non-Starch
Vegetables, Cruciferous Vegetables, Sulfur
Rich Vegetables, Alkaline Smoothies,
Juices & Raw Soups

Dark Leafy Greens, Essential Fats &
Oils, Microgreens & Sprouts

4 FOUNDATIONAL PILLARS

3–4 Liters of Filtered, Alkaline Water	Oxygenation & Breathing	Supplements to Resolve Deficiencies	Exercise & Lymphatic Drainage

That averages out to three servings per meal.

With each meal, include two to three servings of healthy fats, ideally in the form of oils (extra virgin olive oil, macadamia nut, avocado, black cumin, or coconut) and/or avocado, raw nuts, and seeds. This adds up to seven to ten total daily servings of healthy oils and fats spread over three meals (1 tablespoon of oil equals one serving).

Over three meals, these two collective groups should comprise 80 percent of your

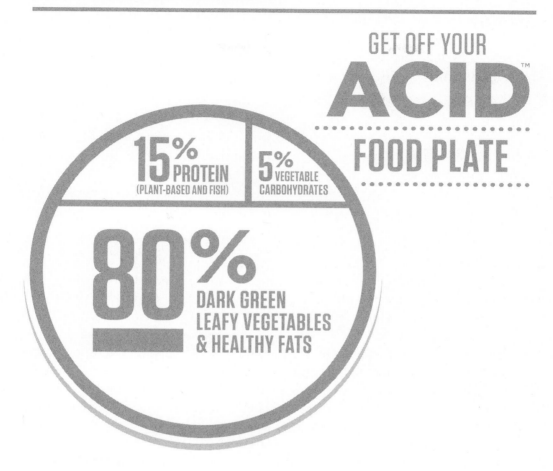

GET OFF YOUR

ACID™

FOOD PLATE

15% PROTEIN
(PLANT-BASED AND FISH)

5% VEGETABLE CARBOHYDRATES

80% DARK GREEN LEAFY VEGETABLES & HEALTHY FATS

food plate. While the vegetables will take up the most physical space, the healthy fats will comprise 50 to 75 percent of the total *calories* on your plate. Fats are much higher in calories compared to vegetables, so the amount of space a fat serving takes up on a plate is quite small (such as extra virgin olive oil on a salad). Vegetables should be the largest portion, visually.

Protein should comprise 10 to 15 percent of the total plate, ideally coming from a plant-based source. If you are going to have any animal-based proteins, the best option is wild-caught fish rich in omega-3 fats. Vegetable carbohydrates make up the smallest percentage of the food plate, comprising no more than 5 to 10 percent.

LEVEL 1 FOODS

Dark-green leafy vegetables, sprouts, and essential fats and oils.

Dark-Green Leafy Vegetables

Arugula, beet greens, cabbage, collard greens, green leaf lettuce, kale, mustard greens, red leaf lettuce, romaine lettuce, spinach, chard, and watercress.*

This is the first category-one list at the base of the pyramid, and for good reason. These vegetables need to be the cornerstone of your diet. If you add more dark-green leafy vegetables to your daily meals, you'll be well on your way to better health. Their rich green color indicates they are rich in chlorophyll, or what I call the "blood" of the plant. Indeed, research from the *Journal of Medical Genetics* states that chlorophyll is almost identical in molecular shape to the hemoglobin in red blood cells, which makes it a very powerful blood cleanser and blood builder.

But that's not all. Green leafy vegetables are especially nutrient dense. They are loaded with health-enhancing phytonutrients such as phenols, indoles, and flavonoids, as well as substances such as sulforaphanes, which are all disease-fighting compounds. Greens are abundant in trace minerals, omega fatty acids, and vitamins

and antioxidants, such as vitamins A, C, K, folate, and E. And greens are high in fiber, which is why they are so supportive of digestion and maintaining a healthy microbiome.

What does this all mean to you? Eat more greens! Dr. Herbert M. Shelton said it well: "A salad a day keeps acidosis away!" The more dark-green leafy salads loaded with colorful vegetables you eat, the more bulletproof your body will be for preventing infections and cancer, detoxifying and cleansing your liver, losing weight, and protecting your skin.

Sprouts

Sprouts are what I consider a "living food," and for that they deserve their own category. Living foods are the most nutritious foods on the planet. Anything you consume sprouted will be on average thirty times more nutrient dense than its full-grown adult counterpart, which is amazing! Along with wheatgrass juice, sprouts are the most powerful alkalizers to the body.

Sprouting is a rewarding process that you can do at home. It involves soaking and germinating just about any type of nut, bean, or seed, as long as it is certified organic and pathogen-free. Sprouts are super easy to grow and require very little space and sunlight (I live in New York City where space is always limited, and sprouts have become an essential part of my diet and my life in general). Alfalfa is perhaps the easiest to grow, and it's very tasty. Other favorites of mine include broccoli,

---

*7–10 servings daily, which can also be combined with the Level 2 foods.

THE STONE COLD FACTS
ABOUT KIDNEY STONES

About 85 percent of all kidney stones contain calcium salts, known as calcium oxalate. It seems logical to connect the formation of kidney stones with oxalic acid, which is contained in spinach, cabbage, broccoli, and Brussels sprouts. Those with kidney disorders, kidney stones, gout, and rheumatoid arthritis are typically advised to avoid these vegetables.

First, I certainly wouldn't avoid spinach or other leafy greens because of the oxalic acid effect. Not only do these veggies have so much to offer nutritionally, a normal, healthy person developing kidney stones from a high volume of oxalic acid in foods is very unlikely. But if you have challenges with kidney stones, you need to know is it's neither a calcium problem nor a vegetable problem—it's an *acid* problem!

Dietary oxalate accounts for only 10 to 15 percent of the oxalate found in the urine of individuals who form calcium oxalate stones. In 2007, one of the largest and longest studies (forty-four combined years, 240,681 people, and a total of 4,605 kidney stones) on kidney stones and oxalate vegetables was published in the *Journal of the American Society of Nephrology*. It concluded, "The relation between dietary oxalate and stone risk is unclear. . . . The data does not implicate dietary oxalate as a major risk factor for kidney stones." Some studies suggest people with recent antibiotic use may be at much greater risk from dietary oxalate. Many antibiotics can kill the flora that degrades oxalate such as oxalobacter, lactobacillus acidophilus, and bifidus. This is why it is so important to maintain a healthy gut microbiota.

Other acidic factors linked to kidney stone formation include the following:

▸ Soft drinks—due to high phosphoric acid content, which reduces levels of citrate in the urine and increases the risk of stone formation

▸ Processed foods particularly high in refined salt

(Continues)

▶ Excess sugar consumption

▶ High animal protein diet

▶ Excess cadmium, which is a heavy metal that increases the conversion of vitamin C into oxalic acid. Excess cadmium can be a problem for people who consume a lot of meat, mushrooms, shellfish, grains, rice, and tobacco.

The solution? A Swiss study found a diet rich in alkaline vegetables is associated with a lower risk of kidney stone formation. If you are prone to kidney stones, follow the 7 Ways to GET OFF YOUR ACID, paying attention to the following:

▶ Drink 3 to 4 liters of filtered alkaline water per day

▶ Consume a high chlorophyll supplement (Daily Greens)

▶ Take an alkaline mineral supplement (Daily Minerals). Maintain your healthy gut flora with probiotics and molecular hydrogen.

▶ Consider doing a micro-nutrient depletion blood test to uncover the cause of why you may have developed kidney stones in the first place, which is usually due to a mineral deficiency, typically brought on by an overly acidic diet.

mung bean, pea, clover, fenugreek, and radish.

It's an easy process. Simply buy a sprout tray (they usually come in two or four packs) and stagger the sprouts in the trays so you'll always have sprouts growing at different intervals. I recommend having four small trays with 2 tablespoons of sprouts per tray. Keep them in constant rotation, and you'll always have a supply ready to add to salads and sprouted wraps. I rinse them (or soak overnight for optimal sprouting) and let them sit out, then rinse and drain every night and morning. Within five to eight days, you will have sprouts ready to eat!

Plants, nuts, seeds, and legumes all contain special agents such as anti-nutrients, enzyme inhibitors, polyphenols and lectins that act like a suit of armor to protect them from their predators, thus ensuring their continued survival. This "armor" poisons any animals or predators that eat them and prevents them from being able to be fully absorbed, even by humans! Raw almonds have become quite popular, but if they are not soaked and sprouted beforehand, they will not fully develop, and you will receive minimal nutrition. When you soak, strain, and sprout whatever it is you choose to eat, you are removing the poisons that were protecting the plant, nut, or seed, while at the same time unlocking the nutrient potential that always lies within . . . you just weren't able to access it!

Essential Fats and Oils

7–10 servings daily. Once demonized, fats are now considered an essential part of a healthy diet. Since the 1950s, fats have been maligned thanks to some junk studies funded by the sugar industry that have blamed fat for ill health. However, research has shown that these perceptions were misguided. The key is knowing the difference between healthy and unhealthy fats. There are two kinds of polyunsaturated fats: omega-6 "bad" fats, which are pro-inflammatory, and omega-3 "good" fats, which are anti-inflammatory and found in wild-caught fish—salmon, sardines, anchovies, herring, and trout—and chia, hemp, and flax seeds. The omega-3 fats are a-linolenic acid (ALA), which are plant-based, and docosahexaenoic acid (DHA) and eicosapentaenoic acid (EPA), which are animal based (for example, fish oil).

Next, there are the monounsaturated omega-9 fats—avocados and olives, extra virgin olive oil, sesame oil, macadamia nuts, pistachios, and almonds. These are excellent sources of fat.

And, finally, there are the healthy saturated fats such as medium-chain triglycerides (MCTs), which are found in coconut oil and MCT oil. These are the best of all. They are anti-inflammatory, antioxidant buffers of acid that help reset your body's metabolism to burn fat and move away from burning sugar as the primary source of fuel.

Cold-pressed coconut oil is by far my favorite MCT because it's truly a perfect food. These healthy fats are highly alkaline and can be consumed in its raw, butter-like form and used for cooking, even at high temperatures. Coconut oil contains medium-chain triglycerides, which is a good-for-you kind of saturated fat, unlike artery-clogging fats found in cheese and steak.

MCTs are unique fatty acids that are easily digested and have numerous health benefits. Our body sends these types of fats straight to the liver where they can be easily converted into energy or ketone bodies, which are actually great fuel for the brain, and they've been proven to have a therapeutic impact on brain disorders such as Alzheimer's.

Coconut oil is rich in capric, caprylic, and lauric acids—three fatty acids that have unique properties: they're antimicrobial and disinfectant. In other words, they help create a strong, healthy immune system. As a result, coconut oil staves off infections both externally and internally. Externally, it protects the skin from absorbing microbes that cause infections. Internally, the fatty acids are converted to monocaprins

ESSENTAIL FATS & OILS (Including Raw Nuts and Seeds)

RAW ORGANIC NUTS: Almonds *(in moderation due to high protein count and moderate amount of Omega-6)*, Pecans, Macadamia Nuts, Pine Nuts, Hazelnuts, Pistachio Nuts (in moderation due to their potential to mold), Brazil Nuts *(high in Selenium)*, Coconuts, Pecans, Cashews *(in moderation due to potential to mold)*, Walnuts *(in moderation because high in Omega-6 fats)*

RAW ORGANIC SEEDS: Psyllium Seed Husks, Chia Seeds, Flax Seeds and Flax Meal *(small amounts)*, Hulled Hemp Seeds *(non-irradiated)*, Pumpkin Seeds, Sesame Seeds, Black Seeds *(Black Cumin)*, Sunflower Seeds *(in small amounts due to high Omega-6 Content)*, Safflower Seeds *(in small amounts due to high Omega-6 Content)*

RAW NUT BUTTERS: Almond Butter, Coconut Butter, Hemp Butter, Cacao Butter, Macadamia Butter, Tahini

NUT MILKS: Coconut Milk *(from a carton, which is my favorite option for smoothies, and full-fat from BPA-free can)*, Hemp Milk, Almond Milk *(in moderation)*

NOTE: *When store bought, be sure the nut milk ingredient panel does NOT contain the carcinogenic filler carrageenan, or cane sugar (or juice/syrup)—both highly acid-forming to your body. When possible, make your nut milks at home where you know every ingredient*

RAW OILS: Extra Virgin Olive Oil, Avocado Oil, Black Cumin Oil, Macadamia Oil, Sesame Oil *(in moderation)*, Cold-Pressed Coconut Oil, MCT oil

NOTE – *Most oils get oxidized very quickly, which is why this list is very short (for example, flax oil will get oxidized the second you open the container, if not before in manufacturing). When choosing oils, be sure to choose oils packaged in a dark bottle and from a refutable source. When in doubt, err in the side of caution.*

OTHER: Avocados, Olives, Purslane *(popular weed used in salads)*, Microalgae *(marine base source of DHA)*, Cacao Nibbs, Coconut Meat

TRANSITIONAL FATS *(good source of healthy fats, BUT still from animal source, so use as a transitional food or in moderation)*: Ghee *(Clarified Butter)*, Grass-Fed Butter *(Kerrygold brand)*

OTHER Omega-3 FATS: Wild-Caught Salmon, Herring, Anchovies, Sardines, Trout and monolaurin, which boost the immune system.

While I like olive oil, a report from *60 Minutes* revealed that many varieties have actually been diluted with inferior oils or allowed to sit too long in warehouses, thus becoming rancid. I recommend trying to find extra virgin olive oil from a domestic provider or a trusted importer or, best of all, a local producer. Farmers markets are the best place to locate good, fresh oil made with real olives.

Most oils oxidize by being exposed to air, which can cause rancidity. That's why the list of recommended oils in Table 6.1 is short (for example, flax oil will oxidize the second the container is opened, if not before during manufacturing). When choosing oils, be sure to pick dark bottles from a reputable source. When in doubt, err on the side of caution.

Avocado is probably my favorite food of all, and not just in the good-fat category. There is a reason why avocados have been nicknamed "God's butter." They are rich in vitamins K, C, B_5, and B_6 as well as some key minerals such as calcium, manganese, phosphorus, potassium, zinc, magnesium, and iron. In fact, avocados contain more potassium than bananas without all the sugar. They're also surprisingly high in fiber, so they help maintain digestive health. And they contain two antioxidants that keep eyes healthy.

With more than 77 percent of an avocado's calories coming from monounsaturated fat, this is one of the highest-fat foods, and that's a good thing because this type of fat, oleic acid, reduces inflammation and has been shown to have heart disease and cancer-preventing effects. Besides being one of the best foods you can eat, it's utterly delicious and filling. When people are transitioning to an alkaline lifestyle, I let them know up front that one of the benefits is eating as many avocados as you like.

LEVEL 2 FOODS

Low-sugar fruits, low- and non-starchy vegetables, cruciferous vegetables, and sulfur-rich vegetables (plus alkaline smoothies, juices, and raw soups). *

Low-Sugar Fruits

Lemons, limes, grapefruit, avocado, tomatoes, coconut meat, pomegranate, and watermelon (a neutral fruit)

Most fruits are high in minerals and fiber but are loaded with sugar, which, of course, is acidic. When it comes to choosing fruits to eat more frequently, go for those low in sugar. That's what separates these alkaline fruit powerhouses from the rest of the pack. Lemons, limes, and grapefruits are especially low in sugar (2 percent, 2 percent, and 5 percent sugar, respectively), while oranges, on the other hand, are high in sugar (12 percent), which you *can* detect because they taste sweet. Watermelon has a neutral pH, so that's a fine choice. Stick to

---

*Can be included in the requirement for 7 to 10 servings of veggies.

VEGANS TAKE NOTE!

Vegans are often heavily deficient in two of the most important nutrients—omega-3 fatty acids in the form of DHA and EPA. These are primarily found in certain fish and fish oil (with a few small plant-based exceptions). The third omega-3, ALA, is found in plant sources such as dark-green leafy vegetables, oils, nuts, and seeds.

Many vegans think they get plenty of omega-3 fatty acids from chia, hemp, and flax, but this is not the case. In order to be utilized, plant-based omega-3s in the form of ALA must be converted to DHA and EPA in the body through a complicated process that requires enzymes (it is specifically governed by the enzyme delta-6-denaturase, which gets completely used up by the pro-inflammatory omega-6 fats). Research shows the maximum they will convert is 5 percent, and that's being conservative, as many studies show conversion rates of less than 1 percent.

However, there is a plant-based source of DHA—a weed known as purslane. I first discovered purslane at our local organic farmers market and became an instant fan. It is a perfect addition to supercharge salads! However, there are no plant-based dietary sources of EPA, which is a necessary nutrient to decrease inflammation and properly balance the omega-6 to omega-3 ratio. This is why I say a vegan diet can never be truly healthy.

---

tart citrus and those forgotten fruits: avocados and tomatoes.

Low- and Non-Starchy Vegetables

Asparagus, beets, bell pepper, carrots, celery, chicory, chives, cucumber, eggplant, endive, escarole, fennel, garlic, green onions (scallions), leek, okra, onions, parsley, rhubarb, squash (cushaw, summer, crookneck, and spaghetti squash), turnip greens, water chestnuts, and zucchini.*

When you're trying to supercharge your diet, mix it up with low- and non-starchy vegetables. "Rainbow" salads are ideal ways to increase veggie intake, and the different colors all represent different nutrients in the ingredients. Even if you're not making a whole salad, cut up some veggies and use them as a bed under the protein source. Vegetables should be consumed either

---

*Can be included in the requirement for 7 to 10 servings of veggies.

raw, flash steamed, or sautéed, when they are cooked for no more than four minutes to preserve enzymes and avoid nutritional degradation.

Cruciferous Vegetables

Broccoli/Chinese broccoli, cauliflower, Brussels sprouts, radish, daikon radish, turnip, bok choy, rapeseed, arugula, maca, rutabaga, kohlrabi, rapini, and wasabi.*

I'm going to give a special shout-out to cruciferous vegetables such as broccoli, cabbage, cauliflower, and Brussels sprouts. Here's the deal: cruciferous vegetables have incredible properties that aid in DNA repair and help slow cancer cell growth by stimulating Phase II enzymes from the liver to protect the body under attack. These aid digestion, promote detoxification, support eye health, reduce inflammation, regulate blood sugar levels, fight allergies and aging, and prevent thickening of the arteries. It's hard to imagine a category of foods that works as hard as these guys.

Cruciferous veggies also contain something called goitrogens, which can inhibit the body's iodine uptake. That said, it would take an inordinate amount of these veggies to impact the body significantly.

The verdict? Eat plenty of cruciferous veggies and prepare them flash steamed or cooked rather than raw. The enzymes involved in the formation of goitrogenic materials in plants will be partially destroyed by heat.

Sulfur-Rich Vegetables

Cabbage family (broccoli, Brussels sprouts, cabbage, cauliflower, collard greens, kale, radishes, rutabaga, turnips). Onion family (onions, garlic, chives, leeks, and shallots).**

Sulfur-rich vegetables are foods that contain the highly beneficial sulfur compound. They are anti-inflammatory, antioxidant, and alkaline—what I call the triple A of health. Sulfur is an important compound for helping your body build protein and collagen, which makes it a phenomenal repairer of connective tissue. I highly recommend organic sulfur for anyone recovering from an injury or surgery or suffering with back and joint pain.

After I dislocated my shoulder for the twelfth time, I finally learned about sulfur as a connective tissue healing food. In addition to taking a methylsulfonylmethane supplement (MSM), which is sulfur based, I also focused on eating foods rich in the sulfur compound. In addition, it is a great food and supplement for anyone who has cancer. As a powerful strengthener of collagen and the connective tissue matrix, it can help prevent or slow down cancer metastasis.

---

*Can be included in the requirement for 7 to 10 servings of veggies.
**Can be included in the requirement for 7 to 10 servings of veggies.

POWERHOUSE FRUITS AND VEGETABLES

A study published in the Centers for Disease Control and Prevention's *Preventing Chronic Disease* journal aimed to find the most nutrient-dense foods. Dr. Jennifer Di Noia of William Paterson University developed the criteria for classifying and ranking the foods. In order to be considered a powerhouse, a 100-calorie serving of the food had to supply 10 percent or more of the daily recommended value of seventeen key nutrients we all need to stay healthy: potassium, fiber, protein, calcium, iron, thiamin, riboflavin, niacin, folate, zinc, and vitamins A, B_6, B_{12}, C, D, E, and K.

Of the top 41 nutrient-dense foods, 38 are alkaline-forming foods (leafy organic greens, cruciferous vegetables, and low-sugar fruits). The remaining three—strawberries, oranges, and blackberries—while offering many healing nutrients, are mildly acidic because of their sugar content. Other foods long considered "super foods," such as blueberries, raspberries, and garlic, did not make the cut because they did not meet the 10 percent threshold for all the key nutrients.

Here's a list of the forty-one powerhouse foods and their density of nutrients:

watercress, 100.00%

Chinese cabbage, 91.99%

chard, 89.27%

beet greens, 87.08%

spinach, 86.43%

chicory, 73.36%

leaf lettuce, 70.73%

parsley, 65.59%

romaine lettuce, 63.48%

collard greens, 62.49%

turnip greens, 62.12%

mustard greens, 61.39%

endive, 60.44%

chive, 54.80%

kale, 49.07%

dandelion greens, 46.34%

red pepper, 41.26%

arugula, 37.65%

broccoli, 34.89%

pumpkin, 33.82%

Brussels sprouts, 32.23%

scallions, 27.35%

kohlrabi, 25.92%

cauliflower, 25.13%

cabbage, 24.51%

carrot, 22.60%

tomato, 20.37%

lemon, 18.72%

iceberg lettuce, 18.28%

strawberry, 17.59%

radish, 16.91%

winter squash (all varieties), 13.89%

orange, 12.91%

lime, 12.23%

grapefruit (pink and red), 11.64%

rutabaga, 11.58%

turnip, 11.43%

blackberry, 11.39%

leek, 10.69%

sweet potato, 10.51%

grapefruit (white), 10.47%

LEVEL 3 FOODS

Raw organic nuts and seeds, sea vegetables, herbs and spices, and grasses such as wheatgrass (1–2 servings daily).

Raw Organic Nuts and Nut Butters

Almonds (in moderation due to high protein count and moderate amount of omega-6 fats), cashews and pistachios (in moderation due to potential to mold), hazelnuts, macadamia nuts, pine nuts, pecans, pistachios, Brazil nuts (high in selenium), walnuts (in moderation because high in omega-6 fats).

Almond butter, coconut butter, hemp seed butter, cacao butter, macadamia butter, and tahini.

Raw, organic nuts are some of the healthiest foods and can be amazing as you transition to an alkaline lifestyle. They are great as snacks, can go in a healthy trail mix, can be used in alkaline desserts, and can be added to your favorite alkaline breakfast smoothie! Nuts are nutritional powerhouses that can help regulate blood sugar levels, fight inflammation, decrease hunger urges, help weight loss, and lower your risk of cardiovascular disease. They also contain large amounts of fiber, which helps you sustain high energy levels and acts as a powerful neutralizer, as they bind to bile acids and sugars that are passing through the digestive tract.

My favorite nuts are raw almonds, pistachios, and macadamias because these varieties are particularly high in phytosterols, which have been shown to block estrogen receptors in breast cancer cells, possibly preventing cancer cell growth and decreasing the likelihood of prostate cancer. If you choose to eat almonds, walnuts, or pecans, I recommend soaking them first and then dehydrating them to bring back the crunch. This will wash away the toxins and provide a superior healthy fat to eat raw or to use to make nut milk.

Nut Milks

Homemade almond milk (in moderation), coconut milk (from the carton, which is my favorite option for smoothies, and full-fat from a BPA-free can), hemp milk, and hazelnut milk.

While almond, cashew, and coconut milks are much better alternatives to cow's milk, not all nut milks are created equal! Check labels to avoid carrageenan, a known carcinogen that studies have shown to be linked to inflammation and ulceration of the colon. Also, many nut milks contain cane sugar, which is highly acidic; look for unsweetened milks. If going with store-bought, coconut milk is always better than almond milk. Of course, my preference is always to make nut milks at home when I have the time (it takes only ten minutes and a blender). Look at the recipe section (page 191) to find my easy home instructions.

Raw Organic Seeds

Black seeds (black cumin), chia seeds, hemp seeds, flax seeds and flax meal, pumpkin seeds, sesame seeds, safflower seeds (in small amounts due to high omega-6 content), sunflower seeds (in small amounts due to high omega-6 fatty acids), and psyllium seed husk.

Seeds such as flax, chia, and hemp are great cancer preventers. By delivering the all-important omega-3 fatty acids and fighting the toxic build-up of the standard American diet (SAD), these good fats keep your cells healthy. Plus, they're so easy to integrate into your diet. Sprinkle them in smoothies, on an avocado half, in granola, and in trail mix. If you're not going to give up yogurt, be sure to add 1 tablespoon to help metabolize the sugar and neutralize the acid. Adding seeds is one of the easiest ways to introduce more alkaline foods that deliver a significant power boost.

Herbs and Spices

Ginger/ginger root powder, turmeric, parsley, chives, tarragon, rosemary, fennel, thyme, basil, bay leaves, rosemary, peppermint, oregano, paprika/smoked paprika, cinnamon, ground cumin, garlic powder, oregano, onion powder, nutmeg, red pepper flakes, coriander, cayenne pepper, ground cloves, curry, mustard seeds, sea salt, black pepper, cardamom, allspice, chili powder, chipotle, anise seed, dill weed, dill seed, and saffron.

Herbs and spices are highly alkaline, and they contain many health benefits, not to mention they improve the taste of so many foods. Use them liberally. They are powerful in that many are antibacterial, antiviral, antioxidant, and are loaded with B vitamins and trace minerals. My favorites of these spices are turmeric and ginger. These are known as the power spices. They're as healthy as they are delicious. Did you know that if you add black pepper to turmeric, it increases the potency of turmeric by 2,000 percent! Add to smoothies or make my two favorite recipes: Detox Tea with turmeric, ginger, lemon, and black pepper (page 153) or Golden Coconut Mylk in the Healing Tonic recipe section (page 191).

Wheatgrass

I also include wheatgrass in this grouping. This alkaline, detoxifying herb is so potent, you can actually gain health benefits from soaking in a bath with it. Out of the 102 minerals found in soil, guess how many wheatgrass has? Yes, 102! Wheatgrass also has more vitamin C than oranges and more vitamin A than carrots. Include one serving daily.

Wheatgrass has been shown to

- stimulate thyroid hormone production;
- increase red blood cell count, which cleanses the blood and organs;
- reduce gastrointestinal issues such as acid reflux, constipation, diarrhea, and even ulcers;

- lessen the side effects of radiation because of an anti-inflammatory compound;
- cleanse the liver; and
- neutralize toxins and environmental pollutants in the body.

There is a caveat about wheatgrass, however. It should be consumed in moderation—no more than a couple of ounces per day. If used excessively, it can make you feel sick.

Sea Vegetables

Arame, blue-green algae, chlorella, dulse, E3Live, kelp, seaweed (green, brown, and red), and spirulina.*

The earth is 70 percent water, and so is your body. The ocean is loaded with minerals, and it's one of the most healing environments for your body because the health of our blood is dependent on those same minerals. Sea vegetables are high in all the essential minerals and omega-3 fats. In addition, they are a great source of iodine, which is essential for healthy thyroid function.

You Need Vitamin Sea

Over the years, I've seen thyroid cases in my wellness clinic skyrocket. While hypothyroidism and Hashimoto's cases are rising, iodine intake, the chief nutrient necessary for thyroid health, is declining. This is important because physicians have been telling patients to cut back on iodized salt. Most Americans consume refined table salt, which lacks healthy alkaline minerals compared to mineral salts like Celtic Grey Sea Salt, that contains small traces of iodine and are loaded with trace minerals..

If you have thyroid concerns, carefully start to increase sources of iodine into your diet. If you are *not* on thyroid medication, begin by adding different kinds of fresh and dried seaweeds into your diet. Fresh is always best, but if seaweeds are scarce, alternate between kelp powder (brown algae) and dulse flakes (sea lettuce), which are both highly alkaline sea vegetables. Start with ⅛ teaspoon daily for one month and see how you feel, and then go up steadily from there. If you are on medications, speak with your health care practitioner before implementing any changes.

Urine pH needs to be in a range of 6.3 to 6.6 for iodine uptake to occur; otherwise, it's a perfect recipe for thyroid imbalance. Increase sea vegetables along with more dark-green leafy vegetables, and healthy alkaline fats. These will make a big difference. Try this along with the rest of the Get Off Your Acid protocol, and your thyroid can naturally reset to a healthier state.

---

*Can be included in the requirement for 7 to 10 servings of veggies.

LEVEL 4

Plant-based protein and fish protein
(1 to 2 servings daily).

Plant-Based Protein

Beans and peas (adzuki, mung,
garbanzo or chickpea, butter beans,
lentils, green beans, green peas, sugar
snap peas, snow peas, lima beans—
ideally soaked overnight), and quinoa.

Beans and peas are high in protein, fiber, and antioxidants and are relatively inexpensive if you're on a budget. Plus, their shelf life goes a long way. But the fear of eating beans because they'll give you gas is valid. Beans have specific types of sugar that we don't have enzymes to process. When the beans reach the colon, bacteria in the colon begin to ferment these sugars, producing gas in the process. To overcome this, make sure to chew beans very well because digestion starts in the mouth. Lean toward smaller beans such as lentils and adzuki and avoid sugary and dairy foods with your beans.

Beans also contain *lectins*—carbohydrate-binding proteins that have the potential to be toxic and inflammatory to the gut lining. Plant-lectins are designed to protect the lectin-containing plant by "poisoning" any potential plant-eating predators. In addition to beans, lectins are found in potatoes, wheat, rye, rice, and peanuts—most of which are acidic and should be avoided anyway. But that doesn't mean we should stay away from *all* lectin-containing plants.

Avocados contain the lectin agglutinin and are what I consider one of the healthiest foods on the planet!

Let's not focus on whether a particular food is lectin-containing but more on how your body reacts to the specific food once consumed. Is your digestive tract healthy enough to break down the proteins it's consuming in the first place? If you happen to have a symptomatic reaction to a specific food such as beans, either avoid them all together, or add a digestive enzyme. Remember, we all respond to foods differently. When cooking beans, I add some kombu (another sea vegetable). Listen to your body, and if you want to add beans to your diet, do so in moderation (no more than a couple times per week).

Fish Protein

Omega-3 fish: wild-caught salmon,
anchovies, sardines, herring, and
trout.

The most important thing to know about fish protein is where it is coming from. When you're shopping for fish, remember a few things: always look for wild, not farmed, salmon. Farmed fish are fed GMO soy, corn, and other grains, which is the last thing you want to be eating. Atlantic salmon is farm-fished and fed with grains, and Pacific salmon, once touted as the best, has been contaminated by the radiation accident in Fukushima, Japan. Good sources of fish are New Zealand, Spain, and Norway. Also, the smaller and oilier the fish, the safer it is. Sardines and anchovies are lower on the food chain and eat more plant matter, so they're higher in omega-3 fatty acids and less contaminated with toxic chemicals and metals such as mercury. Larger fish will have a higher level of contamination, heavy metals, metastatic tumors, and parasites. Stay away from the huge ones with a long lifespan—swordfish and grouper.

MY TOP SEVEN ALKALINE PROTEINS

If you're worried about where to get protein once you go alkaline, have no fear. As long as you're eating a few good, plant-based protein sources throughout the day, you're going to be in great shape. I do love salmon as a protein source, but the following seven are plant-based and accessible to everyone.

Alkaline Protein #1: Chia Seeds

Protein per 2 tablespoons: 5 grams

Chia seeds are one of my favorite foods, and I use them all the time, as they are so versatile. Chia seeds are considered a complete protein because they contain all nine essential amino acids that the body needs. Thanks to chia seeds' blood-sugar stabilizing ratio of protein, fats, and fiber, they're the perfect hunger-busting addition to your diet, and they can help you lose inches in your waistline. These seeds fuel me during all of my running and marathon training. But that's not all . . . Chia seeds are one of

the highest plant-based source of omega-3 fatty acids (although it is minimal), which research shows can decrease the risk of heart disease, and they contain more fiber than flax seeds or nuts. They are 50 percent omega-3 fatty acid and 20 percent protein. Chia seeds are also a powerhouse of iron, calcium, zinc, and antioxidants.

How to Eat It: The best thing about these little seeds is that they form a gel when combined with nut milks or water. This makes them fantastic for making healthy puddings, thickening smoothies, or replacing eggs in baking. For constipation, add 2 tablespoons of chia to 6 ounces of water, let them soak for ten minutes, and drink daily. I add chia to every smoothie, coconut water, and green drink I make. One of my favorite healthy desserts is chia pudding, which is easy to make and will become a household favorite, guaranteed! (See recipe on page 227.)

Alkaline Protein #2: Hemp Seeds

Protein per 2 tablespoons: 10 grams

Studies show that hemp, the kind you eat and not smoke (yes, there is a difference), can fight heart disease, obesity, and metabolic syndrome, likely because it's rich in protein and fiber.

Hemp seeds contain significant amounts of all nine essential amino acids, as well as plenty of alkaline minerals—magnesium, zinc, iron, and calcium. They're also a rare vegetarian source of essential fatty acids (omega-3s), which can help fight chronic inflammation and depression as well.

How to Eat It: Simply sprinkle the hemp seeds into salads and cereals, on top of avocado with lime juice, or add to your post-workout shake, morning smoothie, or to my Alkamind Organic Daily Protein Powder to jump-start your day. My formulation uses three powerful plant-based, alkaline proteins, (hemp, pea, and sachi inchi) plus coconut oil to turn the protein into slow-burning fuel that will burn fat and build lean muscle. It also uses zero acidic ingredients (dairy (whey), sugar, artificial sweeteners, or fillers).

Alkaline Protein #3: Quinoa

Protein per cup: 8 grams

Quinoa is not a grain like most people think but a seed from a plant related to spinach, chard, and beets. Quinoa comes to us from South America where the ancient Incas and the Indians of the Andes Mountains cultivated and revered it, calling it "the mother grain."

Not only is quinoa higher in protein than other whole grains, but it provides a complete protein—again, meaning all nine of the essential amino acids we must obtain through our diet are present.

Quinoa is a brilliant food and one of my absolute favorites! It's versatile and can be used to make breakfast porridge, soups, and salads. It can be used to thicken stir-fries and is a much better option than rice.

PLANT-BASED POWER PROTEIN SMOOTHIE

Serves 2

3 tablespoons hemp seeds

3 tablespoons chia seeds, soaked for at least ten minutes

1 tablespoon coconut butter

1 tablespoon coconut oil

8 ounces coconut milk

Blend and enjoy!

How to Eat It: Quinoa works great with some adzuki beans and avocado to create a well-balanced meal packed with protein and healthy fat (see Quinoa Burrito Bowl recipe on page 220). You can increase the flavor and nutrient content of your favorite green salad with a scoop of quinoa. I also love to use sprouted quinoa in healthy granolas. I've even sprouted quinoa to make raw food paella in my Excalibur dehydrator!

Alkaline Protein #4: Hummus

Protein per 2 tablespoons: 3 grams

Hummus is a classic, and when it's made fresh, not only is it packed with protein with 3 grams for every 2 tablespoons, but it's also alkaline.

Garbanzo beans or chickpeas are high in lysine, and tahini is a rich source of the amino acid methionine. Individually, these foods are incomplete proteins, but when you combine them to make hummus, they create a complete protein. Just be aware that not all store-bought hummus brands contain tahini, and they can potentially contain many other acidic ingredients.

How to Eat It: Spread hummus onto sandwiches and wraps in lieu of mustard, mayo, and other spreads, or use it as a dip for raw veggies.

Alkaline Protein #5:
Beans

Mung (14g), adzuki (17g), lentils (18g), navy (16g), black (15g), white (17g), and kidney (15g)

Besides their obvious high protein count, here is why beans are so great. They are high in fiber and antioxidants and are relatively inexpensive if you are on a budget, and their shelf life goes a long way. If we have any preppers out there, add this one to the list.

Beans contain iron, zinc, calcium, selenium, and folate and are low on the glycemic index, which makes them alkaline. But similar to all other ingredients on this list, beans should be consumed in moderation.

How to Eat It: Beans are delicious and nutritious. If you are new to eating beans, start with a small amount and increase gradually by eating them once a week, then twice a week, and then continue eating beans regularly so your body will learn to digest them. Add a large strip of dried

kombu seaweed, a slice of ginger, fennel, and/or cumin to the pot of boiling water with beans when cooking, as this decreases the gas (remove once cooking is finished). Chew beans very well before swallowing (as you should do with all food). The smallest beans are the easiest to digest (mung, adzuki, lentils), and they should always be eaten with lots of vegetables.

Alkaline Protein #6:
Vegetables

Don't forget that you can get protein from vegetables! We don't always associate veggies as being protein sources, but some in particular are great in this regard.

▸ **1 cup broccoli (5 grams)**
▸ **1 cup spinach (5 grams)**
▸ **2 cups cooked kale (5 grams)**
▸ **1 avocado (10 grams/cup)**

Alkaline Protein #7:
Ezekiel Bread

Protein per 2 slices: 8 grams

As I've mentioned, Ezekiel bread does have some gluten in it, but it's good food for anyone who needs to swap out white or whole wheat bread when transitioning to an alkaline diet (the only reason why it made the list). It's made with sprouted healthy grains, which absolutely increases the bread's fiber and nutritious vitamin content, and makes it much easier on your digestive system compared to most other breads. For those who are sensitive to gluten, when the grains are sprouted, it greatly reduces its gluten and antinutrient content. Some examples of the sprouted grains are barley, beans, lentils, millet, wheat, and spelt. Ezekiel also contains an impressive eighteen amino acids. This includes all of the nine essential amino acids, making it a complete protein, something most other bread products can't claim.

I recommend Ezekiel bread as a good swap for regular toast and as your new go-to sandwich base instead of white bread. It will also ensure you get at least 8 grams of complete protein every time you sit down for breakfast or lunch.

How to Eat It: Use Ezekiel Bread any way you'd use traditional bread; it's extremely versatile. You can have it as toast with some raw almond, cacao, or coconut butter, a drizzle of Manuka honey and some cinnamon to top, OR you can have some Ezekiel toast with some sliced avocado, drizzle of extra virgin olive oil, cumin, sea salt, lime juice, cilantro, tomato, and some jalapeño if you want a kick.

LEVEL 5 FOODS

Starchy vegetables and acidic fruits (1 serving daily)

Starchy Vegetables

Artichokes, dried beans, green peas, jicama, lentils, legumes, parsnips, potatoes (new potatoes best choice), pumpkin, squash (acorn, banana, butternut, hubbard, winter), sweet potatoes, and yams

Starchy vegetables are complex carbohydrates, and should be consumed in moderation (no more than two to three times per week). These foods should never be more than 5 to 10 percent of your daily diet. When eating them, be sure they are fresh as opposed to stored. (For example, red new potatoes would be far better than Idaho potatoes). Also, be attentive to what you eat with starchy vegetables.

Fruit

Apples, apricot, blueberries, raspberries, bananas, strawberries, acai, melon, cantaloupe, peaches, blackberries, Clementine oranges, cranberry, guava, honeydew, kiwi, kumquat, lychee, mango, nectarine, persimmon, papaya, passion fruit, pear, plum, grapes, and tangerine

A piece of acidic fruit is a much better option than a bag of chips. Most are high-water content fruits, high in minerals, vitamins, and fiber. However, the sugar content is what makes these acid-forming. If you are healthy, then limit fruit intake to once daily and preferably buy in season and always organic. Always try to combine these fruits with some form of healthy fat, as this will slow down the metabolization of the sugars and prevent your insulin from spiking. (For example, try green apple with raw almond butter, or a banana with coconut butter). If you are having any health challenges, these fruits need to be eliminated 100 percent from the diet, as they will fuel the fire of any acidic condition.

08

Feel pHenomenal!
My 7 Ways to GET OFF YOUR ACID

Now that you understand what acid is and why it's so bad for you, the foods we categorize as acidic versus alkaline, and how to eat to balance your body's pH while burning fat at the same time, it's time to learn the key lifestyle strategies to GET OFF YOUR ACID. These can be incorporated into regular routines to revamp your health, stave off illness, and gain more energy.

So without further ado, ladies and gentlemen, here they are, the top seven lifestyle changes you can make to feel *pHenomenal*:

1. Oxygenate

2. Alkaline hydration

3. Chlorophyll

4. Mineral salts and supplements

5. Lymphatic system drainage

6. Daily detox

7. Alkaline exercise

OXYGENATE

Oxygen is the most important nutrient. You can go without food for forty days and without water for four days, but you can go without oxygen for only four minutes. Breathing is an essential element to life, and yet we continually use less and less of our lung capacity. Think about it—when you're stressed, is your breath slow and deep, or fast and shallow? Remember earlier when I said the effect of stress outweighs any dietary acid? That's because increased mental and emotional stress has a *huge* impact on the oxygen levels in your body.

When you are stressed, exhausted, and tired, there is a very good chance you have low oxygen levels. But how does this happen? The number one cause of lack of oxygen is from insufficient carbon dioxide (CO_2) to help transfer it! Insufficient means you are exhaling too much, which happens when you are stressed. I'm going to get a little technical here, but it's important that you get this.

> ## Oxygen is the giver of life.
> —OTTO WARBURG, M.D.

There is something known as the Bohr effect: when there is a drop in the CO_2 in the blood due to stressed breathing patterns (fast, shallow breathing), the bond between oxygen and the hemoglobin in the red blood cells becomes stronger (the body holds onto whatever oxygen it can get). And with that stronger bond, oxygen doesn't transfer easily to the cells. As this happens, blood actually becomes more alkaline! You may be asking right about now, "Wait a minute, that's good because you've been telling me alkaline is good?" Generally, this is true, but not in this case.

Having a balanced pH of 7.4 is ideal, and if something shifts blood to becoming too acidic or too alkaline, that's bad. Here is a case of blood becoming too alkaline. To adjust for this abnormally high pH, the kidneys will release magnesium, calcium, potassium, and phosphorous from the body via the urine. This will stress your body and, ultimately, deplete core mineral reserves. As a result, without enough oxygen in the body, blood cells will fill up with toxins and acids rather quickly. While blood becomes too alkaline, your body becomes too acidic.

In the absence of oxygen to stay alive, the cells begin fermenting glucose to make energy. The byproduct of fermentation is lactic acid. As toxins build up in the cells, there is an even greater lack of oxygen, which leads to fermentation and the buildup of lactic acid, which results in an even bigger deficiency of oxygen. This vicious cycle spreads from cell to cell, driving pH down, which results in chronic, low-grade acidosis.

Remember what I said earlier: cancer requires oxygen deficiency in the cells. As the toxicity piles up in the cells and reaches a threshold where it denies cells of 60 percent or more of its oxygen, the cells starve. At that point, cells have two options—die or they can mutate to stay alive.

This is why oxygenating your body with proper breathing is one of the most important and powerful ways to alkalize and detoxify your body.

Did you know that 70 percent of the toxins inside of your body are removed through the lungs? Breathing is also one of the major acid buffers. The acids and toxins cannot leave your body without first combining with oxygen. Oxygenating your body will be the most powerful detoxification strategy.

How do we improve the oxygen levels in our bodies? By consciously focusing on breath! Do you want to know what a proper breath should look like? Try this: close your mouth, and pinch your nose closed for

3 seconds (holding your breath), then remove your hand and watch what happens. Did you notice how your breath changed? It may have been a few seconds later, but you naturally took a breath in the way that you are supposed to: light, deep, slow, relaxed, and with your diaphragm, not your chest, leading the way.

With proper breathing, in time you will recalibrate and reset your respiratory center to adapt to a higher CO_2 level in your blood, which in turn will allow red blood cells (hemoglobin) to release oxygen to the rest of your body. This will balance blood pH, and the increase in oxygen will help your body detoxify the acids from its tissues! Here are some of my favorite breaths to help you find the right breathing pattern:

Sounding Breath

This method is done lying on the ground in the supine pose (the yoga asana called *shavasana*), letting all your limbs relax. Exhale completely, and then slowly draw in your breath through the nose. As you inhale, feel how your lungs and abdomen fill up. As you exhale, contract your throat to make a slight hissing sound and completely exhale and empty your lungs. Let your breath be long and slow.

Sitting Breath

Sitting breath is done while sitting, so it can be done anywhere. Exhale with a deep sigh in order to reset your diaphragm. Then breathe in slowly through your nose for a count of seven and hold your breath for a count of seven. Then for another count of seven, exhale through your nose. Repeat this three times to help calm your spirit and relax your nerves. The benefits of doing breathing exercises every morning (or evening) for 20 to 25 minutes include the following:

- increasing lung capacity and improving breathing efficiency;

- improving circulation, blood pressure, and cardiovascular efficiency;

- boosting the immune system and enhancing immunity;

- increasing energy levels and giving lots of positive energy;

- strengthening and toning the nervous system;

- combating anxiety and depression and improving sleep;

- improving digestion and excretory functions;

- providing massage to the internal organs, stimulating the glands, and enhancing endocrine functions; and

- normalizing body weight and providing great conditioning for weight loss.

High Altitude Oxygen Training Masks

Due to the effects of high altitude, the 1968 Olympics held in Mexico City (7,380 feet above sea level) saw dramatically lower than

3 · 6 · 5 POWER BREATH

This is my favorite and most alkalizing breathing exercise, and the one that I do when I get up in the morning to jump-start my day.

HERE'S HOW IT WORKS:

1. Breathe in through your nose for 3 seconds

2. Hold breath for 6 seconds

3. Breathe out your mouth for 5 seconds

Do 10 repetitions, at least once, ideally three times daily. At the very least, I recommend practicing this deep breathing exercise in the morning to energize your lymphatic system and jump-start your day.

INHALE
3 SECONDS

10x

EXHALE
5 SECONDS

HOLD
6 SECONDS

record performances in endurance-based events, while sprint-based events continued to break records. From this, high-altitude training masks were born. The masks simulate high-altitude living, where there is less oxygen available.

When wearing a mask, kidney cells recognize there is deceased oxygen in the bloodstream, and, in response, the body stimulates production of erythropoietin (EPO). EPO is a glycoprotein that, in turn, makes more red blood cells—the hemoglobin molecules that carry oxygen through your body. Just breathing into the mask for 10 to 20 minutes can improve the oxygen efficiency.

A study published in 2011 in the *Journal of Epidemiology and Community Health* found that living at a high altitude might protect you from ischemic heart disease. Researchers note that Colorado has the nation's lowest death rate from heart disease and has lower rates of obesity, lung, and colon cancers. What Colorado has that those other states don't is an average altitude of 6,800 feet above sea level—it's the highest state in the United States (pun indended).

Hyperbaric Oxygen Therapy

Hyperbaric Oxygen Therapy (HBOT) is the science of restoring one's health by utilizing an increased pressure of gases, primarily oxygen. Oxygen is delivered in a pressurized vessel or chamber, as well as through a facemask. Under normal atmospheric pressure, oxygen transport in the body is limited by the oxygen-binding capacity of hemoglobin in the red blood cells, while very little oxygen is transported by blood plasma. With HBOT, oxygen transport by the red blood cells *and* plasma is significantly increased, facilitating a higher level of healing at the cellular level. Oxygen is the most powerful way to alkalize your blood and your body, which is why HBOT is also a pHenomonal detoxification protocol, especially if you are dealing with chronic disease such as cancer.

ALKALINE HYDRATION

Drink alkaline water fortified with minerals and molecular hydrogen. There may be naysayers who claim alkaline water doesn't work and claim it's nothing more than a marketing ploy. The reasoning behind these statements is this: as water travels into the stomach, the alkaline nature of the water gets canceled out by hydrochloric acid (HCL) in the stomach, rendering it virtually useless. This couldn't be further from the truth.

Here's what happens once mineral-rich alkaline water is consumed. First, there isn't a pool of acid sitting in your stomach waiting for food to digest. HCL is made on demand and in different amounts based on the specific food you eat. For example, if you eat high-water-content vegetables loaded with minerals, vitamins, and enzymes, your stomach will require very little acid to break them down. Likewise, if you eat a steak with a lot of protein, your stomach will need to produce a lot of HCL to digest it. So the first rule of thumb is this: never drink water when eating because the water will flush away any potentially healthy enzymes that assist in digestion. Instead, drink water before or after your meal.

Consume Alkaline Water on an Empty Stomach

This way, there is no food being digested to block its path. Without any obstructions, water bypasses what little acid that may be in your stomach, quickly emptying into your small and large intestines, where most liquids are absorbed.

Any water that does reach your stomach acid will have an alkalizing effect on stomach pH. For example, the ideal pH of your stomach is strongly acid, ranging from a pH of 1 to 3. The reason why you need such a strong acid environment is twofold: first, the acid is necessary to kill on demand any bacteria found in food, which will make food safer as it passes into the small intestine. This is where all food and the respective nutrients are absorbed. Second, you need stomach acid to help digest any heavy proteins that you may be eating.

The following is perhaps the most important effect of drinking alkaline water. When alkaline water reaches the strong acid environment of your stomach, the already acidic pH will become more alkaline. But remember, it is *necessary* for your stomach to maintain an acidic pH for the reasons I just mentioned. As the stomach pH becomes less acidic, in turn, your stomach has to produce more HCL. It does so to bring the pH back down into its ideal range of 1 to 3.

Here's the special part. **A byproduct of a stomach that produces more HCL is a highly alkaline mineral salt known as sodium bicarbonate, or baking soda.** The stomach creates this with the help of salt, water, and carbon dioxide gas:

NaCl (mineral salt) + CO_2 (carbon dioxide) + H_2O (water) = HCL (hydrochloric acid produced) + $NaHCO_3$ (baking soda by-product)

Your stomach, and particularly the pyloric sphincter (the valve between the stomach and small intestine), rapidly pushes the baking soda into the small intestines and directly into the blood, where it does three important things:

1. it acts as a powerful neutralizer of acid in your blood, helping you maintain a balanced pH of 7.4;

2. it protects digestive enzymes; and

3. it increases the oxygen-carrying capacity of red blood cells, and as we just learned, oxygen is the *most* important nutrient for your body!

I can't emphasize enough how important water is. *Be sure the number of ounces of water you drink per day is equal to at least half of your body weight (i.e., 150 pounds body weight equals 75 ounces of water per day).*

The Most Powerful Antioxidant Ever

In addition to alkaline water, there is another component necessary for water to make it an antioxidant powerhouse: molecular hydrogen or diatomic hydrogen (H_2). Antioxidants, such as vitamin C, glutathione, and alpha lipoic acid are vital to your health and well being, as they go after and stop the spread of free radicals.

What are free radicals, and why are they so bad? Free radicals are aggressive oxygen compounds in the body that not only attack surrounding tissues, but also play a significant role in the development of chronic diseases such as heart disease, cancer, and autoimmune disease. Free radicals cause your body to rust from the inside out and accelerate the aging process. Anything that can bind to these free radicals can stop them from doing the damage they inflict, and as a result, you can age more gracefully.

That is *exactly* why antioxidants are so important. And, molecular hydrogen is what I would consider the master antioxidant.

There are more than 700 scientific studies and publications, including more than 40 human studies in more than 170 different human disease models on the therapeutic benefits of H_2. Here are the three most important benefits, explained by my friend, colleague, and foremost authority on H_2, Paul Barattiero, C.Ped., founder and CEO of Synergy Science/Echo H_2 Water:

REDUCES ROS
(REDUCTIVE OXYGEN SPECIES)

Free radicals are "oxidizers," and hydrogen is what is known as a "reducer." For example, when you cut into an apple and it begins to brown, oxygen has oxidized the apple. When you are acidic, much the same can happen inside your body because of something called a "free radical." Some free radicals are good, but many speed up the aging process, and these are known as reactive oxygen species (ROS). ROS are cytotoxic, which means they are cell damaging or toxic to our cells. So when there are too many ROS free radicals, you age faster than your true chronological age because you are rusting from the inside out.

The most dangerous free radical is the hydroxyl free radical, or OH. It wreaks havoc in the mitochondria, the energy powerhouse of your cells. The reason molecular hydrogen is a strategic antioxidant is that one H_2 can convert two hydroxyl radicals in your cells into two water molecules.

OH (hydroxyl free radical) + OH (hydroxyl free radical) + H_2 (molecular hydrogen) = H_2O + H_2O

REDUCES INFLAMMATION

Everybody has inflammation in the body. In the short run, inflammation heals, but when it becomes chronic, it becomes detrimental to your health. There are many obvious signs of inflammation, but two less obvious signs are bad breath and the buildup of excess plaque on teeth.

The body is designed to develop hydrogen on its own, and it does so in the gut. In fact, your body has the ability to produce 10 liters of hydrogen every day in the gut as a byproduct of healthy digestion. But an acidic diet will wreak havoc on the microbiota and the digestive tract. And if the digestive process is not working correctly, and you don't have the appropriate bacteria strains, oxidative stress increases. As a result, inflammation ensues. This is why using water with molecular hydrogen is so important—it addresses one of the true causes of inflammation, which is reducing oxidative stress.

If you happen to be in a situation where there is a legitimate need for antibiotics, using molecular hydrogen can help heal your gut by outpacing the damaging effects of the antibiotics. So many people are prescribed antibiotics for viral infections, which is completely ineffective, or to keep inflammation down in the body, but as I talked about earlier, taking one dose of antibiotics is like dropping a bomb in your gut. It will wipe out all the good bacteria, and it may take up to two years for your gut to recover.

Molecular hydrogen can stimulate anaerobic microflora, which can quickly reestablish the good bacteria and gut health. This is beneficial for inflammatory bowel disorders, such as irritable bowel syndrome (IBS), Crohn's disease, celiac, and diverticulitis. In other words, it repairs your gut faster than the antibiotics can kill it. Gut health is directly tied to your immune system and level of susceptibility to sickness.

INCREASES COGNITIVE FUNCTION

Hydrogen is number one on the periodic table of elements, which means it is very small. Being a tiny element, it can go anywhere in the body where it is needed, and it can do so within thirty minutes. It is so small it can even traverse the blood-brain barrier, where it has a very powerful effect on brain and cognitive function.

When drinking water with dissolved molecular hydrogen, gastric ghrelin and leptin secretions are stimulated. Ghrelin is the hunger hormone the stomach produces that triggers eating. Leptin is the hormone that tells you you're satiated. They work together, and when they are stimulated, they affect the hippocampus, hypothalamus, and brainstem for increased cognitive function. Therefore, anyone suffering from Parkinson's, Alzheimer's, or other neurologic issues (diseases of the brain) can experience immediate symptomatic improvement because of drinking water with molecular hydrogen dissolved in it.

In a 2015 study from PeerJ, researchers concluded that high-content hydrogen water can inhibit colon cancer (particularly in combination with 5-fluorouracil, a medication used in the treatment of cancer). The study confirmed, "Oxidative stress is involved in cancer development. Hydrogen (H_2) is a potent antioxidant and exhibits anti-inflammatory and potentially anticancer-like activities." The study further revealed that hydrogen water administration improved the survival of mice with colon 26-induced cancer, as well as enhanced cell apoptosis (cancer cell death) in cancer cells.

Water Filtration Systems

By now, you can see the power of adding molecular hydrogen combined with mineral-rich alkaline water. Paul Baratierro and Synergy Science created the only system that produces neutral pH water with hydrogen, alkaline pH water with hydrogen in one machine. His Echo® H_2 Water systems have anti-scale technology that cause the machine to always dissolve molecular hydrogen in the water. Other alkaline machines will dissolve molecular hydrogen for only a few weeks. You would have to clean the electrolysis chamber every week or two to continue to have dissolved H_2 again (what are the chances of that!).

The Echo® H_2 machine does not require this constant cleaning. This machine produces water with the three most important aspects I want you to have in water:

▸ **Robust filtration that removes chlorine, chloramines, heavy metals, pesticides, pharmaceuticals, chromium 6, VOCs, etc. . . . but does not remove minerals.**

- Neutral 7 pH water with H_2 dissolved, four levels of alkaline pH water with H_2 dissolved, and 4 levels of acid pH water with hypochlorous acid for disinfection and skin conditions.

- Patented system that ensures molecular hydrogen (H_2) is always dissolved in the water.

Echo has molecular hydrogen units that can fit under the counter or over the counter, and installation is free. The unit I have is the Echo 9 Under Sink System with Digital Faucet. Here is what I like about it. First, it looks nice. More importantly as I just mentioned, you can choose on the digital faucet from four alkaline pH settings:

- Neutral pH 7, which can be used for drinking

- Alkaline pH 8 and 9, which are great for drinking

- Alkaline pH 10, which can be used for drinking sparingly (though my opinion, I'd stick with pH 9)

- Alkaline pH 11, which works better than any detergent as a surfactant and cleaning off dirt, as well as water for cooking and cleaning your produce before eating. Unbelievably, alkaline water is sweeter than any other water you have tasted.

There is also a setting for acid water with hypochlorous, which works great to kill bacteria. For example, I use the alkaline pH 9 for my drinking water, pH 11 to wash my produce and cook with, and the acid water with hypochlorous in a spray bottle to clean countertops to kill bacteria minus any chemicals. You can even combine the acid water with hypochlorous and pH 11 to wash your fruits and vegetables, as the combination will clean the dirt and kill the bacteria. All settings deliver a therapeutic concentration of molecular hydrogen.

Now, if these units are beyond your budget for you, there are also molecular hydrogen tablets and drops that you can add to your water, giving you 1.5 ppm of H_2.

CHLOROPHYLL

A US government survey found that out of twenty-one thousand people surveyed, none (0 percent) ate the recommended daily average of basic nutrients. ZERO percent of us! And that's not all. It takes sixty servings of spinach in 2017 to get the same amount of iron that was in one serving in 1948! Additionally, nutrient levels in broccoli have decreased by more than 50 percent in just twenty-one years. These are some crazy stats!

This is why supplementing has become a necessity and why it's so important to start every morning with a chlorophyll-rich alkaline green juice. Drinking a concentrated, green, alkaline super food powder dissolved in water is the very first thing you should think about doing when you wake up. There is no better way to energize and kick start your day. One scoop will give you five servings of organic greens, and the chlorophyll is a powerful blood builder and cleanser.

HOW TO HYDRATE
Make sure water is:

▶ **Filtered.** Tap water is usually untrustworthy and contains traces of bacteria, heavy metals, and other toxins. There are 327 known contaminants in tap water. In fact, in a recent study traces of Prozac were found in tap water from the urinary discharge of people taking the drug!

▶ **Alkaline pH.** The ideal pH should be between 8.0 and 9.5

▶ **Room temperature (ideally).** Cold, chilled water is harder for your body to use, and it burns vital energy.

▶ **Not bottled.** Bottled water is usually acidic and filled with BPA, which is a known carcinogen. Use a glass bottle or BPA-free bottle whenever possible. In a study by German researchers, nearly 24,500 chemicals were found lurking in a single bottle of water. The researchers were shocked to learn that most of the bottled water revealed interference with the estrogen and androgen hormone receptors in the body; amounts as little as 0.1 ounces inhibited estrogenic activity by 60 percent and androgenic activity by 90 percent.

▶ **Boosted with lemon or lime, pH drops, trace minerals, Alkamind Daily Greens, or Daily Minerals.** These boosts will alkalize and neutralize acids.

▶ **Boosted with molecular hydrogen.** Turn your water into an antioxidant machine with molecular hydrogen (H_2).

Follow These Guidelines

▶ Drink 3 to 4 liters daily. The average person loses 2.5 liters daily, so anything less than that will cause dehydration.

▶ Sip, don't chug, and stay consistent all day.

▶ Out of sight, out of mind. Always have a glass or stainless steel bottle filled with water at all times.

▶ Think progress, not perfection. If you are drinking only one glass of water daily, going from one glass to three liters is going to be far too big a jump.

Increase slowly. You want these habits to sustain themselves. Attach drinking water to a habit you do every day such as brushing your teeth. For example, you can make a rule that every time you brush your teeth, drink a glass of water first. That's extra water right there.

▸ Coffee doesn't count! In fact, coffee has a dehydrating effect, and you will have to subtract the ounces you drink from the total amount. The same goes for caffeinated teas (astringents) and carbonated water (which has a pH of 6.0, ten times more acidic than tap water). Herbal teas, alkaline green juices and smoothies, and raw soups count toward the 3- to 4-liter goal.

While I love making fresh juices at home and highly recommend them, not everyone has time for the mess and hassle involved. As soon as fresh produce is juiced, the cell walls of these nutrient-rich organic greens and fruits begin breaking open. If the juice is not consumed immediately, it will grow bacteria and degrade over time. This is why it's important to get a good quality alkaline green powder—it's quick, convenient, inexpensive, easy-to-use, and most importantly, packed with super food nutrition. Just stir it into water and sip!

What's Better, Juicing or Blending?

This is one of the most common questions I get. The answer is they are both equally important in alkalizing your body, and you should try to consume drinks both ways every day. However, they are not the same, and it's important to know the differences.

JUICING

Juicing removes the insoluble fiber—the pulp. This allows the nutrients to pass quickly and more easily into the bloodstream, easing digestion. Juicing extracts up to 70 percent (and depending on the juicer, even more) of the nutrition from the produce, and without the insoluble fiber your body will absorb close to 100 percent of these nutrients, giving you quick energy.

Now don't get me wrong—we all need fiber in our diets. It is important for the health of the digestive system, and it slows down the metabolizing of sugars in the body, helping to prevent insulin levels from spiking. But it also slows down the absorption of nutrients, and some nutrients stay in the fiber.

Why is this important? If you tend to have a sensitive digestive system that has any problems processing fiber, juicing becomes a fantastic way to deliver nutrient-dense,

> **❝** *I came across Alkamind in November 2014, when I was feeling my worst, dealing with type 2 diabetes and liver disease. That is when I learned about the Alkamind Daily Greens supplement and started drinking it on a regular basis. When I started drinking Alkamind, my fasting blood sugar in the morning was in the mid-200s. I was having liver dumps almost daily, and it was quite scary. Between November 2014 and March 2015, my fasting blood sugar went all the way down to the ideal range. My endocrinologist was elated that my results were so good. My body responded so positively to the alkaline greens almost immediately.*
>
> *I am so thankful for Alkamind. I'm not sure what else to say other than you should give it a try and see for yourself what happens when you GET OFF YOUR ACID!* **❞**
>
> —Gretchen L.

alkaline sustenance quickly into your body. One caveat is you must be careful about which ingredients you choose to use. Avoid juicing moderate- to high-sugar fruits such as pineapple, as they will cause a massive spike in your blood sugar levels. The low sugar alkaline fruits I recommend for juicing are lemons, limes, grapefruit, and even tomatoes.

Here is a list of my top ten veggies I love to juice with:

- cucumber
- celery
- carrots
- beets
- ginger
- herbs (parsley, mint, cilantro)
- kale or spinach
- chard
- leaf lettuce (i.e., romaine)
- cabbage

For anyone transitioning to an alkaline diet, I want you to succeed, and having a green juice that uses only veggies may be a little hard at first, so the last thing I want is for you to become discouraged. If you are starting out, I recommend adding a green apple or a pear to your juice to make it more palatable, if you so desire.

BLENDING

Blending, on the other hand, includes the whole fruit or vegetable. Both the insoluble (pulp) and soluble fiber remain in the blended smoothie, which slows down digestion, giving you a more sustained release of the nutrients and keeping you fuller longer.

Having a blended smoothie can be a great way to start the morning, as is a good breakfast replacement meal that can be loaded with all of your favorite super foods and healthy fats (i.e., chia, flax, or hemp seeds, coconut oil, raw almond butter, etc.). When clients ask me what the best blender is (or juicer), while I love the Vitamix or the NutriBullet, my answer is always emphatically, "The one you will use!"

Both juicing and blending are simple and effective ways of increasing your daily intake of vegetables and low sugar fruits. You can sneak five to nine servings of organic greens into a single juice or smoothie! Think about how long that would take you to consume otherwise.

Note: it is important to drink your juice or smoothie right away. The longer you wait, the elements such as light, heat, and oxygen (oxidation) will begin to degrade the nutrition in the smoothie. However, juice can last up to twenty-four hours in the fridge, and a smoothie will last up to forty-eight hours in an airtight container.

MINERAL SALTS AND SUPPLEMENTS

Your body doesn't run on calories, proteins, fats, or carbs. Your body is electrical and runs on salt. In fact, salt water (blood) constitutes 70 percent of your body. Mineral salts are one of the most important acid buffers, and we are all woefully

deficient in them. They are simply the fastest way to neutralize damaging acids in the body.

Magnesium. It's one of the most critical, yet deficient minerals, and controls more than six hundred chemical reactions in your body.

Potassium. When your body needs electrolytes to promote recovery from a workout, take potassium. When you're deficient, muscles cramp up, spasm, and contract. And what's the most important muscle? The heart.

Calcium. Acid robs calcium from your bones. It is critical in maintaining healthy bone density and a strong nervous system.

Sodium. Sodium bicarbonate is only 28 percent sodium (which actually decreases blood pressure, unlike table salt). Bicarbonate is the most powerful mineral for neutralizing acid and slowing the aging process. But don't fret; there are so many natural ways to get the minerals (especially magnesium) your body needs on a daily basis.

In Veggies

First, organic is always better, and you must demand it. When available, go to the farmers market, as research shows their produce's mineral levels are 50 percent higher than what you buy in the plastic containers in conventional grocery stores. Aim for high alkaline foods loaded with magnesium such as spinach, kale, chard, watercress, avocados, collard greens, and turnip greens.

As a Topical Treatment

I like using magnesium oil on my skin. For sore muscles, wrinkled skin, or any buildup of lactic acid from a workout, applying magnesium transdermally is effective and it works fast.

In a Healing Bath

To prevent your body from having to self-regulate and further deplete its supply of minerals, take an Epsom salt bath before bed. Check out the detox bath "recipes" in the detox section on page 154.

Before Bed

Finally, about thirty minutes before sleep, take my Alkamind Daily Mineral supplement of magnesium, calcium, potassium, and sodium bicarbonate. Not only will you get a good night's sleep, but you will also wake up with amazing energy levels. Most importantly, you will be giving your body the magnesium it needs to have a healthy body full of vitality. In addition to mineral salts, I recommend adding supplements to balance nutrients overall.

No matter how healthy we eat, we are all nutrient-deficient in some way. It is impossible to get all the nutrients we need from food because our soil is so depleted. That's why I recommend supplements. Some folks believe they don't need supplements, while others take everything but the kitchen sink,

as the saying goes. It's a complex and confusing subject, but we are all deficient in some key areas, so there are some supplements I recommend across the board.

Of course everyone is different biochemically, so talk about supplements with your health practitioner. Someone who already takes a blood thinner medication would not want to add fish oil, as it is also a blood thinner. That's a conversation to have with your doctor.

There are certain daily supplements I universally recommend because most people are deficient in them. In each case, take them in liquid form (or powder to liquid) whenever possible, rather than as a tablet. When you take a tablet, research shows you will absorb only 10 to 30 percent of it. You will absorb only 50 percent of a capsule. But liquid supplements will go straight to your blood, virtually bypassing the digestive system. With liquids, absorption is 98 percent and higher. Liquid supplements are also absorbed more rapidly, in one to four minutes, instead of many hours. Remember, you're not what you eat; you're what you absorb!

Fish Oil

Fish oil (3g) is one of the most crucial health supplements, as it will ensure you get the essential omega-3 fatty acids your body requires. It will help you narrow whatever your omega 6:3 ratio may be (ideally you want it to be 1:1, and no more than 4:1).

Fish oil is the only reliable and sufficiently potent source of EPA and DHA.

Research shows the average adult should take 3,000 mg per day. This quantity provides maximum protection from cardiovascular disease as well as a variety of anti-inflammatory benefits.

At Alkamind, we created the world's premier fish oil, which has two key features you won't find in any other brand. Every serving contains the ideal 2:1 ratio of EPA to DHA and is organically filtered and triple purified by a process called molecular distillation. Not only does this process give you the purest fish oil free of all heavy metals and contaminants, but it also concentrates the supplement so you need to take less to get more.

I prefer fish oil to krill oil, which, while interesting for its astaxanthin content (a carotenoid similar to beta carotene), provides only a trivial amount of EPA and DHA. Krill is often marketed as having a more highly absorbed phospholipid form of omega-3s, which is true, but it contains so little that you'd have to consume an entire bottle every day to yield a sufficient quantity of EPA and DHA.

Probiotics

Probiotics play a crucial role in regulating proper intestinal and digestive function. The word itself is derived from the Greek and literally means "for life." Aim for about 30 billion CFUs every day, which usually amounts to two capsules. I recommend a refrigerated brand because it's live bacteria and because it decreases the moisture in the supplement, causing less degradation.

FISH OIL REPEATING ON YOU?

I can't tell you how many of my clients worry about fish oil burps. Seriously, it's a thing. So here are my tips for beating the burps.

1. Choose high-quality oil. Burping is often a reaction to low-quality oil that has become oxidized and gone rancid.

2. Take fish oil before a meal; otherwise, it will sit on top of the undigested food (oil and water don't mix well!).

3. Freeze fish oil to keep it super fresh.

I also recommend changing it up every thirty days—using a different probiotic brand, giving you alternating bacterial strains. For example, I keep two different brands of probiotics in my refrigerator and rotate them every month.

Vitamin D$_3$

One of the biggest "D-ficiencies" I see across the board is vitamin D. In fact, the research shows that 90 percent of Americans are deficient. It's so critical because it's required for the absorption of calcium in the large intestines, and a lack of calcium can result in osteoporosis as well as acid buildup. Research shows that deficiency in vitamin D is an underlying cause of falling victim to the flu. Even more evidence comes from a study in PLOS ONE, which showed that having a serum vitamin D level of at least 40 ng/ml can reduce your risk of cancer by 67 percent, compared to having a level of 20 ng/ml or less.

When you look at vitamin D levels on a blood test, most doctors consider the healthy range to be 30 ng/ml to 100 ng/ml, anything below 20 is deficient, and 20 to 29 is insufficient. So if I score a 29, my levels are insufficient, but if I score one point higher, would my levels be optimal? Here's the deal: I don't want you to be at the bottom of that zone; I want you to be at the top. In regards to vitamin D, 30 ng/ml is dangerously low, yet many doctors would not say a word about that because it is still in the "normal" range. To be healthy, aim for that number to be above 50 ng/ml and ideally closer to 70 ng/ml.

Your body can produce vitamin D when skin is exposed to sunlight, but most people don't get enough sunshine to produce enough, especially if they live in northern climates like I do in New York City. For that reason, I recommend supplementing 5,000 IUs from a liquid-based supplement. The RDA for vitamin D is 600 IU. In my opinion, this amount is the bare minimum needed to avoid severe diseases such as rickets. In this case, the RDA is actually the RDI—recommended daily insufficiency. You follow that advice, and you will be deficient.

Vitamin D is fat-soluble, which means you must take it with a fat for it to absorb properly. Because of this, you should choose one that is combined with a fat-based oil such as olive oil, coconut oil, or MCT. People have become scared of the sun, slapping on all of these toxic sunscreens and lotions. Sunshine is so important, but like everything else, I say, take it in moderation. Know your numbers and get blood work done every year. If you haven't tested vitamin D levels in more than one year, make an appointment today.

If I were to meet with you personally, I might advise other particular supplements to you, but the supplements on this list, I can tell you, will make anyone leaps and bounds ahead of someone who doesn't take them.

LYMPHATIC SYSTEM DRAINING

The lymphatic system is the vacuum cleaner of the body, drawing all the bad stuff out. It's one of your body's most important systems because its primary function is detoxification. To keep blood pH at 7.4, accumulated acids and toxins are dumped into the tissues of the body for safekeeping. It's then up to the lymphatic system, the garbage collectors of the body, to draw acids out of the tissues (when the body has enough energy and resources to do so) and put them back into the blood to be eliminated from the body.

Blood circulates because of the pumping mechanism of the heart. But the lymphatic system doesn't have a heart to pump and move its fluid. It relies on movement to drain it. We need to ensure the lymph system is free flowing and doing its job. When I look at patients' live blood cells in my office, very often I see clogged and backed up lymphatic systems. It's always a good indicator about why there's weight gain, bad skin, flagging energy, and weak immunity. When the lymphatic system is clogged, nothing works as it should.

Since the lymphatic system is responsible for getting rid of acids and toxins, acids begin to accumulate in the body if you become too sedentary, which disrupts the body's capability of maintaining a proper pH balance. When you are not moving and thus, not "lymphasizing," your body and all its elimination pathways must work harder to get these acids out. Not only does this sap your energy, but it can also produce common over-acidic conditions such as reflux, different skin conditions (acne, psoriasis, dermatitis), and digestive issues, to name a few.

How to Rebound for Lymphatic Drainage

I recommend using a rebounder (mini trampoline) to drain your lymph. When rebounding to move lymph, you must do it in a very specific, mindful way. This doesn't involve jumping all over the place, jogging, or kicking. That will come later, when we talk about rebounding for exercise. When lymphasizing, you want to keep the balls of your feet on the surface of the rebounder and bounce gently up and down for ten to twelve minutes. That's it. You won't believe

how effective this is for moving the lymph and stimulating weight loss at the same time!

Other equipment can be used for this purpose. In addition to rebounding, there's something called whole body vibration, which can be thought of as a rebounder on steroids. It removes toxins like wringing out a sponge. There's also the chi machine, in which you lie on your back and the device swings your body back and forth—a motion that gently stimulates the lymph.

Dry Skin Brushing

Dry skin brushing is one of the best ways to stimulate the lymphatic system, keeping blood and other vital tissues detoxified. It is energizing, assists in breaking up cellulite, removes dead skin, stimulates circulation, and strengthens the immune system.

To do this technique, take a natural bristle brush, which can be purchased at most natural food stores or pharmacies. Using long strokes on your skin, start at your feet and work up the body toward your heart. Be sure to cover the whole body but skip the face and the breasts. Do not feel as though you need to spend a tremendous amount of time on this, two to three minutes before your shower is fine.

DAILY DETOX

Toxicity is a big factor in disease as well as premature aging. The way your body holds up or degrades is heavily based on toxicity. In addition to eating a more alkaline diet,

SKIP THE ANTIPERSPIRANT

Antiperspirant is one of the most toxic things you can use, and it's a major contributor to women getting breast cancer. Antiperspirant prevents toxins from getting out of your body. These products contain aluminum, which is one of the worst heavy metals because it's seven times more toxic than mercury.

---

we can all take steps toward detoxification as part of a regular routine to further alkalize the body. Here are my favorite practices for detoxing on a daily basis. These are powerful, and they'll make you feel amazing, with a fresh burst of energy, especially when practiced regularly. I suggest going through this list of detox protocols and determining which ones will work best with your lifestyle. Your goal should be to do at least one daily (ideally two).

Cleansing

A cleanse is an awesome way to jumpstart health, energy, and metabolism, but cleansing should be a lifestyle, ideally incorporated into a daily routine. Some people like to do a cleanse once or twice a year. I do a seven-day alkaline cleanse every season, and I believe it's important that everyone does this at least once a year. Sometimes

after a big event such as a birthday or a holiday like Thanksgiving or New Year's Eve, I'll do a two-day detox, which is a full-body reboot.

Optimally, though, you should do *something* to detox every day because the world is so toxic. It's impossible to escape the toxicity. Detoxification is not just a one-off; it's a lifestyle. If you'd like to try my *7-Day Alkaline Cleanse* or *2-Day Detox Challenge*, you can learn more and order the materials on my website at www.getoffyouracid.com. It's a great way to kick off your new commitment to a less acidic lifestyle.

Lemon Water

I recommend drinking lemon water any time of day, and all day. This is a gentle, yet effective way to support and cleanse the liver, kidneys, and colon, and help alkalize the body. It assists in breaking up mucus and provides energy via enzymes, vitamin C, potassium, and trace minerals. Please use fresh, ripe lemons, not prepared lemon juice.

One serving of lemon contains 51 percent of daily vitamin C needs as well as other vitamins and minerals. Lemons help combat stroke, cancer, and asthma. They also help with maintaining a healthy complexion, increasing iron absorption, and boosting the immune system. While lemons contain citric acid, they are very alkaline-forming in the body due to their high mineral and low sugar content.

Always try to buy organic lemons and limes, and feel free to drop the entire slice into the glass of water. If nonorganic, you

> **66** *The* Get Off Your Acid 7-Day Alkaline Cleanse *is a game changer in regards to how you view food and the food choices you make. I have never cleansed before and ventured into this because I had been recently diagnosed with high cholesterol, was gaining weight, and felt sluggish. My husband, Dan, who has a high cardiovascular risk profile and is also overweight and was eating the same things I ate on the cleanse. After completing it, I lost 7 pounds and became caffeine free, and my husband dropped 9 pounds—we both have more energy than ever! We were nothing less than amazed! Thank you, Dr. Daryl, for making a real actionable difference in our health and eating habits! Update: After four cleanses, I have reached my ideal goal weight, and my husband has lost more than 50 pounds!* **99**
>
> —Lou P.

won't want the pesticides, herbicides, and fungicides in your water, so squeeze the juice and discard the rest. Lemons are probably not organic at restaurants, so you know what to do.

Lemon and Olive Oil Shot

Help cleanse the liver and gallbladder with this powerful morning cocktail. It's simply 1 tablespoon of organic extra virgin olive oil and half a squeezed lemon. If you can get in the habit of doing this regularly, it will be a huge boost to an invigorating morning routine. Drink this on an empty stomach. Remember, it takes fat to burn fat!

Acid Crusher Detox Tea

This tea is one of the most alkaline beverages you will find. I also call this the "anti-inflammatory tea," as it massively lowers

system inflammation that results from an overly acidic lifestyle. This is a great tea to begin your day and can be a good alkaline substitute for coffee drinkers. Black pepper activates turmeric's healing properties, increasing its power by 2,000 percent, so be sure to include it. Buy organic turmeric root for effectiveness. (It can be hard to find, so I buy 1 pound from Amazon and freeze it.) This tea is easy to make, can be used daily, and leftovers can be stored in the fridge for a healthy iced tea.

- ▸ **16 to 20 ounces filtered water**
- ▸ **1-inch piece of fresh, organic turmeric root**
- ▸ **1-inch piece of fresh, organic ginger root**
- ▸ **pinch of black pepper**
- ▸ **1 lemon slice**

Bring water to a boil. While water is heating, peel the turmeric and ginger and dice it (the smaller the pieces, the better). Once the water boils, remove it from the heat and add the turmeric, ginger, and black pepper to the pot. Simmer for at least 10 minutes (the longer it simmers, the more potent and concentrated the tea will be). Pour the tea into a cup, squeeze a lemon slice over it, and enjoy!

Detox Bath

Skin is the largest organ of the body and a big part of your detoxification system. An Epsom salt bath helps create a more alkaline state through absorption, and the ritual feels great.

Directions: Each evening, place 2 cups of Epsom salt and 1 cup of baking soda in the tub, run the hottest water you can stand, and add 8 drops of your favorite essential oil (lavender, eucalyptus, or lemon oils are great). Soak for twenty minutes and allow yourself to sweat. When you are finished bathing, wrap up in towels, go under the covers, and sweat some more. You should feel very relaxed and sleep soundly.

Chia Shot (Constipation Reliever)

Getting additional fiber as we cleanse is vital to supporting the colon in its role of toxin elimination. In addition to lots of fresh vegetables, ground flax seeds and chia seeds are recommended. You should be eliminating at least two times per day.

Put 1 tablespoon of chia seeds in every green juice drink, smoothie, and coconut water (stir with a cappuccino frother for 30 seconds to avoid chia floating to the top of the drink). For the chia shot, add 2 tablespoons of chia or ground flax to 6 ounces of water every night after dinner. Let it sit for 10 minutes before drinking.

Castor Oil Packs

Castor oil packs are an inexpensive way to nurture and support the liver while you cleanse. That's because castor oil is said to be able to penetrate deeply through the skin—as much as 4 inches—into the body! These packs can be used to stimulate and detox the liver and gall bladder. One caveat: it can get a little messy.

Directions: You will need 100 percent pure, cold-pressed castor oil, wool (not cotton) flannel, and a hot water bottle (or heating pad).

1. Fold the wool flannel into three or four layers, and soak it with castor oil.

2. Put the flannel in a baking dish and heat slowly in the oven until it becomes hot, but not hot enough to scald or injure your skin.

3. Rub castor oil on your stomach, lie down, and place the hot flannel on top of your stomach.

4. Seal off the flannel with plastic wrap.

5. Cover with a hot water bottle or heating pad for one hour, keeping the flannel as hot as safely and comfortably possible.

After you are finished, wash the oil from your abdomen. The oil-soaked flannel can be kept sealed in a glass container until further use, as castor oil does not become rancid as quickly as other oils. It is recommended you use the pack once a day for three days, then take three days off, and then use it for another three days. This is a safe regimen to perform continually, especially if you suffer from liver-based symptoms such as eye problems, PMS, pre-menopausal symptoms and menopausal irritability, mood swings, bloating, tender breasts, hot flashes, anxiety, migraines, skin rashes and breakouts, angry outbursts, or tension between the shoulders.

Many people report a remarkable sense of well-being and tranquility while applying the castor oil pack. Because the emotion of anger is closely tied to the liver, angry feelings may resurface. Stay with your feelings and try to channel them constructively. You may try to transform this anger into forgiveness, first for yourself and then for others.

Infrared Sauna

This is probably the most powerful and effective way to clean your blood and detox your body. Sweating in an infrared sauna helps the body release heavy metals such as mercury and lead, and environmental chemicals as well. But the benefits don't stop there. With infrared sauna technology,

---

SAUNA OPTIONS

Good: Sauna. Promotes a detoxifying sweat. Steam is beneficial as well.

Better: Far Infrared Sauna. Penetrates the epidermis about 1.5 inches into the body, healing surface-level wounds and helping to detoxify.

Best: Near Infrared Sauna. Penetrates tissue up to 30 to 40 cm in depth, promoting deep healing at a cellular level. The National Aeronautics and Space Administration (NASA) has confirmed penetration of Near Infrared Saunas of up to 9 inches!

---

you can also lose weight, relax, relieve unwanted pain, increase circulation, and purify skin.

I suggest working up a sweat with a light jog or a session on the rebounder, then head right to the sauna. Take water with you, stay well hydrated, and add some minerals, as you may lose some electrolytes in the process. If you have access to a nearby cold shower, do hot, then cold. Mixing it up brings your core temperature back down so that you can enjoy the benefits of the sauna longer. Length of time and temperature is for you to determine. Speak with a healthcare provider, and always err on the side of caution.

Colonics

Did you know that the average American has 10 to 15 pounds of impacted fecal matter lodged in their intestines? When the bowel becomes unnaturally acidic from undigested meat, sugar, white flour, caffeine, alcohol, dairy, and gluten, it attempts to protect itself by secreting a glycoprotein substance that lines the entire intestinal wall with mucus. This is known as a mucoid plaque, which makes it extremely hard for the body to absorb vitamins, minerals, and nutrients and results in toxicity build-up and deficiency, leading to malnutrition.

This buildup produces toxins, which enter the blood's circulation and poisons the body. The colonic is a tool used to create a clean and healthy colon and remove this mucoid plaque, resulting in better digestion and elimination and proper absorption of food. The average colonic takes between 30 to 45 minutes and is a very safe, natural process.

You can also do wheatgrass juice (preferred method) and organic coffee enemas for extra detoxification. Although taking coffee through the mouth is a liver suppressor, doing it the other way, it's an enhancer. If you wish to try one of these methods, bring your own organic wheatgrass juice to a hydro therapist. Ask your clinician about what sort of coffee can be used (preferably organic) and always follow his professional advice to the letter. When you're going to have a colonic performed, be sure to avoid all proteins immediately before or after the procedure, and take probiotics to replace the good flora that will be washed away—in fact, double up the day before, on, and after.

While lying on a table, a low-pressure pump or a gravity-based reservoir flushes several gallons of water through a small tube inserted into the rectum. After the water is in the colon, the therapist may massage your abdomen. Then you release the water like a regular bowel movement; the process flushes out the fluids and waste. It took me a long time before I had the courage to do my first colonic, and looking back, I can't believe I was so afraid! It is a gentle and harmless experience, and I highly recommend it during or after a cleanse. You will feel like a million bucks!

How often? A hydro therapist will make specific recommendations, and everyone is different. My first time, I did three colonics in a row (over a three-day period). Now, I do them quarterly for maintenance.

Contraindications: Colonics are never to be performed on a person with active ulcerative colitis, colon cancer, or following colon surgery.

Salt Magnesium Oxide Flush

The Salt Magnesium Flush is a procedure that gives the small intestine a shower from the inside. By ingesting magnesium oxide, which has a pH of 10, you'll create a highly alkaline environment where your body needs to adjust again to the pH of the digestive tract, which is 8.4. In order to remove the highly charged pH substance, your small intestine will flush itself with water to dilute and lower the pH, taking with it all kinds of toxins and clogging substances.

As a result, you will oxygenate and detoxify the small intestine, improving the health and function of the digestive tract. With this method of cleaning the small intestine, and by using colonics to clean the large intestine, you will feel lighter than ever before and brim with energy.

I recommend performing a salt flush on an empty stomach, starting with 1 tablespoon of magnesium oxide (available at natural food stores), 8 ounces of water, and the juice of one lemon. After drinking this concoction, stay well hydrated. The process is harmless, but it results in many frequent bowel movements, so plan to be at home when attempting this cleansing ritual. If you are looking for a more gentle small intestine cleanse, add 1 teaspoon magnesium oxide to 8 ounces of water with the juice from one lemon slice just before sleep (on an empty stomach).

When you decide to do a salt magnesium flush, take probiotics the day before, during, and after to replenish the good bacteria in your system.

Coconut Oil Pulling

Have you heard of oil pulling? It's a traditional, Ayurvedic way to clean, antibacterialize, and detoxify the teeth and gums using coconut oil. It's highly effective at curing tooth decay, gingivitis, and bad breath, as well as preventing cavities. Dental research has connected the health of your teeth and gums to the health of your body, but ancient Indian cultures were way ahead of us on this. They used oil pulling for health, and you can do the same.

Directions: Use 2 teaspoons of only organic virgin coconut oil. It is best to do this in the morning before brushing your teeth. Or it can be done later in the day. Work the oil in the mouth, sucking, pushing, and pulling it through the teeth and around the gums for 15 to 20 minutes. Do not gargle the oil, and do not swallow the oil, as it will be full of bacteria. When finished, spit it into the trash (not into the plumbing), and rinse your mouth thoroughly with water.

If you have active gum disease, tooth decay, or any serious health problem, follow the therapeutic protocol. Oil pull at least once daily, ideally three times per day.

ALKALINE EXERCISE: SLOW AND STEADY

You might think any exercise you do will fight acid and keep you more alkaline. That's a common misconception, and I wouldn't blame you for thinking it. After all, working out *is* a great way to GET OFF YOUR ACID. However, not all workouts are equal. While some workouts fight acid, others actually create more acid in your body!

When it comes to balancing pH, the best workout is a low-intensity exercise such as rebounding, yoga, tai chi, or brisk walking, followed by a sweat in the sauna. I love the book *Slow Burn* by Stu Mittleman, who is a friend and mentor. He points out that years of high-intensity workouts can create a toxic state in the body. The rule of thumb is, if you are able to have a conversation while working out, that's a good thing.

You're creating minimal amounts of lactic acid. Your body will be aerobic, not anaerobic; alkaline, not acid.

Working out, if done incorrectly, can be as acidic for you as an ice cream sundae with all the toppings! And all that acid will have a negative effect on energy, on the immune system's ability to fight illness, and on longevity and long-term health. That doesn't mean you can't ever enjoy the more acidic forms of exercise; it means you need to be careful about *how* they are done, and you must be very diligent about arming your body with the right nutrients to deal with the acid. So before we discuss the best workouts, let's talk about the three worst (and what to do if you actually like them).

Three Bad Workouts That Build Up Acid Quickly

SPINNING

Love spinning? I do, too! But the high-intensity of a spin class starves your body of oxygen and causes major buildup of lactic acid. Once you hit about 75 to 85 percent of your aerobic capacity, or the moment in the spin workout when you feel you've topped out, your body starts producing and accumulating more and more lactic acid. So, what can you do about it?

You can neutralize that acid to improve the workout and speed up recovery by taking a mineral supplement, such as Alkamind Daily Minerals, either during or immediately after class with a huge glass of water. I bring single-serve packets with me when I'm cycling (remember, there is a window of 10 to 15 minutes to get these alkaline nutrients back into your cells once your workout is complete).

SPRINTING

Sprinting is an activity that utilizes short bursts of energy, and the primary sources of that energy result in lactic acid buildup. As an alternative workout, jogging is a lower-intensity workout that doesn't cause such high production of lactic acid. Here's how you can know whether you're building up lactic acid or not: if you can hold a conversation when running, you are aerobically training, you are burning fat (not sugar), and you are alkalizing your body!

In addition, when you sprint, your body *thinks* it's in danger. For all it knows, you could be running away from that old saber-toothed tiger. When you are in fight or flight mode, the stress hormone cortisol increases and completely shuts down the digestive and immune systems as well as the production of hydrochloric acid in your stomach. Once digestion is thrown off, the vicious cycle begins.

To avoid this, *always* warm up with a ten-minute walk. This tells your body you are not in danger. You are moving for the sake of moving. After the ten minutes, gradually increase your stride to a nice, comfortable pace.

WEIGHT TRAINING

Weightlifting is a high-effort, short-term activity that requires bodies to produce energy faster than they can deliver oxygen to muscles. Where does the necessary energy come from? Your body gets the extra energy by fermenting glucose (sugar), which produces, you got it, lactic acid. That sticks around in muscles if you don't do something about it quickly. Interestingly, this is the same exact method that cancer goes through to keep cells alive, as it get its energy in the form of ATP by fermenting sugar.

Again, a lower-intensity weightlifting experience can prevent muscles from shifting into anaerobic mode, and when you do push it hard, take a mineral supplement so you can still enjoy a workout without the acidic effects on your body.

So now that we've covered the worst exercises, let's talk about the best.

Three Good Workouts for Fighting Acid
REBOUNDING

We've talked about rebounding in terms of moving lymph around, which is a slow, gentle activity in which you keep the balls of your feet planted. But when you're ready to increase heart rate up and sweat, the rebounder doubles as a fantastic exercise option. In fact, if I could do only one form of exercise for the rest of my life, it would be rebounding—that's coming from a dedicated die-hard runner.

Why is rebounding also good? The G-force (gravity) at the top of the bounce is eliminated, and the body becomes weightless for a fraction of a second. At the bottom of the bounce, the G-force suddenly

doubles over what is ordinary gravity on earth, and internal organs are put under pressure. Their cellular stimulation is increased accordingly so waste materials within cells are squeezed out. This makes it one of the most powerful forms of exercise to detoxify your body.

▸ **Rebounding is a true cellular exercise. It builds physical cellular strength by challenging the structure of each cell. This strengthening of the cells helps to protect against degenerative disease.**

▸ **It leads to improved posture, increased vascularity, better muscle tone, enhanced timing, sharper vision, greater coordination, better balance, more rhythm, and elevated energy levels.**

▸ **It improves the tone and quality of the heart muscle.**

▸ **It provides the stimulus for a free-flowing lymphatic drainage system, which helps rid your body of toxins, cancer cells, trapped protein, bacteria viruses, and other waste the cells cast off.**

▸ **It floods the cells with oxygen, and it can actually increase your ability to convert glucose into glycogen. Further, it may be possible to train your body (through consistent lymphasizing) to store this glycogen and have it released when you need it for a sudden burst of energy.**

Rebounding Exercises

On a rebounder, you can actually do more than just run in place. Here are a few different exercises to perform on a rebounder.

WARM-UP: Just do small micro-bounces without actually having your feet leave the mat. Do this by engaging your core, using the toes and calves to push the mat down.

BOUNCE: Keeping shoulders over your back, hands at your sides, and your core engaged, and begin making bigger bounces.

STAR JUMPS: Now you can begin adding in the arms by reaching them up above your head when you jump up, then putting them back down at sides when you hit the mat. The motion of the arms is similar to a jumping jack.

JOGGING IN PLACE: It looks like what it sounds like. Gently jog in place on the rebounder.

BUTT KICKS: To add a little oomph to the jogging in place, begin stretching your quads by trying to touch your heel to buttocks when it is coming up from the mat.

SCISSOR JUMPS: Jump up in the air, then try to cross your ankles by engaging your inner thighs, then uncrossing them as you come back down to the mat.

Classes on rebounders and trampoline parks are springing up all over, so be on the lookout for jumping fitness options in your area. The rebounder is the most powerful exercise to keep cells healthy. This exercise increases circulation and metabolism, aids in fat burning, and is much more fun than an average jog. The rebounder simply melts the fat off your body. Best of all, you don't need to go to a class to participate! You can buy an inexpensive rebounder to use in the comfort of your own home. Success with this lifestyle is all about convenience.

What to Look for When Buying a Rebounder

▸ **Minimum 40-inch diameter, but you can use one as big as 53 inches**

▸ **U-bar recommended, but not required**

▸ **Rebounders with springers are less expensive but noisier and give a little more of a rigid bounce. Rebounders with bungee cords are more expensive, slightly softer on your back, and are so silent I can bounce with my children sleeping in the same room!**

▸ **Legs can be foldable (more costly) or non-foldable.**

That's my take on rebounders. When people ask me which is the best one, I say it's the one you are going to use *every* day for at least ten minutes. Don't worry about all the bells and whistles; they all function pretty much the same.

YOGA

Practicing yoga relieves stress that can cause a build-up of acid in the body, and it also encourages deep breathing—a naturally detoxifying, alkalizing practice. Regular yoga practice improves muscle and joint flexibility and encourages healthy blood flood. At the same time, it builds strength without shifting muscles into the anaerobic exercise that many workouts do, which leads to acid buildup. Less lactic acid in the muscles means less acid to fight after completing your workout.

SWIMMING

Swimming is another great aerobic workout that is low-impact and amazing for staying in shape. It also works wonders on your lungs. Your body learns to use oxygen more efficiently, breathing in more fresh air and breathing out more carbon dioxide. And deep breathing is one of the best ways to fight acid. Many people find swimming to be a major stress reliever, so it fights acid on multiple fronts.

I hope these exercise options inspire you to find a way to work out in a way you enjoy and your body can thank you for. Even if you mix in tougher, more-acidic workouts with gentler forms of exercise, the result is that you'll be in better shape and you're going to prevent acid from building up.

How to Fuel a Workout
BEFORE YOUR WORKOUT

Stay very well hydrated before, during, and after a workout. Your body will lose an extra liter of water while working out, so that liquid must be replaced. The average person loses 2.5 liters of water daily, which means if you are exercising, that loss becomes 3.5 liters. Your goal should be to drink 3 to 4 liters of water not only on the day of the workout, but also on the days leading into your workouts. The same goes for nutrition. Unbelievably, what you eat right before a workout is not as important as what you eat the night before, or even two days before. What you eat two days before a workout will have a massive impact on your performance that day, so you need to be proactive, not reactive about what you put into your body on an ongoing, regular basis.

About thirty minutes before a workout, eat something that is easy to digest. Try a green juice for energy, as there is nothing easier on the digestive system. Green juice will deliver vitamins and minerals to your body right away, which will give you a healthy energetic kick-start. If you want something besides juice, go with something light such as raw vegetable soup, pureed vegetables, or raw nut butter. The lower intensity the workout, the more fat you should eat.

Remember, if you eat fat, you will burn fat, and then your body will crave fat, and that is the cycle you want. If you eat sugar, you'll be more likely to burn sugar, and then you will crave sugar. Therefore, the very worst thing you can ever do is carb load before working out or the night before a big race. It's amazing; I participate in many marathons, and the night before, I see most people throwing big pasta parties. And what are the most common foods on the actual marathon course? Bananas, oranges, candy, and sports drinks. All bad. When exercising, again, always avoid sugar.

Avoid a lot of protein right before a workout as well, as this can cause cramping since protein is acidic and requires more fluids to be metabolized than carbs and fat do. Cramping occurs when the body is less hydrated, and when the body has to use its mineral reserves to neutralize any acidic foods or toxins entering the body. Protein is for building muscles, not for fueling them.

DURING YOUR WORKOUT

You might be asking, "What does Dr. Daryl eat during a workout?" Good question. First, I drink. And I have a feeling you already know what I drink. Water! Lots of it!

I try to drink a liter of water while I'm working out. That might sound like a lot, but that's what your body is losing as it sweats. Replenishing as you go is essential to preventing dehydration. I like to add a few slices of lemon or lime to the water bottle before I hit the gym because it tastes delicious and it has extra alkalizing effects.

If I exercise for more than ninety minutes, I eat a small snack that is more fat-oriented. A sprouted tortilla, for example, can be spread with raw almond butter, a drizzle of Manuka honey, some chia seeds, and cinnamon to prevent an insulin spike from the honey. Cut it into tiny slices, wrap them individually in plastic, and put them

in your pocket. Or eat a spoonful of homemade energy gel—you can make your own by combining 1 cup water and 2 to 4 tablespoons of chia seeds (store the gel in mini plastic bags, the kind used for packing vitamins). This is a great healthy fat and full-workout energizer if needed.

AFTER YOUR WORKOUT

After a workout, alkalizing foods are an integral part of the body's post-repair process. If you don't alkalize, the lactic acid will build up in your body and joints. You want to get something into your body quickly, and the window to do this is about 10 to 15 minutes. The first thing to do after a workout, before even leaving the gym, is take a single-serve pack of Alkamind Daily Minerals (not to sound like a broken record, but I hope you are beginning to sense the importance) and add it to 16 ounces of water. That way, you will start refilling the tank right away with the minerals that have been depleted: calcium, magnesium, potassium, and sodium bicarbonate.

Then, for your next meal (wait at least thirty minutes), prepare a plant-based protein smoothie with some greens and some healthy omega-3 fats such as chia, flax, and/or hemp seeds, a scoop of coconut oil, and a scoop of my plant-based Organic Daily Protein smoothie powder. This will help keep your body in fat-burning mode and will build lean muscle mass.

Plant-based omega-3 fatty acids are very helpful for repairing body tissue. I also like nut butters such as raw almond butter and, yes, even dark-green leafy veggies such as spinach and kale. These are all packed with protein. Forty-five or more minutes after a workout, eat some solid proteins, whether it's a salad with some salmon and/or avocado, slivered raw almonds and hemp seeds, or sprouts. Avoid all grains and sugars (even from fruit) for several hours after a run or the gym. The reason is that the exercise combined with sugar will throw off the body's blood sugar balance and send a signal that the body has entered starvation mode, holding on to all of the sugar, carbs, and fat that it can.

THE TAKEAWAY
ON EXERCISE

▸ Find something you love to do.

▸ Be consistent with it.

▸ Slow and steady wins the race. Don't kill yourself in workouts. That's

creating stress and lactic acid. If you can "hold a conversation" while working out, you are most likely burning fat, not sugar, and aerobically alkalizing your body.

▸ Love the rebounder. It's easy. It's quick. It's detoxifying. If you can do only one form of exercise for the rest of your life, make it rebounding at home for 10 to 15 minutes. Everybody has 10 minutes. Make it a priority, and set the tone for the day.

▸ Exercise has a ripple effect for all other choices you'll make in your life. Usually during the times when I have been exercising, I ate better, felt better, and looked better. Likewise, when I wasn't exercising, I had less energy and motivation and made unhealthier food choices. If you are looking to kick-start your health, start exercising and all else will follow.

09

Stress—The #1 Cause of Acid

Often when people think about an alkaline lifestyle, they are focused only on food and exercise. I am here to tell you that stress outweighs all that a million to one. Any time you experience stress, your adrenal glands produce the hormones epinephrine, norepinephrine, and cortisol, which puts your body into a state of "fight or flight," and you become more acidic.

Stress deactivates the parasympathetic nervous system—the system responsible for "rest and digest." Ideally, these two systems will live in harmony and balance with each other, which is significant for your health because if you are living in chronic stress, like so many people are, your digestive system (and immune system) will shut down.

Why does the body do this? Your body assumes you need energy and you need it fast, so you will be able to *run* to safety! The last thing it needs is to focus on digesting! Your body doesn't know if stress is coming from a relationship or something at work or a sick family member. All it knows is *I am in danger, and I need to get out of this dangerous situation NOW.*

To your body, stress is stress, and as a result, digestion remains shut down as you continue to become more acidic. Decreased digestion means increased leaky gut, and undigested food particles, bacteria, yeast, and toxins are getting into the blood where they don't belong, which kicks the buffering system into full gear. Over time, locked in this mode, you become tired, exhausted, and completely depleted of mineral reserves.

The body also produces a hormone called aldosterone, which stimulates the kidneys to excrete acid ($H+$ ions). Here is another reason why pH testing is so important: chronic stress will produce an acidic urine pH, just as an acidic diet would. If you recall, urine pH directly reflects adrenal glands, kidneys, and water, and the body has to eliminate the acids that result from the digestion of fats, carbohydrates, and proteins, as well as other metabolic and toxic waste.

With all that said, stress is something we will always have in our lives in one form or another—sometimes less and sometimes more. Of course, we want to minimize stress, but many times the levels of stress can be unavoidable. You never know when life is going to throw a curve ball, and when it happens, you need to be ready. Being healthy is not about how *much* stress you have; it's about how you *adapt* to stress. It's about keeping your body in peak state and having a balanced pH with plenty of mineral reserves so that if a stressful situation arises, you will be ready and it will not take you down.

Meditation is one of my favorite daily practices to help combat stress. Here's the deal: you don't have to be on a mountaintop in the Himalayas sitting in lotus position to meditate. You can do it every day, wherever you are. And it has benefits far beyond relaxing your body and mind. I'd go so far as to say, if you meditate, everything in your life will improve: your mental state, levels of stress, relationships, and, yes, even your job. Now is a great time to pick up a simple meditation habit.

However, I know many people who resist the idea of meditating. Or they've tried it and found it too hard to sit still and keep their minds from wandering, so they tell me they aren't "any good at meditation." Well, there's no such thing as being "bad" at meditating! As with so many things, it just takes practice—and that's the point. The patience and the commitment is part of what makes it work. While resistance to meditation is understandable and normal, there are likewise so many great reasons to meditate!

▶ It lowers stress levels.

▶ It can decrease anxiety and the tendency for depression.

▶ It can decrease blood pressure.

▶ It eases your body into more restful sleep.

▶ It can prevent muscle tension.

▶ It helps your body eliminate toxins.

▶ It can increase nitric oxide levels.

▶ It can strengthen the immune system.

▶ It changes the way the brain responds to stressors.

▶ Long-term meditation changes the physical structure of the brain in ways that improve memory and focus.

▶ Finally, it helps you GET OFF YOUR ACID! Since it reduces stress levels, and stress causes more acid than any food, meditation goes a long way toward alkalizing your body!

When you meditate, you become a much better breather, and there is nothing more powerful for alkalizing your body than oxygenation through slow, deep breathing. Once you start practicing, you'll see the benefits. If you don't believe me, take it from Ray Dalio, founder of Bridgewater Associates, the world's biggest hedge fund. He swears that meditation is the secret to his remarkable success.

This week, challenge yourself to try an easy meditation. Even if you hate it, try it again the next day. Set a timer for five or ten minutes the first time you try it. A short amount of time will take away the intimidation factor. You can do just about anything for five minutes, right?

PACE YOUR BREATH

BreathPacer is a pretty cool iPhone app that not only calculates your ideal breath rate based on your height, but also helps you find and implement your natural therapeutic breathing pattern. The app states that people have different optimal breathing rates, and height is a very good predictor of this because blood volume circulated through the cardiovascular system varies based on height. Your ideal breathing rate should fall between five and six breaths per minute.

The app also has a great feature that allows you to breathe to the sound of rain in order to time your breaths. Inhale as the bar rises (and the rain gets louder), exhale as the bar falls (and rain gets softer), and hold your breath while the bar is not moving. It is a phenomenal tool to teach you how to slow your breathing and stimulate your parasympathetic nervous system.

CALMING MEDITATION

This wonderful practice will calm and center you in any situation. It can also be used when you feel overwhelmed by a craving. Very often, the craving will pass by the end of ten to twenty breaths.

To practice this, close your eyes, place your hands on your belly, and tune in to the sensations around you, as you inhale and exhale. Gradually begin to deepen the breath, taking ten to twenty slow, conscious breaths deeply into and out of the belly. You can do this meditation several times in a row or frequently throughout your day.

ATTITUDE OF GRATITUDE MEDITATION

This is so simple, yet immensely powerful. If I have one favorite meditation, the gratitude meditation is probably it. It is especially important if you find yourself spiraling down the hole of negative thinking and negative manifestations in your life.

This can be done anytime, but it can be particularly good first thing in the morning or last thing at night. Sit quietly with your eyes closed and meditate on all that is good in your life. If you are having trouble finding something good, simply feel gratitude for the gift of breath and a healthy body. Your objects of gratitude can be as big or as small as you want. What is one thing you are grateful for today that made this day worth living? You may choose to write down these items after or before meditating on them. Do this for as long as you want.

Meditation is an important part of detoxifying your body, as it helps take you away from the state of fight or flight, which breeds acid. I recommend it as part of any attempt to remove acids and toxins from your body—you'll be left feeling more energetic and younger than you've felt in years!

CHIROPRACTIC CARE

This is at the core of what I do. I look at health like a wheel, and the spokes on that wheel are the healthy lifestyle habits that should be part of your daily life: alkaline nutrition, exercise, stress management, good sleeping habits, and a positive mental attitude (PMA). At the center of this wheel, most importantly, is a properly functioning nervous system.

For you to be healthy, your brain needs to send signals down the spinal cord and out the nerves through every system, organ, muscle, tissue, and cell. When that pathway is clear, you can express your true, innate health potential. On the other hand, anything that interferes with the nervous system is bad and is going to interfere with your quality of life. An acidic diet, being sedentary, and having toxic thoughts (chemical, physical, and emotional stress) can all cause interference with your nerve system.

Chiropractic care reduces stress on the entire nervous system, freeing up the nerves so digestion and other bodily functions improve for greater overall health. When you receive a chiropractic adjustment, circulation and oxygenation increases, breathing is better, and the stimulation of the parasympathetic nervous system inhibits the production of cortisol, a hormone that shuts down digestion and immune function, making you more acidic.

Think of a kink in the garden hose and how it interferes with water flow. In your body, you need everything to be free flowing. Your chiropractic doctor will check you for nerve stress (80 percent of the time, you can't feel it building up, just like a cavity) and will remove any nerve interference in your system with an adjustment. It is safe, and it works.

Chiropractic care has changed my life and the lives of my family and countless patients. Most people think chiropractors are back doctors, and while chiropractic care has been proven to be the most effective at treating back pain, this is scratching the surface in terms of what regular chiropractic care can do for your health and the health of your family. Whether you are experiencing headaches, back pain, sinus trouble, stress and anxiety, asthma, or digestive issues, there is always a nerve system component to those issues, and chiropractic care can help. I see my chiropractor every week (yes, I have a chiropractor, as you can't adjust yourself), which helps to keep me in peak condition.

I highly recommend, whether you have back pain or not, to go see a chiropractor to have your nerve system evaluated. I didn't say adjusted; go get checked first. Gather information, and then go from there. Don't wait for back pain to happen before considering going.

Remember, too, that any pain you experience is not the beginning of the problem. Like a toothache, the problem has been developing most likely for quite some time, and the pain is merely the warning signal. If you don't listen to the signal and do something about it, you may lose the tooth. While you can always replace your teeth, you have only one spine and nerve system, which are *not* replaceable. This is why you need to be proactive with your spinal care—if you take care of your spine, it will take care of you.

SITTING IS THE NEW SMOKING

American adults are sedentary more than three-fifths of their waking hours, and four out of five of us don't get the recommended amount of exercise each week. The same holds true for our children. They sit all day long at school, and the 40-pound backpack on their shoulders is adding gasoline to the fire. Research has shown that 10 percent of ten-year-olds have degeneration and arthritis in their L5 vertebrae— that's crazy! Arthritis is not normal at any age, especially if you're 10!

Most people sit all day at work and then come home and sit some more. Sitting has become the new smoking: research shows that for every hour we spend watching TV, 22 minutes is eliminated from our lifespan.

For that reason, we need to move more! The more you move, the more energy you will have and the better you will feel. Our metabolism slows by 5 percent each decade, and our lack of mobility and the effect it has in our lymphatic system isn't helping. At age 35, you'll burn 100 fewer calories per day than you did at age 25, and 200 fewer calories than you did at age 45. That could translate to 8 to 12 extra pounds each year. The more we move, the better your lymphatic system will function, and the less acidic and toxic your body will be.

Every half hour, get up and move your body, and set a reminder on your phone, if that's what it will take. Standing desks can help you get up out of that chair, but standing all day may cause a different problem. You still need to move. Invest in the desk that can do both—a sit/stand desk—so your body will never be in one position for too long.

Get creative and come up with new ways to work that don't revolve around the chair. Put a rebounder in your office and take short breaks throughout the day to bounce the stress away. Here is the takeaway: motion is life!

10

The Get Off Your Acid
7-Day Challenge

> Knowledge is not power.
> It is only potential power.
> Action is power.
>
> —TONY ROBBINS

Now that I've given you strategies for eating alkaline and my favorite detox protocols, my challenge to you is to go 80/20 in favor of alkaline eating, following the GET OFF YOUR ACID food pyramid, *and* try all seven of the lifestyle changes for a full week. This chapter includes a few tips to help you get through the 7-Day Challenge and make fit it into your life—not make your life fit into it. At the end of one week, go back to that very first quiz you took and see if your numbers increased. Taking the

quiz before and after the week should yield some exciting results.

All I am asking is that you do this for seven days, and I believe you'll want to keep going. As long as you're making progress, I think you're going to find this is a great lifestyle choice. Other diets are all about deprivation—this isn't. I think you're going to want to keep feeling this good. If you have an off moment, don't beat yourself up, just hop back on the plan. The biggest challenge for most is consistency. Something may come up, such as a birthday party, and you'll feel pressure to drink champagne or eat cake. I suggest having a small glass or a couple bites. You don't have to deny yourself entirely if you want to partake. But if you can exercise a little control, you'll find it easy to keep charging ahead.

The program is really about adding the greens and the minerals, eating more healthy fats, hydrating with more water, conscious breathing, low-impact exercise, adding some supplements you may not be taking at this moment, de-stress techniques, and at least one daily detox protocol. It really is simple, and you're going to see results. Cutting things out is fantastic, but you don't have to be 100 percent all the time. Remember 80/20 is the goal. Think progress, not perfection.

Envision what your life will be like if you do these things, and envision the way your life will be if you don't make changes. What will your weight be? What will your energy be? What will your visible signs of aging be? If you have a compelling enough reason for wanting to change, nothing will stop you. That reason might be living longer for your grandkids, fitting into your old jeans, clearing up skin conditions, or battling a more serious ailment. But the main reason should be for a better quality of life every day.

The top reasons I hear from people about why they want to do the 7-Day Challenge is they want to look better and they want to lose weight. That's fine by me because these are powerful drivers. The great thing is, this program does these things for you while also doing the critical work of improving health by making your body more alkaline. Not only will you look better, but you'll feel better and live better!

MAKE SURE YOUR GOALS ARE SMART

SPECIFIC. "I want to lose weight" is not specific. "I want to lose 5 pounds a week with the ultimate outcome of 15 pounds," that's specific.

MEASURABLE. How will you measure your goal? Tracking progress is important and will hold you accountable.

ATTAINABLE. Goals should push you, but you also need to choose a goal that you know you can achieve.

REALISTIC. Is your goal and time frame realistic for the established goal? Five pounds a week is less realistic for certain people.

TIMEBOUND. Give yourself a deadline. If you don't have that, the goal is just a wish.

" *I will keep this short and sweet. My wife challenged me to do the* Get Off Your Acid *7-Day Challenge. I immediately thought, NO WAY. I can't eat like that, I could never go cold turkey from sugar, caffeine, processed foods, etc. . . . Well, not only did I do it, but I lost 15 pounds, am off two separate medications for reflux, and feel huge amounts of new energy and vitality. The support of this program is undeniable. It's easy, cost effective, and needs no gimmicks because it simply works.* "

—*Louis G.*

" *I have been struggling for the last four years to lose the weight I gained after a year of chemotherapy to eradicate the stage 3 breast cancer I had. How was it that I could fight breast cancer twice but not control my long-standing addiction to sugar and food, which most likely was a major contributing cause to the cancer in the first place?*

I came across Dr. Daryl and the Get Off Your Acid *program, and my God, it has made such a huge difference in my life. The seven-day program was so easy to do and follow, the recipes are so delicious, and I wasn't hungry once. It made such a difference in my day-to-day life that I decided to continue! I'm on my fourth week right now and feel so energetic with no more cravings. Best of all, I'm finally shedding my weight (down 22 pounds!) and feel healthier than ever! I recommend this program to everyone! Thanks again, Dr. Daryl!* "

—*Carine V.*

QUIZ: WHAT'S MAKING YOU ACIDIC?

▶ To take this quiz online, go to http://getoffyouracid.com/five-acid-sources-quiz

As you GET OFF YOUR ACID, to help target which steps you may want especially focus on, take this quiz to find out which sources of acid are most problematic for you. Place a check mark in front of any sentence that describes you. At the end, you will add up how many check marks you have in each acid category.

Dietary Acids

_____ 1. Do you frequently eat simple carbohydrates like bread, pasta, sweets, or processed snack foods?

_____ 2. Do you drink fruit juice, soda, carbonated water, or coffee more than once per week?

_____ 3. Do you consume dairy on a regular basis (milk, yogurt, ice cream, whey, etc.)?

_____ 4. Do you eat or drink anything made with artificial sweeteners (diet soda, sugar-free desserts, yogurt, sugarless gum, etc.)?

_____ 5. Do you suffer from constipation, bloating, gas, diarrhea, or acid reflux regularly?

Metabolic Acids

_____ 1. Do you prefer spinning, CrossFit, High-Intensity Interval Training (HIIT), or similar workouts that push your muscles as far as possible?

_____ 2. Do you eat animal-based proteins and/or fructose (high fructose corn syrup, moderate-to high-sugar fruits) at least three times or more per week?

_____ 3. Do you regularly participate in intense training that leaves you huffing and puffing and feeling depleted afterward?

_____ 4. Are you a shallow chest breather and/or yawn on an occasional basis?

_____ 5. Do you often feel too tired to work out, even first thing in the morning?

Emotional Acids

_____ 1. Do you often lose sleep because your mind is too active or you're worrying?

_____ 2. Are you frequently very stressed, either from work or your personal life?

_____ 3. Do you have moments where you suffer from lack of confidence or insecurity at least a couple times a week?

_____ 4. Are you currently dealing with anxiety or depression?

_____ 5. Do you find yourself responding to others with frustration or anger (do you have a short fuse)?

Environmental Acids

_____ 1. Do you buy standard (non-organic) cleaning products or bath and beauty products for your home?

_____ 2. Do you drink from plastic water bottles or use other products made with Bisphenol A (BPA) once a week or more?

_____ 3. Do you use a microwave to heat your food?

_____ 4. Does your shopping cart contain many non-organic choices that may contain GMOs or pesticides (check this if you tend to buy non-organic)?

_____ 5. Do you keep a cell phone in your pocket throughout your day, make cell phone calls without a headset, or keep a laptop on your lap when working?

Consumed Chemical Acids (Consumed or Transdermal)

_____ 1. Have you taken antibiotics, birth control pills, or prescription medications within the past year?

_____ 2. Do you eat farmed, not wild-caught, or Atlantic-caught fish or seafood (and if you don't know, you can assume that is a yes)?

_____ 3. Do you drink wine, beer, or liquor more than once per week?

_____ 4. Do you smoke cigarettes or use recreational drugs?

_____ 5. IDo you have any dental fillings with mercury or use a standard deodorant (containing aluminum in the ingredients panel)?

YOUR RESULTS

Add up how many check marks you have in each acid category. The category with the most is your dominant acid type and the most significant source of toxicity in your body; the category with the least (or none) may not be making you as acidic; the others fall somewhere in between.

DIETARY ACIDS

The foods you eat and the beverages you drink are the primary cause of acid buildup in your body. Sugar, gluten, artificial sweeteners, dairy, meat, caffeine, carbonation, and processed foods are the primary drivers of this type of acid.

Follow my 80/20 alkaline rule to replace acidic foods with nutrient-rich alkaline ones. Reduce (or even cut out) the acidic foods mentioned above as quickly as you can, but keep in mind they are addictive so it can take some time to wean off them. At the same time, add more dark green leafy vegetables and healthy fats. These mineral-rich alkaline foods will energize your body, help your digestive system heal, and minimize cravings as you transition to a healthier alkaline lifestyle. For more info, see Chapter 8.

METABOLIC ACIDS

If you have a high score in this category, metabolic acids such as lactic acid, carbonic acid, or uric acid has built up in your body.

Lactic acid. You could be getting too much intense exercise without replenishing minerals properly. Also, when your body is poorly oxygenated from being toxic and over-acidic, the cells mode of respiration (the way they breath and produce ATP— the energy currency of the body) can change from *aerobic* to *anaerobic* metabolism. The byproduct of this change in metabolism is lactic acid.

Carbonic acid. You might be getting little to no exercise or are most likely a shallow chest breather.

Uric acid. Your diet might be too high in protein and/or fructose (from moderate- to high-sugar fruits and/or high fructose corn syrup). For more info, see Chapter 4.

EMOTIONAL ACIDS

Stress is a primary cause of acid buildup in your body, and it may be sabotaging your efforts to eat well, feel well, and get yourself into a regular exercise protocol. Keep an arsenal of stress-relieving techniques ready to go for any time you're feeling tense or overwhelmed.

Do the 3:6:5 power breath (see page 138) every morning when you wake up to increase oxygen in your blood and endorphins in your body. Even incorporating five minutes of exercise (on a rebounder, for example) or daily meditation will make a difference, as a little bit of stress relief every day adds up over time. When you are feeling stressed, make sure you drink water. For more info, see Chapter 9.

ENVIRONMENTAL ACIDS

Much of the acid that builds up in your body is caused by toxic chemicals and acids from the environment. Where does it come from? The United States imports and/or produces 42 billion pounds of chemicals per day. The average home has more than 1,000 chemicals on hand at any given time,

DR. DARYL'S 80/20 DAY: MY GO-TO REGIMEN

6:30 a.m., rise and shine: Alkamind Daily Greens drink

Morning exercise: rebounder 12 minutes Lymphatic Drainage

Detox protocol while rebounding: 3:6:5 power breath

7 a.m., breakfast: alkaline smoothie loaded with greens and at least 2 healthy fats (coconut oil, chia seeds) (see recipes on page 194).

Supplements: omega-3 fatty acid (fish oil) 2,000mg; probiotic x 1; vitamin D_3 5,000 IU drops on tongue; antioxidant: molecular hydrogen or glutathione

8 a.m., detox protocol: Acid Crusher Detox Tea (see recipe on page 153)

10 a.m.: Alkamind Daily Greens drink

Midmorning snack: celery stick with nut butter (only if hunger arises, otherwise avoid to keep insulin levels down)

11 a.m.: urine pH and/or saliva pH test

12:30 p.m., lunch: rainbow salad with avocado, and raw soup

3 p.m.: Alkamind Daily Greens drink

Mid-afternoon snack: garlic hummus with veggie sticks (see recipe on page 200), only if hunger arises, otherwise avoid to keep insulin levels down

6:45 p.m., post-work workout: 10-minute walk or lymphatic drainage on rebounder; 30-minute run or 30-minute rebounder aerobic workout; Alkamind Daily Greens drink during or post workout; Alkamind Organic Daily Protein (vanilla coconut) post workout with spinach,
1 tablespoon of hemp or chia seeds,
1 tablespoon of coconut oil, and 8 ounces coconut milk

7:30 p.m., dinner: rainbow salad (kale/watercress/romaine/spinach) with extra virgin olive oil and lemon; cauliflower steak with turmeric and ginger; avocado with 1 tablespoon macadamia oil, black pepper, cumin, and sea salt; optional protein: small piece of wild-caught baked salmon or slivered nuts and seeds in salad

Supplements: omega-3 fatty acid (fish oil) 1,000mg; probiotic x 1; digestive enzyme; antioxidant: molecular hydrogen or glutathione; B_{12} shot twice weekly (my wife, Chelsea, opts for a daily liquid or sublingual B_{12})

Dessert (optional): Vanilla Coconut Chia Pudding (see recipe on page 227)

9 p.m., evening detox protocol: Detox Bath (see page 154)

10 p.m., before bed (30 minutes before sleep): Alkamind Daily Greens drink and the average person is exposed to 167 chemicals per day just using standard personal care products—and it's not limited to this. Because of all this environmental toxicity, you may have experienced some autoimmune, hormonal, thyroid, or adrenal issues.

Check your home for sources of exposure and switch to organics. Replace cleaning products, bath and body products, linens, and cosmetics with toxin-free organic versions recommended by the Environmental Working Group (EWG). Get an electromagnetic field (EMF) protector for your bedroom, office, and cell phone, and never use your phone directly against your ear (use the speaker or a headset). Use glass instead of plastic whenever possible, eliminating common sources of BPA. For more info, see Chapter 1.

CHEMICAL ACIDS (CONSUMED OR TRANSDERMAL)

Chemicals affect our hormones and the delicate microbiome within the gut. Drink well-filtered water as much as possible. Buy organic at the grocery, especially in the produce department. If you eat meat, be sure that it is organically grass-fed. Fish should be wild caught. If you have mercury fillings, find a dentist who is skilled in removing them the appropriate way. Switch from an aluminum-based deodorant to one that is natural and aluminum free. Avoid drugs, smoking, and alcohol, and take prescription medication only if necessary. For more info, see Chapter 1.

THE BATTLE IS WON AT THE GROCERY STORE

The most daunting part about changing your diet is that first trip to the grocery store when you find yourself standing in the middle of the aisle with an empty cart; it's sad because you feel like things you're not allowed to eat surround you.

Luckily, going alkaline doesn't mean you have to eliminate anything—at all. Eat what you love, but in moderation. Remember, your daily diet should consist of 80 percent high-alkaline foods, which means 20 percent can be acidic. Don't aim for perfection to start, only for improvement. Even so, your first trip to the store after deciding to go alkaline might be scary. I'm here to help. The following are my favorite tips for grocery shopping.

Never Shop Hungry

The most important rule I can share with you about the grocery store is never go to the supermarket hungry! Who's guilty of that one? I know I am.

Shop the Perimeter

You should be spending most (if not all) of your time shopping the perimeter of the grocery store, not the center aisles where most processed food resides.

Use My Quick Alkaline Shopping List

Eating alkaline is easy if you have the right ingredients in the cupboards and fridge. Once you adapt to eating this way, it will become second nature, but to begin, you can rely on this shopping list to stock up on alkaline foods.

GREENS

Going alkaline also means going green. Arugula is good, but spinach is even better to use as the base for salads. Asparagus and Brussels sprouts are great as side dishes, while zucchini can be used as an entree (veggie pasta, anyone?) and avocado can be put on, well, almost everything! And don't forget watercress, the king of greens, at the top of the list of the forty-one most powerful foods!

HERBS, SPICES, OILS, AND FATS

Garlic is highly alkaline, and who doesn't love a dose of the stinking rose? And despite what you might have heard about saturated fats, coconut oil is the good guy. Coconut oil contains 90 percent of the fatty acids that are great for the brain and the body. Remember, to lose fat, you need to eat fat, and don't be afraid of it. My favorite fat burners are chia seeds, hemp seeds, flax seeds, raw almonds, macadamia nuts, and avocados. Throw them in your favorite smoothie, salad, or dessert!

FRUITS

Here's where so many people go wrong—they think all fruit is good, and therein lies one of the biggest misconceptions. There are three components to look for in fruit to determine if it's alkaline or acidic: the mineral content, fiber content, and the sugar content. Alkaline fruits (lemons, limes, grapefruit, tomatoes, pomegranates, coconut, and to some degree, watermelon) are high in minerals and fiber and, you guessed it, low in sugar, because sugar equals acid!

STARCHES

Passing on the pasta is a hard thing to do. If you crave starches or need something a little

THE DIRTY DOZEN

Apples
Domestic blueberries
Grapes
Imported nectarines
Peaches
Strawberries
Bell peppers
Celery
Cucumbers
Lettuce
Potatoes
Spinach

heavier to feel full, choose quinoa instead. Sweet potatoes are not only alkaline but also high in vitamin A and fiber, and new potatoes are alkaline-approved, too. Starchy foods in moderation are quite okay.

PROTEINS

Alkaline is primarily a plant-based lifestyle, but if you fancy yourself a carnivore, opt for seafood such as wild-caught salmon, sardines or anchovies. If you can't source it from New Zealand or Spain, go for the Pacific Ocean. I often order from a great company called Vital Choice Wild Seafood and Organics for fresh, wild-caught, flash-frozen seafood. Even better, choose hummus, adzuki beans, lentils, and chickpeas (you're allowed in the center aisles for those).

(NON)DAIRY

Dairy is a highly acid-forming food; stay away at all costs! Choose unsweetened, unflavored almond milk and coconut milk to help lower cholesterol, lose weight, and make smoothies taste great. Better yet, make your own at home.

Buy Organic and Avoid Pesticides

I hear from a lot of you that although you buy lots of fresh fruits and vegetables, you don't always, or even often, choose organic produce. Well, in just one statistic, I want to show how important it is to buy organic: 68 percent of food samples

PESTICIDE HANGOVERS

Have you ever woken up with a hangover after only one glass of wine and wondered why? Or maybe wine gives you a headache? More often than not, it's not because of the alcohol content (although alcohol is acidic and contains yeast and sugar). It's actually from all the pesticides and sulfates that are being put into grapes. So if you want to drink wine periodically or as part of the 20 percent acid-forming foods and drinks you consume, choose a good, sustainable, organic wine that has no sulfates, no herbicides, no pesticides, and no fungicides.

measured by the Environmental Working Group (EWG) had detectable pesticide residues, even after they were washed and peeled! That means that more than two-thirds of the nonorganic produce you're eating has pesticide residue, which is dangerous and harmful to your body and your health.

Many of you have probably heard of the Dirty Dozen, which is a great resource. These twelve foods must always be organic. An easy way to think about it is the thinner the skin on the fruit or veggie, the higher the amount of contaminants. For example, bananas are less likely to contain pesticides than apples.

Read the Codes

Here's a great bit of information on how to read codes to know what's organic. Every single fruit and vegetable has an SKU sticker on it. You've seen them, right?

- If a sticker begins with the number 9, it means it's organic. Remember this: *nine is fine.*

- If a sticker begins with a number 8, it means that it's genetically modified. Remember this: *eight, I hate.*

- If the sticker begins with any other number, it means that it was conventionally grown and is neither GMO or organic. Most likely it was grown with herbicides, pesticides, fungicides, and synthetic fertilizers.

Another option that's even better is to shop for produce at the local farmer's market. Certified organic farmers proudly advertise their status, and you can talk to the growers to find out more information.

PREPARATION IS KEY: TIPS FOR FOOD PREP AND STORAGE

Maximize produce by learning how to store food. Produce longevity is the best way to save money and reduce waste in a world where so many are underfed. Take avocados, for example. I buy the hardest, least ripe ones and put them in the fridge, where they'll last up to three weeks. When you take them out, they'll ripen within three days on the counter. This way you will always have them on hand, and they will be ripe when you're ready to use them.

- Put baking soda in the fridge to absorb moisture.

- Use smoothie bags. I cut fruit and freeze it for simple, one-step smoothies in the morning. I put in everything in the bag that would go in the smoothie, but without the liquids and nut butters: spinach, kale, chia seeds, etc. Dump it all in the blender with the liquid and/or the nut butter, and an ice-cold smoothie will be ready to go. If I'm really under the gun, I put everything in the blender, then put that in the freezer the night before.

- If herbs are looking a little wilty and sad, just trim the stems and pop them in a glass of water, and they'll perk right up.

- At the farmers market, buy organic tomatoes and raw, organic ginger in bulk. Freeze them in airtight, BPA-free plastic bags.

- Wash produce just before using it, not before storing, to keep it from becoming moldy.

- Keep berries, citrus, melons, and peas in the front of the fridge, which tends to be colder.

- When storing leafy greens, spread them across a paper towel. Roll the towel tightly, secure with a rubber band, and place it in an open plastic bag. This keeps the leaves dry, even while being stored, and allows the ethylene gas to escape. Ethylene is the enemy of freshness. If it's allowed to build up in a bag, it produces enzymes that speed spoilage, so leave a little opening for air to flow.

- At our house, Sundays are prep days. I love to make a large batch of quinoa in my steamer or on stovetop. That will last all week for salads or breakfast bowls or wraps. It's so versatile.

- I also make a huge salad on Sundays. I cut up all kinds of ingredients from red onion to red bell peppers, broccoli, etc. I keep the greens separate and make a few jars of salad dressing and veggie dips. Then, for the next couple of days, I can grab handfuls of stuff and make superfast salads on the go.

- Make raw soups and freeze them. Any time you freeze anything, there should be very little oxygen/airspace in the container. That makes food items degrade.

- Metal knives are oxidizing, so I prefer ceramic knives. An apple slice with a metal knife browns faster than if it were sliced by a ceramic knife.

- Can't forget about desserts! My famous Vanilla Coconut Chia Pudding takes ten minutes to make in the blender, then place in the fridge for at least five hours. This is also true for Avocado Chocolate Mousse. Make these on Sunday, and you will have delicious desserts loaded with healthy fats for the entire week.

EATING OUT THE ALKALINE WAY

Maintaining an alkaline lifestyle can be challenging when eating out in restaurants. But it is possible, especially if you follow these tips:

- Avoid bread before the meal and avoid dessert after.

- Chew slowly to eat less and better digest what you do eat. Chew everything, even smoothies!

- Drink water with a squeeze of fresh lemon, but don't drop in the slice, as they are usually non-organic.

- Smaller portions are your friend, so opt for multiple sides, appetizers, and salads.

- Order dressings and sauces on the side.

- Choose dishes that are steamed, broiled, baked, grilled, roasted, or sautéed instead of fried.

- Bring your own salt: Redmond Real Salt, Himalayan, or Celtic Grey Sea Salt.

SWAP THIS OUT FOR THAT

SWAP THIS OUT	BETTER CHOICE	BEST CHOICE
White Rice	Brown Rice	Quinoa
Milk / Soy Milk	Almond Milk	Coconut Milk or Homemade Almond/Hemp Milk
Vegetable Oils (Canola, Soybean, Sunflower)	Flaxseed Oil	Coconut/Olive Oils
Pasta	Gluten-Free Pasta	Zucchini Noodles / Kelp Noodles
Balsamic Vinegar	Apple Cider Vinegar	Lemon & Olive Oil
Coffee	Green Tea	Herbal Tea
Milk Chocolate	Dark Chocolate	Raw Cacao
Table Salt	Sea Salt / Kosher Salt	Celtic Grey Sea Salt / Himalayan
Margarine / Butter	Ghee / Kerrygold (grass-fed)	Coconut Butters / Raw Nut Butters
Soy Sauce	Tamari / Braggs Liquid Aminos	Coconut Aminos
Sugar / Agave / Brown Sugar	Coconut Sugar / Nectar, Manuka Honey	Stevia, Lo Han (Monk Fruit)
Peanuts	Cashews	Raw Almonds/Macadamia Nuts
Carbonated/Bottled/Tap Water	Filtered Water	Alkaline Water w/ Minerals & H2
Fruit Juice	Freshly Squeezed Fruit Juice	Cold-Pressed Green Juice
Granola	Oatmeal	Gluten-Free Oats/Quinoa
White Bread	Gluten-Free Bread	Sprouted Bread/Ezekial
Animal Proteins / Farmed Fish	Grass Fed Animal Proteins / Wild-Caught Fish	Plant-Based Proteins
Beer / Cider	Wine	Vodka (Chopin or Ciroc)

REMEMBER SWAP OUT
> BETTER > BEST

If you've been following me for a while, you know my **Swap > Better > Best** philosophy. For almost any acidic ingredient, you can find a better alternative out there. This is the best way to approach travel. You can't eat 100 percent alkaline all the time, but you can try to cut back on the acid you consume.

MINDSET
IS EVERYTHING

And now, my friend, you've arrived. You have all the information you need to move or transition from an acidic to an alkaline lifestyle and to improve your quality and longevity of life in the process. Armed with all this powerful knowledge, the last (and most important thing) you need is the right mindset. I named my company Alkamind because I believe that you can't get alkaline without your *mind* in the game. Remember this: if your *why* is big enough—your reason for wanting to improve your life—the *how* will come easily.

To put yourself in the right headspace, remember a few key pointers.

Stress is a killer. It is the worst, most acidic factor there is, so do whatever you must to remove stresses from your life. Creating more health in your life will naturally ease the stress you may be experiencing.

Always remember to breathe. Good, deep, quality, mindful breath is medicine.

Set SMART attainable goals. Make these goals and take the time you need, applying an 80/20 philosophy.

Little, modest shifts in everyday habits add up to huge geometric changes of major proportion over time for our health and happiness.

Have fun with the process. Start by adding, not subtracting. Bring in the good stuff before cutting out the bad stuff. Make it a gradual process so the transition is easier and more enjoyable.

That's it. Now you know how to GET OFF YOUR ACID, with all the tools, strategies and tips you'll need to guide you. Are you ready to feel refreshed and energized? To clear your mind, deepen your sleep, drop that extra weight, brighten your skin, and sharpen your mind?

I'm challenging you because you deserve happiness and the healthiest life. Your life counts. Einstein said, "You can't solve a problem with the same mindset that created it." We cannot invoke change until WE change. Everyday is a new opportunity to change your life, and here's the best part, you have the power and information to rewrite your destiny. The question is, what are you going to do with it?

There's nothing to wait for . . . you've got this!

11

Coming Full Circle

> ### If I knew I was going to live this long, I'd have taken better care of myself.
>
> —GEORGE BURNS

Since we've arrived at the end of the book, it feels important to bring some closure to my personal tale. As you recall, I opened the book with my father's story. As I complete the final edits of this project, it pains me to share the news that we lost my father one week ago, on August 15, 2017. As devastating an event as it was, I can't help but acknowledge the timing of his death, with his journey paralleling my work on this project.

I opened the book with the recollection of his own battle with acid to impart just how important it is to take care of your health now, before it's too late. Health is a gift. It is our birthright and our most prized possession, but many of us wait too long to assess, nurture, and protect it. If you wait until you feel pain or discover a disease to make changes, you've lost your best fighting chances. You don't have to be perfect in your efforts—not at all. The important thing is that you make the effort. Unfortunately, my father's condition was revealed too late to reverse it permanently, though I was grateful that we were able to extend his life beyond professional expectations. His medical team told me that, without question, my work with him helped prolong his life and fight back against what was already severe and ultimately irreversible damage.

My message to you is, don't wait. Be proactive, Find your purpose. Take control of your health, and help your loved ones make positive changes at the same time. We can all support each other in a move toward better health. And if the information in this book isn't enough to incentivize you, let my father's story inspire you. I know now that this project, and the overlap with my father's experience, defines my purpose. When my father left us, I was holding his hand. In that moment, I thanked him for being the most incredible father, for being a role model, for providing me the life and opportunities that he did, and for all the sacrifices he made so that I could have a better life. Then I made a vow to him. The last thing I told him was that I would make it my life's mission to do whatever I can with the information I've learned to prevent as many people as possible from suffering as he did—no matter what it takes.

B. J. Palmer, the developer of chiropractic, said this, "You never know how far reaching something you think, say, or do today will affect the lives of millions tomorrow." I know he is right. And I know my sharing all I've learned has the power to heal millions. Please consider the teachings of this book and do what you can to cherish and protect your health. It would be the greatest honor to my father's memory and the greatest commitment to your own long and happy future.

PART III
Alkaline Recipes to
GET OFF YOUR ACID

Let food be thy medicine, and medicine be thy food.

—HIPPOCRATES

RECITES

Entrees

Desserts

ALMOND-HEMP MYLK

Serves 2 to 4

HEMP SEEDS are a great source of omega-3 fatty acid, which is very important for your growing child's brain and nervous system. It is also considered a complete protein, containing all nine essential amino acids. We used this recipe when it was time to transition our son, Brayden, off breastfeeding. But this recipe is not only for babies. We use this all the time as a foundation in our smoothies or as a healthy nut mylk that is always in the refrigerator. Keep it in an airtight glass container, and it will last for about three days (if it lasts that long!).

1 cup raw almonds, ideally soaked overnight

½ cup raw hemp seeds, ideally soaked overnight

3½ cups filtered water, divided (or 1½ cups filtered water, and 2 cups of coconut water)

1 teaspoon vanilla (I prefer to use 3 drops Medicine Flower Vanilla)

½ teaspoon salt (Celtic Grey, Himalayan, or Redmond Real Salt)

1 tablespoon cold-pressed coconut oil

1 pitted date (optional)

1 frozen banana (optional)

Soak almonds and hemp seeds overnight separately in a large bowl. In the morning, strain this to get rid of the excess water. Next, add the soaked almonds and hemp seeds into your blender. Add 1½ cups of filtered water and blend on high speed. After thoroughly blending, pour the nut mylk mixture though a cheesecloth or nut bag strainer to filter (strain the cloth inside out, as it's easier to discard contents left in nut bag when done).

Place the filtered nut mylk in the blender again and add the remaining 2 cups of filtered water (or coconut water), vanilla, sea salt, coconut oil, and optional, date and/or the frozen banana. Blend on high until you have a smooth, creamy texture. Place in an airtight container in the refrigerator. Enjoy!

MACADAMIA CHAI NUT MYLK

Serves 2 to 4

MACADAMIA NUTS are an extremely healthy fat rich in omega-7 fatty acids. That's because 80 percent of the fats in macadamia nuts are monounsaturated, like olive oil. Macadamias are also rich in palmitoleic acid, which provides the building blocks for the enzymes that control the burning of fat.

1 cup macadamia nuts

2 cups filtered water

1 cup coconut water

2 teaspoons cinnamon

1 teaspoon cardamom

½ teaspoon fresh ginger

¼ teaspoon black pepper

½ teaspoon salt (Celtic Grey, Himalayan, or Redmond Real Salt)

1 vanilla bean or 4 drops of Medicine Flower Vanilla (optional)

Using your high-speed blender, process all ingredients until creamy and smooth. After thoroughly blending, pour macadamia chai nut mylk mixture though a cheesecloth or nut bag strainer to filter (strain the cloth inside out, as it's easier to discard contents left in nut bag when done).

GOLDEN COCONUT MYLK

Serves 2 to 3

THIS SOOTHING hot drink is a wonderful alkaline replacement for morning coffee. It has phenomenal spices, both for flavor and for health. The primary health ingredient, turmeric, is anti-inflammatory, anti-bacterial, anti-fungal, and alkaline. The combination of the turmeric with ginger and black pepper is very powerful: energizing and detoxifying, fighting inflammation, and slashing cravings for sugar.

1 cup unsweetened coconut milk

1 cup filtered water

1 tablespoon fresh turmeric, grated

1 tablespoon fresh ginger, grated

½ teaspoon vanilla extract (I use 2 drops of Medicine Flower Vanilla)

½ teaspoon cinnamon

Pinch of freshly ground black pepper

Pinch of nutmeg

Pinch of ground cardamom

Pinch of ground clove

Pinch of cayenne pepper (optional)

Organic liquid stevia to sweeten, as desired (optional)

Simmer all the ingredients on the stove for 10 minutes. Strain and drink!

CHIA FRESCA

Serves 1

THIS DRINK'S known in South America as agua fresca. Many high-endurance athletes use it because it's full of alkaline minerals, or electrolytes. In addition, chia is a slow-burning fuel that provides energy all day long. It's also great for healing and recovery after exertion. It's important to note that most store-bought coconut waters are pasteurized, which destroys the bacteria, as well as the good minerals. When shopping for coconut water, look for it to be raw, straight out of the coconut. Or look for packaged brands that include cold-pressed coconut water with no other ingredients.

1 fresh lemon slice	Coconut water	4 tablespoons chia seeds

Squeeze the lemon and put the slice in the coconut water. Add the chia. Stir with a spoon and let sit for 5 to 10 minutes, or use a small handheld electric mixer to stir the chia in for 1 minute.

ALKALINE LEMONADE

Serves 4 (Makes 1 pitcher)

THIS "LEMONADE" is loaded with healthy fats that help you to burn fat. Additionally, the lemons are highly detoxifying and alkalizing. Plus, the grated ginger and cayenne are a great combination to boost metabolism, further aiding your fat-burning process.

3 lemons, peeled, seeds removed	1 teaspoon salt (Celtic Grey, Himalayan, or Redmond Real Salt)	1 teaspoon grated ginger (optional)
3 tablespoons coconut oil or extra virgin olive oil	A few drops of organic liquid stevia, to taste	Pinch of cayenne pepper (optional)
1 green apple, cored		
6 cups filtered water		

Add all the ingredients to the blender and blend on high speed. Keep refrigerated, serve, and enjoy!

DR. GREEN DETOX SMOOTHIE

Serves 1 to 2

THIS IS ONE of my favorite smoothies, as it's a pure alkaline recipe with no fruit added. When you need a real power punch of energy and cleansing vitality, you can't do better than a straight-up green smoothie. I especially love the fresh grassy flavors of the cilantro and the parsley.

1 handful of spinach

½ lemon, peeled

1-inch ginger, fresh

½ cucumber, peeled

1 small handful of cilantro

1 small handful of parsley

1 cup coconut water (or filtered water)

Optional: organic liquid stevia or 1 date

Optional: handful of ice

Blend and enjoy!

CHUNKY MONKEY SMOOTHIE

Serves 1

THIS DELICIOUS smoothie uses the powerful antioxidant cacao to create a rich, chocolaty flavor. Add in the hemp seeds and almond butter, and you have many healthy fats. If you didn't know better, you'd think it was a "guilty pleasure" milkshake. Despite all its health benefits, this is a kid pleaser—they love everything about it from the name to the taste. It even sneaks in kale—one of the planet's most powerful super foods—which is high in those ultra-essential minerals.

1 cup unsweetened coconut milk (or almond milk or hemp milk)

1 banana, peeled and frozen

½ cup kale

2 tablespoons raw almond butter

2 tablespoons raw cacao

1 tablespoon hemp seeds or chia seeds

5 mint leaves (optional)

Blend and enjoy!

OMEGA MORNING BLAST SMOOTHIE

Serves 1

I DEVELOPED this delicious sipper specifically to help increase your intake of omega-3 fatty acids. The average American diet has a 19:1 omega-6 to omega-3 ratio, which is very unbalanced. In fact, that disproportionate amount of omega-6 fatty acids consumed leads to inflammation, which, in turn, leads to disease. Start taking control of your health by integrating more of these crucial fatty acids into your diet.

1 large handful of spinach

½ cup blueberries

1 tablespoon raw almond butter

1 tablespoon chia seeds

1 tablespoon ground flaxseed

1 tablespoon hemp seeds

1 tablespoon coconut oil

1 cup coconut milk (or almond milk)

Blend and enjoy!

BLOODY MARY SMOOTHIE

Serves 2

I MUST START by telling you this is Kelly Ripa's favorite morning smoothie, and she's tried almost all of my recipes. A while back, she had a "smoothie-off" with John Leguizamo, and she made this one on "Live with Kelly." It's savory and tasty without the alcohol (so it's alkaline, not acidic), and you can even punch it up with a little extra cayenne.

4 small tomatoes (Roma tomatoes work well)

1 stalk celery

½ cucumber

1 lemon, freshly juiced

½ teaspoon cayenne pepper

¼ teaspoon salt (Celtic Grey, Himalayan, or Redmond Real Salt)

½ teaspoon black pepper

Put all the ingredients into a blender and mix well. Pour into a glass with ice, and enjoy your alkaline morning mocktail!

CARROT CAKE PROTEIN SMOOTHIE

Serves 1

THIS IS, hands-down, everyone's favorite smoothie. I once conducted an online poll, and this won by a mile. You just can't argue with something super healthy that tastes like a classic dessert. The carrots are great for your vision, thanks to the vitamin C and beta-carotene, and they're also antioxidant, so they help slow premature aging. Add a scoop of my Organic Daily Protein and you have a morning boost that tastes like a glorious treat.

1 cup unsweetened coconut milk (or almond milk)

1 tablespoon raw almond butter

½ banana, peeled and frozen

1 handful of spinach

3 carrots, shredded

1 teaspoon cinnamon

1 scoop plant protein powder (optional) (can add a scoop of Alkamind Organic Daily Protein in Creamy Chocolate or Vanilla Coconut flavors, or use

2 tablespoons of hemp seeds or chia seeds for added fats and protein)

Blend and enjoy!

CINNAMON BUN SMOOTHIE

Serves 2

WHEN I was growing up, cinnamon buns were my biggest vice. And really, they are some of the worst foods you could eat because they are loaded with gluten, sugar, and trans-fats. You can't imagine how psyched I was when I realized I could substitute something so smart that satisfies my sweet tooth craving.

1 cup almond or coconut milk

1 large handful of spinach

1 banana, peeled and frozen

2 tablespoons of raw almond butter

1 date, pitted

¾ teaspoon cinnamon

1 tablespoon hemp seeds

½ teaspoon vanilla (optional) (I prefer 2 drops of Medicine Flower Vanilla)

Ice cubes (optional)

Put all the ingredients into a blender and mix until smooth.

GREEN MINT DETOX SMOOTHIE

Serves 1 to 2

YOU WOULDN'T necessarily think to put romaine in a smoothie, but this combo is a delicious green blend that focuses on the flavors of mint and ginger, which are very healing for the gut, as they fight nausea, sooth upset stomachs, and are powerful anti-inflammatories. The lime also adds a touch of acid for a balanced and satisfying taste.

1 cucumber, peeled

6–8 leaves romaine (or large bunch spinach)

1 cup coconut water (or filtered water)

1 lime, freshly squeezed

1-inch ginger, fresh

1 bunch fresh mint leaves

Optional: organic liquid stevia or 1 date

Optional: handful of ice

Blend and enjoy!

WARRIOR CHIA BREAKFAST

Serves 2 to 3

THE TRUTH IS, I'll put chia seeds in almost anything. They're hydrophilic, which means they can expand up to twenty times in water. That gives them an interesting texture. They are also effective at cleaning the small intestine. Think of them as micro beads that move through and slough your system. In addition to providing a good amount of protein, chia is a great remedy for constipation.

This can be prepared in minutes each night and popped in the fridge. Then, it will be ready for you the next morning. In fact, the longer it sits, the thicker and richer it gets.

1 cup of almond or coconut milk, unsweetened

4 tablespoons of chia seeds

½ teaspoon vanilla (or 2 drops Medicine Flower Vanilla)

½ teaspoon cinnamon

1 tablespoon unsweetened shredded coconut flakes

¼ cup chopped nuts (raw almonds, macadamia nuts, or hemp seeds)

Fresh fruit (pomegranate seeds, strawberries, or blueberries) for topping (optional)

The night before you plan to eat this breakfast bowl, combine the almond milk and chia seeds in a mason jar. Add vanilla, cinnamon, and chopped nuts. Cover with a tight lid and shake the mixture until it's well combined. Refrigerate overnight (or for at least 5 hours).

The next morning, shake or stir the mixture and divide between two to three bowls to serve. Top with fresh fruit, coconut shreds, more chopped nuts, hemp, and/or chia seeds. This recipe makes a portion big enough to last two days (and it's even better on the second day).

WARM WINTER PORRIDGE

Serves 2

THIS RECIPE calls for full-fat coconut milk, the kind you get in the (BPA-free) can—not the one from the carton. This stuff is truly nature's gift. Loaded with healthy saturated fat, it's one of the healthiest things you can put in your body. Besides the health benefits, it's rich and creamy, with that luscious tropical flavor. The healthy fats make you feel full by satiating the brain receptors that control your appetite. Plus, they increase metabolism, which is yet another way to increase weight loss.

½ cup quinoa, rinsed

1 15-ounce can of full-fat coconut milk (I recommend Native Forest)

1 teaspoon cinnamon

1 teaspoon chia seeds

1 tablespoon sliced raw almonds

1 tablespoon hemp seeds

Combine all the ingredients in a saucepan, except the almonds and hemp seeds, and simmer for 10 to 15 minutes, or until liquid is absorbed. Place in a serving bowl and sprinkle with almonds and hemp seeds. Enjoy!

PECAN BREAKFAST BOWL

Serves 2 to 4

2 cups pecans, soaked

1 cup coconut water

½ teaspoon cinnamon

½ teaspoon salt (Celtic Grey, Himalayan, or Redmond Real Salt)

½ vanilla bean
(or 2 drops of Medicine Flower Vanilla)

Place all ingredients in a blender, and process on high speed until a smooth and creamy consistency is reached. Serve in a bowl and garnish with pieces of macadamia nuts, pecans, and/or slivered almonds.

GARLIC HUMMUS

Serves Many

2 cups garbanzo beans

5 cloves garlic

½ cup lemon juice, fresh squeezed

¼ cup raw sesame oil

¼ cup extra virgin olive oil

½ cup raw tahini

¾ cup filtered water

1 teaspoon salt (Celtic Grey, Himalayan, or Redmond Real Salt)

Paprika or smoked paprika, for garnish (optional)

To sprout garbanzo beans: soak the beans overnight in plenty of filtered water. In the morning, strain the beans, rinse in the strainer, and let them sit for a minimum of 10 to 12 hours before eating. (They may swell to almost twice their original size).

To make hummus: mix together all the ingredients in a blender or a food processor and blend until smooth. Garnish with paprika, if using. Serve with raw vegetables (radish, celery, red or yellow pepper, cucumber, broccoli, etc.) and enjoy!

TOASTED CURRY KALE CHIPS

Serves 2

I LOVE to use a dehydrator for these chips because it makes them super crispy when they dehydrate at a low heat over a long period. The process also retains all the phytonutrients, which don't cook off. Baking them in the oven on the lowest temperature will work too. Just remember to do this slow and low for the best results.

1 head of kale torn into large pieces

2 teaspoons extra virgin olive oil

1 teaspoon curry powder (or seasoning of your choice)

Salt (Celtic Grey, Himalayan, or Redmond Real Salt)

Black pepper (optional)

Toss the kale with the oil and season with curry powder, sea salt, and black pepper if you choose.

Baking method: bake for 8 to 10 minutes at 375°F or until crispy, being careful not to burn.

(Continues)

Dehydrate method: using an Excalibur dehydrator, dehydrate the kale at 115°F for about 8 hours or until the desired crispiness is reached.

Quick dehydrate method: in an Excalibur dehydrator, dry the kale at 145°F for 1 hour. Reduce the heat to 115°F and dehydrate for an additional 3 to 4 hours until crispy.

Transfer the kale chips to an airtight container, or vacuum seal for longer storage.

SAUTÉED SHISHITO PEPPERS, TWO WAYS

Serves 2 to 4

THIS APPETIZER is served at some top restaurants such as Nobu and Tao in Manhattan. You can't beat the flavor and the kick, and yet it's an easy, healthy recipe to make. If it's good enough to be served at some of the world's best restaurants, I think you're going to find it's a winner as a regular rotation. But heed my warning, one in ten will be quite spicy, so have fun playing a game of pepper roulette. However, the stakes are low, for if you lose, grab a drink of lemon water and play again!

Sautéed Peppers

10–20 Shishito peppers (depending on how many you want to serve)

1 tablespoon coconut oil

Salt (Celtic Grey, Himalayan, or Redmond Real Salt)

Peppers in Sesame Garlic Sauce

2 teaspoons toasted sesame oil

1 tablespoon coconut oil

Pinch crushed red pepper flakes

1 clove garlic, minced

1½ tablespoons wheat-free tamari (or add Braggs Liquid Aminos or Coconut Aminos)

Raw sesame seeds, for topping

For peppers: heat the oil in a pan on a medium flame. Add the Shishito peppers to the skillet and sauté, tossing frequently, until blistered and tender, roughly 3 to 4 minutes on each side. Place on a serving dish, generously add sea salt, and serve!

For peppers in sesame garlic sauce: heat the toasted sesame oil and coconut oil in a pan. Add the Shishito peppers to the skillet and sauté, tossing frequently, until blistered and tender, roughly 3 to 4 minutes each side or until slightly browned on both sides.

Add the crushed red pepper flakes and minced garlic, then cook, stirring constantly, for an additional 30 seconds. Add the tamari and cook, stirring to coat the peppers evenly, for 1 minute. Sprinkle with raw sesame seeds, serve, and enjoy!

BAKED ZUCCHINI CHIPS
WITH COOL DILL DIP

Serves 2

THERE ARE so many occasions when you want to reach for chips to nosh or dip, but as you well know, that's a terrible choice. These are my best substitute for potato chips, which are generally loaded with pro-inflammatory omega-6 fatty acids. It's a delicious swap that even your kids will love and ask for again.

Baked Zucchini Chips

2 zucchinis, sliced thin

2 tablespoons extra virgin olive oil (or coconut oil)

Salt (Celtic Grey, Himalayan, or Redmond Real Salt)

Dill Dip

½ cup canned coconut milk (I use Native Forest, thick part from top)

2 teaspoons fresh lemon juice

1 tablespoon chopped parsley

2 tablespoons chopped dill

1 clove garlic, minced

Salt (Celtic Grey, Himalayan, or Redmond Real Salt)

Black Pepper, to taste

FOR THE CHIPS: preheat the oven to 225°F and line a baking sheet with parchment paper. Thinly slice the zucchini (using a mandolin, if you like). Blot the zucchini slices with a paper towel to absorb excess water. Place the zucchini on the parchment-lined baking sheet. Brush each slice with olive oil and sprinkle with sea salt. Bake for 2 hours. Alternatively, you can use a dehydrator at 115°F for 12 hours (overnight).

For the dressing: blend all ingredients in a food processor. Add a little water if it's too thick.

HONEYCRISP APPLES WITH WARMED COCONUT BUTTER AND CINNAMON

Serves 2

WHILE HONEYCRISP apples are a good choice, you'll still want to eat a healthy fat to slow down the absorption of the sugars that would otherwise be spiking your insulin. The added fat will also slow the sugars from fermenting and turning to acid in your system. For kids, I cut the apple into a stop sign shape. You'd be amazed how far a whimsical shape goes in getting your kids' attention.

2 honeycrisp apples (or green apples), sliced	¼ cup coconut butter	½ teaspoon cinnamon

Put the apples in two serving bowls. Warm the coconut butter by placing it in a steamer for 10 minutes. Stir and drizzle the melted coconut butter on the apples. Top with cinnamon.

SAVORY AVOCADO WRAPS

Serves 1

THIS RECIPE is similar in concept to a Vietnamese spring roll. Simply roll these up to snack on, share them when entertaining, or pack them up to take on the go.

½ avocado, sliced	½ teaspoon cumin	Small handful of spinach
1 lettuce leaf	Salt (Celtic Grey, Himalayan, or Redmond Real Salt) and pepper, to taste	Green jalapeño pepper, to taste (optional)
½ tomato, diced		Alfalfa sprouts (add some power!) (optional)
1 teaspoon chopped cilantro		
¼ red onion, diced, or to taste		

Smear the avocado on the lettuce leaf and sprinkle with diced tomato, red onion, cilantro, cumin, sea salt, and pepper. Add the spinach. Fold in half and enjoy!

COCONUT OIL FAT BOMBS

Serves 12

YOU KNOW by now that coconut oil is right up there with avocados as my favorite sources of healthy fat. These bite-size bombs are the perfect treat to get a quick hit of the medium-chain triglycerides (MCT) your body needs for optimal performance. Plus, they give you long-lasting energy and taste like the tropics. Enjoy these as a snack or as a simple dessert—there's no guilt in this pleasure.

1 ½ cups unsweetened coconut flakes

¼ cup cold-pressed coconut oil

¼ cup grass-fed butter (Kerrygold) *or* add an additional ¼ cup coconut oil (for vegetarians)

¼ teaspoon cinnamon

¼ teaspoon vanilla bean powder (or 2 drops Medicine Flower Vanilla)

Pinch of salt (Celtic Grey, Himalayan, or Redmond Real Salt)

20 drops organic liquid stevia

extract (or any other low-carb sweetener such as Lo Han or coconut drops from Medicine Flower) (optional)

Preheat the oven to 350°F. Spread the shredded coconut flakes onto a baking sheet. Place in the oven and toast for 5 to 8 minutes until light golden. Mix once or twice during heating to prevent burning. Remove from the oven and carefully transfer the coconut flakes into a blender. Pulse until a smooth and runny consistency is reached.

Next, add the grass-fed butter* (softened at room temperature, chopped into pieces) and coconut oil (in its softened, liquid form, which occurs at room temperature, or above 76°F). In addition, add cinnamon, vanilla, stevia (optional), and sea salt, and blend again.

Once a smooth consistency is obtained, pour 1½ tablespoons of liquid coconut oil fat bombs into each mini muffin paper or an ice cube tray. Place in the fridge for at least 30 minutes to cool and solidify.

Enjoy when cravings for sugar arise or as a healthy snack, and a great off-peak edition when intermittent fasting!

Note: When transitioning to an alkaline diet, it is perfectly fine to use grass-fed butter, as this is a healthy fat. However, it is still a dairy product, which does have some acidifying effects. In its place, feel free to swap it out with an additional ¼ cup of coconut oil (½ cup total if not using grass-fed butter) per the instructions.

ZUCCHINI SUSHI

Serves 2

FOR ALL you sushi lovers out there, this yummy recipe will give you a fix. It's easy finger food for kids, and it's also elegant enough to serve as an impressive treat to share when entertaining. The filling can also be used as a veggie dip—the dip is super flavorful, and you can use it to dress other dishes if the recipe is doubled.

4 zucchinis

¼ cup parsley

1 can artichoke hearts

2 cloves garlic

1 lemon, freshly juiced

1 teaspoon lemon zest

1 can white beans

¼ cup raw cashews or macadamia nuts

1 tablespoon coconut oil

Salt (Celtic Grey, Himalayan, or Redmond Real Salt)

Pepper to taste

Slice the zucchini lengthwise using a mandolin, or slice it very thin with a knife or potato peeler. Brush with olive oil and set aside.

Blend the parsley, artichoke, garlic, lemon juice and zest, white beans, and cashews in a food processor until paste-like. Flash sauté the zucchini slices in the coconut oil for 1 minute on each side, or use them raw. Spread the filling on each zucchini slice. Roll up. Season with sea salt and pepper.

DR. DARYL'S FAVORITE MARINATED KALE SALAD AND DRESSING

Serves 2

This is my favorite salad in the world, and I could eat it every day—in fact, I often do. That's why I named it after myself. This also includes simply the best dressing, and it doubles as a tasty dip for veggie sticks (which is a great alkaline snack on and off the 7-Day Alkaline Cleanse). I always make at least twice the amount so I have extra because I'll put it on anything and everything. Try making it in a blender or mini food processor (the latter makes it a bit thicker). You can also substitute coconut aminos for Braggs if you prefer the flavor.

Dressing

½ cup extra virgin olive oil

2 tablespoons lime juice

2 tablespoons Braggs Liquid Aminos

2 tablespoons red onion, minced

1 clove garlic

½ teaspoon chipotle powder

1½ pitted dates

¼ teaspoon salt (Celtic Grey, Himalayan, or Redmond Real Salt)

Pinch cayenne pepper

Salad

1 bunch kale, Romaine lettuce, or spinach

1 yellow or red bell pepper (no green, as they are acidic) (optional)

1 avocado, sliced or diced (optional)

1 tomato, sliced (optional)

Mix the salad dressing ingredients in a mini blender or food processor on high speed until completely smooth and set aside.

After washing the kale leaves thoroughly, tear out the center ribs, and chop or break apart the leaves into bite-size pieces. Place the kale in a large container where you'll be able to toss the leaves easily. Pour some fresh squeezed lemon juice (½ lemon) and 1 teaspoon sea salt over the leaves and toss, toss, toss (there should be a light coating on each leaf). Cover the kale and refrigerate (30 to 60 minutes is fine).

Slice the red or yellow peppers and add to the kale. Add the dressing and thoroughly mix to soften up the kale even further. Place the kale on a plate and then add the sliced avocado and tomatoes. Add additional sea salt to taste.

GREEN TAHINI KALE SALAD

Serves 4

HAVE YOU ever noticed that sometimes kale isn't as nicely textured as it could be? That's because you need to break up the fibrous veins in the leaves before you use it. When working with kale, I put it in a BPA-free bag with lemon and sea salt and let it sit for 30 minutes to tenderize it. It can also be massaged with olive oil and sea salt to achieve the same tenderizing effect.

Tahini Dressing

⅓ cup extra virgin olive oil

3 tablespoons tahini

2 tablespoons plus ½ teaspoon apple cider vinegar

2 teaspoons gluten-free tamari (or Braggs Liquid Aminos)

2¼ teaspoons lemon juice, freshly squeezed

¾ teaspoon salt (Celtic Grey, Himalayan, or Redmond Real Salt)

1 large clove garlic, minced

1½ teaspoons raw sesame seeds

1 tablespoon parsley, minced

1 tablespoon chives, minced

Salad

1 bunch kale

1 yellow or red bell pepper, diced or strips

1 tomato, diced

1 avocado, cubed

Sprouts, for topping (optional)

For the dressing: combine all the ingredients except the herbs in a small mixing bowl and whisk or blend together. Once thoroughly mixed, add the herbs to the dressing and stir in thoroughly with a spoon.

For the salad: kale can be tough. If you wish to soften it first, add 1 teaspoon of sea salt and ½ lemon juice, massage in with hands and let sit for 30 minutes. Otherwise, place the kale in a large mixing bowl. Add in the diced bell pepper and the tahini dressing, and thoroughly mix with a spoon. Next, add the tomatoes, avocado cubes, and sprouts to top. Season with sea salt and pepper, serve, and enjoy!

THAI QUINOA SALAD

Serves 2

THE SECRET to the punchy flavor here is apple cider vinegar, which I use both for taste and for its alkaline-forming properties, which makes it a tonic for anyone dealing with reflux. This dish combines the apple cider vinegar with lemon, garlic, and tahini for a zesty flavor with a hint of Thai influence.

Thai Dressing

¼ cup plus 2 tablespoons filtered water

1 tablespoon sesame seeds

1 teaspoon garlic, chopped

1 teaspoon lemon juice, freshly squeezed

3 teaspoons apple cider vinegar

2 teaspoons gluten-free tamari

¼ cup raw tahini (sesame butter)

1 date, pitted

½ teaspoon salt (Celtic Grey, Himalayan, or Redmond Real Salt)

½ teaspoon toasted sesame oil

Salad

1 cup quinoa

1 large handful of arugula

1 tomato, sliced

¼ red onion, diced

Steam the quinoa in a steamer or rice cooker and set aside. If cooking on the stovetop, combine 1 cup of quinoa with 2 cups of filtered water or yeast-free vegetable broth, and cook over medium heat for 15 to 20 minutes or until all the liquid is absorbed.

Blend the dressing ingredients in a blender.

Combine the quinoa, arugula, sliced tomatoes, and diced red onion on a serving plate or in a bowl. Add the Thai dressing, hand mix with a spoon, and serve.

AVOCADO, TOMATO, AND RED ONION SALAD

Serves 2

THIS IS a simple, quick, and easy salad to make. I actually have it for breakfast quite often. I know it's unusual, but you should try it sometime. Skip the bacon and eggs and give yourself some healthy fats to start your day; you'll be amazed at how great you feel. It's also a nice side dish or even an entree.

(Continues)

2 avocados, diced

Salt (Celtic Grey, Himalayan, or Redmond Real Salt) and black pepper to taste

1 tomato, diced

½ red onion, diced

1 cucumber, sliced

¼ cup cilantro, finely chopped (or parsley)

2 tablespoons extra virgin olive oil

1 tablespoon lime juice, freshly

squeezed

1 teaspoon cumin

½ jalapeño, diced, to taste

Season the avocado with sea salt and pepper. In a small bowl, combine the tomatoes, onion, cucumber, cilantro, and cumin; season with more sea salt and pepper and arrange over the avocados. Drizzle olive oil and lime juice over the top, and gently mix everything together. Add the jalapeño for a kick!

GREEN SPRING SALAD WITH JALAPEÑO MINT DRESSING

Serves 4

JALAPEÑO IS a great ingredient for metabolism. Be careful, though, because some are much hotter than others. Remember that less is more: start with a little and increase to your taste. I always make more of this dressing and drizzle it or dip in it on everything for the next four days. It's a great strategy to keep you alkaline because salad making is a whiz when the dressings already made.

Salad

1 head of kale, cut into small ribbons

1 cucumber, chopped

1 beet, shredded

2 tablespoons sunflower seeds

2 tablespoons hemp seeds

Dressing

¼ cup lemon juice, freshly squeezed

⅔ cup extra virgin olive oil

1 teaspoon black pepper

1 tablespoon fresh mint

1 small jalapeño, finely chopped (remove seeds for less heat)

Salt (Celtic Grey, Himalayan, or Redmond Real Salt)

For the salad: combine all the ingredients in a large bowl. Dress only the salad you will be eating.

For the dressing: whisk all the ingredients together and season with sea salt. Pour enough onto the salad to coat all the veggies. Feel free to massage the dressing into the kale with your hands, or let the kale marinate in it for 30 minutes to soften its texture.

WATERCRESS GRAPEFRUIT SALAD

Serves 4

MANY OF us think of watercress as this dainty, delicate green that's eaten on finger sandwiches, but that couldn't be further from reality. In a super food nutrient rating, watercress received 100 out of 100 points, unseating the king of all greens, kale. While some citrus is acidic, the citric acid in grapefruit is alkaline once consumed. That means you can enjoy the crisp and refreshing flavors while benefitting from a high-mineral, low-sugar fruit. Combined with these power greens, it's one of the most powerful salads you can eat.

Dressing

½ teaspoon ginger, minced

Juice of 1 lime, freshly squeezed

½ teaspoon salt (Celtic Grey, Himalayan, or Redmond Real Salt)

2 tablespoons extra virgin olive oil

Salad

2 cups watercress leaves, chopped

2 scallions, chopped into small pieces

2 tablespoons cilantro leaves, chopped

2 tablespoons mint leaves, chopped

2 tablespoons basil leaves, torn

1 medium grapefruit, sectioned

2 tablespoons raw almonds, sliced

4 tablespoons pomegranate seeds

1 teaspoons raw sesame seeds

½ teaspoon jalapeño, minced

½ avocado, sliced

For the dressing: in small bowl, whisk together the ginger, lime juice, sea salt, and extra virgin olive oil.

For the salad: in a large mixing bowl, add the chopped watercress, chopped scallions, cilantro, mint, and basil. Cut the grapefruit into bite-size pieces and add to the mixing bowl. Drizzle the ginger dressing over the salad and mix well. Top with sliced almonds, pomegranate seeds, sesame seeds, jalapeño, and avocado.

RAW CHOPPED SALAD WITH LEMON TARRAGON DRESSING

Serves 4

THIS SALAD is colorful, flavorful, and highly recommended for those with arthritis. That's because the celery helps stimulate the lymph system and remove toxins such as uric acid—an acidic byproduct of protein and fructose metabolism. That movement and increased flow can provide relief to inflammation in the joints.

Salad

1 head of kale, cut into small ribbons

2 stalks of celery, diced

1 cucumber, diced

2 carrots, diced

1 fennel, thinly sliced

1 beet, shredded

1 tablespoon sunflower seeds, preferably soaked overnight to sprout

1 15-ounce can garbanzo beans, rinsed and drained (I prefer Eden Organics)

Dressing

¼ cup lime juice, fresh squeezed

2 tablespoons apple cider vinegar

⅔ cup extra virgin olive oil

1 small handful of tarragon leaves, chopped

1 teaspoon black pepper

Salt (Celtic Grey, Himalayan, or Redmond Real Salt)

Combine all the salad ingredients in a large bowl. Dress only what you will eat. Whisk all the dressing ingredients together and season with sea salt. Pour enough onto salad to coat all the veggies. Serve and enjoy!

APPLE CABBAGE SALAD WITH BEETROOT

Serves 4

CABBAGE RANKS up there with broccoli, Brussels sprouts, and cauliflower in its reputation for fighting cancer. It's loaded with fiber and the alkaline mineral potassium, so I recommend cancer patients eat cabbage whenever possible, especially raw and in juices. This salad is surprisingly light and refreshing, and it's great at summer barbecues for a lighter alternative to mayonnaise-laden coleslaw.

(Continues)

Apple Cabbage Salad with Beetroot (Continued)

Salad

1 head of butter lettuce

1 green apple, spiralized

1 small beet, spiralized

1 cup purple cabbage, chopped

2 tablespoons hemp seeds

2 tablespoons sunflower seeds

Dressing

¼ cup lemon juice, fresh squeezed

2 tablespoons apple cider vinegar

⅔ cup extra virgin olive oil

¼ cup cilantro, chopped

1 teaspoon black pepper

Salt (Celtic Grey, Himalayan, or Redmond Real Salt)

For the salad: chop the lettuce and cabbage, and spiralize or use a vegetable peeler for the green apple and beet. Mix all salad ingredients together in a mixing bowl.

For the dressing: whisk all ingredients together and season with sea salt. Dress the salad just before eating. Store salad and dressing separately.

CARROT GINGER AVOCADO SALAD

Serves 4

I LOVE the fresh Asian flavors of this salad, especially because the onion dressing reminds me so much of the common version in sushi restaurants. Plus, the sesame, tahini and tamari flavors give it delicious umami depth.

Salad

1 head of romaine lettuce, chopped

1 avocado, sliced or diced

1 red bell pepper, sliced or diced

½ red onion, chopped

1 tomato, diced, or ½ cup halved cherry tomatoes (optional)

Dressing

¼ cup filtered water

2 tablespoons lemon juice, fresh squeezed

1 tablespoon extra virgin olive oil

1 teaspoon tahini

½ teaspoon sesame oil, toasted

1 tablespoon shoyu or wheat-free tamari or Braggs Liquid Aminos

½ cup carrots, chopped and unpeeled

2 tablespoons ginger, chopped

¼ teaspoon salt (Celtic Grey, Himalayan, or Redmond Real Salt)

1 date, pitted

1 teaspoon apple cider vinegar (optional)

Place all dressing ingredients in blender and blend at high speed. In a mixing bowl, combine dressing with romaine lettuce, red onion, and red bell pepper, and mix well. Place in a serving bowl with sliced avocado on top, and enjoy!

BONELESS BROTH

Serves 2 to 4

THIS ALKALINE vegetable broth can be enjoyed raw, or it can be consumed hot as well. It is a high-potassium mineral broth made by cooking any combination of alkaline vegetables below:

Green leafy vegetables: kale, spinach, chard, watercress, beet greens, collard greens, turnip greens, mustard greens

Green and white vegetables: celery, fennel, cabbage green beans, zucchini, broccoli, fennel, turnip, parsnip, leeks, new potatoes (scrubbed with eyes removed, cut ¼ inch thick. The most nutritious part of the new potato is the peel and the pulp next to it, so you can peel the potato and simmer the peelings with the rest of the broth to maximize the nutrients, vitamins, and minerals)

Red and orange vegetables: carrots, beets, sweet potatoes, squash

Herbs and spices: cumin, turmeric, cayenne pepper, dill, garlic, ginger, parsley, cilantro, and onion. If using onion and garlic or spices such as cumin and turmeric, sautéed them in the pot with a little coconut oil.

My preferred combination:

2 medium zucchinis

2 leeks, chopped

2 celery stalks, chopped

2 bunches of parsley, stems removed and leaves chopped

1 bunch of spinach, stems removed and leaves chopped

½ pound of green beans, trimmed

1 onion, chopped

5 cloves of garlic

1 quart of filtered water

Salt (Celtic Grey, Himalayan, or Redmond Real Salt) to taste

Choose at least four of the vegetables from the list above. Thoroughly wash all of the vegetables, and then chop them into small bite-size pieces, enough for 2 cups.

Place the vegetables in a stockpot with 1 quart of filtered water, adding some sea salt and spices and herbs (I always add garlic).

(Continues)

Boneless Broth (Continued)

Bring the water to a boil, and then lower the heat to low and simmer for about 45 minutes or until the vegetables are soft.

Cool and strain the broth. The remaining vegetables can be pureed with an immersion blender or discarded since most of the nutrients have been extracted. The broth will keep for a few days in the refrigerator in a tightly sealed container. Larger quantities can be frozen for future consumption.

RED LENTIL AND KALE SOUP

Serves 4

THIS DISH is my wife, Chelsea's, favorite because it's very filling, comforting, easy to make, and absolutely delicious. It's also great for weight loss. There are three kinds of lentils: red, green, and brown. I like the red variety for soups because they get soft and have a nice texture. They're also the sweetest and nuttiest. When I tell people to eat beans and legumes, I recommend the small ones, and these lentils fit the bill. They cook quickly (as opposed to green ones, which are firmer and take twice as long). Kale is also great here because it gets soft, unlike in salads when you have to tenderize it with lemon juice. I recommend making a huge batch of this for leftovers—it gets better and better as the flavors meld together.

1 tablespoon coconut oil

1 medium onion, finely chopped

4 garlic cloves, minced

2 large carrots, chopped

2 stalks of celery, chopped

1 bunch of kale, cut into ribbons

6 cups of vegetable broth

1½ cups red lentils, rinsed

Salt (Celtic Grey, Himalayan, or Redmond Real Salt) to taste

Black pepper, to taste

Heat the coconut oil in a large pot over medium heat. Add the onion and sauté until translucent, about 3 to 5 minutes. Add the garlic, carrots, celery, and kale and sauté for 2 to 3 minutes. Add the broth, lentils, sea salt, and pepper. Cook on medium-low heat until the lentils are tender, 20 minutes. Serve and enjoy!

CURRIED CARROT SOUP

Serves 4

FOUR OF my favorite spices come alive in this curry: coriander, cumin, turmeric, and cardamom. And while flavor is king, this dish is hugely healthy. Although curry can be made up of a number of spices, it's often yellow in color because of the turmeric—that lets you know it's usually going to be an anti-inflammatory dish packed with antioxidants. Turmeric is great for memory because of its primary ingredient, curcumin. Studies have shown curcumin may clear the brain of plaque and protein deposits, which can help fight cancers, Alzheimer's, and other life-threatening conditions.

1 tablespoon coconut oil

1½ inch piece of ginger, sliced and crushed

4 cloves garlic, minced

Zest and juice of one lime

2 teaspoons curry powder

1 teaspoon turmeric

3 cups carrots cut into 1-inch pieces

1 15-ounce can of full-fat coconut milk (I recommend Native Forest brand)

2 cups water, filtered

½ bunch cilantro, chopped

Heat the coconut oil in a large saucepan over medium heat. Add the ginger, garlic, and lime zest and cook until slightly browned, about 3 to 4 minutes. Add the curry and cook until fragrant, about 1 minute.

Add the carrots, coconut milk, and water. Bring to a boil, reduce to low and simmer, covered, for 15 minutes. Turn off the heat and leave it on the stove for 30 minutes to allow flavors to meld.

Puree the soup in a blender or a food processor. Garnish with chopped cilantro and lime juice, and enjoy!

HEARTY WINTER VEGGIE SOUP

Serves 4

FLAVOR ABOUNDS in this rustic, Italian-inspired recipe. The robust combination of mineral-rich vegetables makes a satisfying entree with plenty of nutritive power. The white beans deliver a good dose of protein, while the cabbage is full of healthy fiber.

(Continues)

Hearty Winter Veggie Soup (Continued)

3 tablespoons extra virgin olive oil

3 leeks, green parts removed and thinly sliced

2 carrots

1 fennel bulb, thinly sliced

4 cloves of garlic, minced

2 fresh rosemary sprigs, leaves removed and chopped

1 cup savoy cabbage (green cabbage), thinly sliced

6 cups of vegetable stock (yeast free)

1 15-ounce can white beans, drained and rinsed (I use Eden Organics)

Handful of parsley leaves, chopped

Salt (Celtic Grey, Himalayan, or Redmond Real Salt) and pepper, to taste

In a large soup pot, heat the oil over medium low heat, add the leeks, carrots, and fennel and cook until the leeks are soft and slightly browned, about 5 to 8 minutes. Add the garlic and rosemary and cook for another minute. Add the cabbage and sauté another minute. Add stock and bring to a boil. Add the beans and cook on low for 10 to 15 minutes until the veggies are tender. Stir in the parsley and season with sea salt and pepper.

SUMMER GAZPACHO

Serves 2 to 4

THIS IS my favorite summer soup. The ingredients are highly detoxifying and the flavors are just so pronounced and refreshing. It works well as a meal or served in cocktail glasses with spoons as a nice appetizer at a garden party. Even though it's titled "summer," this delicious soup can be enjoyed year round. The longer it sits, the better it tastes!

4 large beefsteak tomatoes

1 red bell pepper

1 cucumber

½ red onion

¼ cup fresh cilantro

¼ cup fresh parsley

2 large cloves garlic

½ lime, freshly squeezed

1 lemon, freshly squeezed

3 tablespoons extra virgin olive oil

1 teaspoon salt (Celtic Grey, Himalayan, or Redmond Real Salt) or to taste

1 teaspoon black pepper, or to taste

Place everything in a food processor with the "S" blade. Pulse blend, leaving it slightly chunky or smooth, whichever you prefer (I prefer slightly chunky).

ULTIMATE CHILLED SUMMER GREENS

Serves 2 to 4

HERE'S A winner for a hot summer day. This recipe is all about combining the most powerful alkaline greens so you get a super dose of chlorophyll—that potent blood cleanser and detoxifier. It's fabulous for the health of your digestive system and highly recommended for anyone who's constipated. You can also kick this up a notch with a little cayenne or smoky paprika.

2 cups of filtered water

2 medium cucumbers, chopped

½ bunch of favorite greens (kale, spinach, arugula, chard)

2 celery stalks

¼ cup freshly squeezed lemon juice (freshly squeezed)

¼ cup extra virgin olive oil

1 clove garlic

1 teaspoon salt (Celtic Grey, Himalayan, or Redmond Real Salt)

Basil, paprika, or cayenne, for garnish

Blend all the ingredients except the herbs together in a blender at high speed to the desired consistency. Eat right away or serve chilled. Garnish with basil, paprika, or cayenne.

RADIANT RAW RED PEPPER BISQUE

Serves 2 to 4

I LOVE this bisque for its smooth texture and savory flavor, but there are plenty of health reasons to celebrate this soup, too. Red bell peppers are commonplace, but their benefits are extraordinary. They contain more than 200 percent of your vitamin C intake, and they're rich in lycopene, which has been shown to fight cancers, including prostate and lung. They're also high in vitamin A and folate. Best of all, red bell peppers help burn more calories, and they stimulate thermogenesis, which speeds up metabolism.

(Continues)

Radiant Raw Red Pepper Bisque (Continued)

3 cups filtered water

¼ cup extra virgin olive oil

1 teaspoon caraway seeds

2 cloves garlic

2 medium red bell peppers, chopped

2 medium cucumbers, chopped

½ medium red onion, chopped

1 teaspoon salt (Celtic Grey, Himalayan, or Redmond Real Salt)

Paprika or cayenne, for garnish

Blend at high speed to desired consistency, eat right away, or serve chilled.

SPICED COLD TOMATO GINGER SOUP

Serves 2 to 4

MOST PEOPLE have tried gazpacho, and it is certainly one of my favorite refreshing summer recipes, but it can be somewhat predictable in its flavor profiles. This version brings some fresh flavor with Asian spices and ginger. You get all the healthful phytonutrients from lycopene in the tomato plus the anti-inflammatory properties of ginger.

3 tomatoes

¼ cup sun-dried tomatoes

4 ounces minced ginger

½ cup tahini

1 teaspoon cardamom

1 teaspoon cumin

½ teaspoon caraway

2 cloves garlic

¼ cup chopped basil

¼ chopped parsley

¼ cup extra virgin olive oil

1 teaspoon salt (Celtic Grey, Himalayan, or Redmond Real Salt)

Place all ingredients in a blender and blend to desired consistency. Add filtered water to reach desired consistency if necessary.

CAULIFLOWER STEAKS WITH GINGER, TURMERIC, AND CUMIN

Serves 4

I HATED cauliflower when I was growing up. What a different story today. I ordered this dish at Morini, a wonderful restaurant in Manhattan, and Chelsea and I both fell in love with it. After much trial and error, we finally re-created it, making an anti-inflammatory version of the steak sauce. Remember to sauté the cauliflower with coconut oil because it holds a high heat—unlike many other kinds of oils that can go rancid and turn into trans fats. You'll notice it doesn't make food taste like coconut; there is only the subtlest hint. I hope you love this one as much as we do!

Cauliflower Steaks

1 large head cauliflower

1 tablespoon coconut oil

Salt (Celtic Grey, Himalayan, or Redmond Real Salt) and pepper to taste

Anti-Inflammatory Steak Sauce

1 tablespoon extra virgin olive oil

1 teaspoon freshly grated ginger

1 teaspoon ground cumin

½ teaspoon ground turmeric

Small handful of cilantro, chopped

For the Steaks: preheat the oven to 400°F. Cut the stem off the cauliflower and remove any leaves. Using a large knife, slice the cauliflower from the top to the base into "steaks" (¾ inch thick or so).

Season each steak on both sides with sea salt and black pepper.

Heat the coconut oil in a pan over medium to high heat. Cook the cauliflower steak until golden brown and crispy, and then turn over and do the same to the other side (about 2 minutes each side, give or take, depending on the size of the cauliflower steak). Then transfer the steaks to a baking sheet.

For the Steak Sauce: in a separate bowl, whisk together 1 tablespoon of olive oil, ginger, cumin, and turmeric. Brush (or place with a spoon) the mixture onto the cauliflower steaks.

Roast in the oven until tender, about 15 minutes. Garnish with cilantro and serve.

QUINOA BURRITO BOWL

Serves 2

THIS ENTREE is easy to make and so delicious. I like adzuki beans not only because they are a complete protein but also because they are smaller and easier to digest than other beans. I soak them overnight or buy them in a BPA-free can. This dish is a weekly staple in our house because our son, Brayden, loves it, too.

1 cup quinoa

2 cups filtered water

2 15-ounce cans of adzuki beans, rinsed and drained (I use Eden Organic)

4 green onions, sliced

2 limes, freshly juiced

4 garlic cloves, minced

1 heaping teaspoon cumin

2 avocados, sliced

Small handful of cilantro, chopped

Cook the quinoa by combining the water and quinoa in a pot over high heat. When the water comes to a boil, cover the pot and turn the heat down to the lowest setting and cook for 15-20 minutes, or until the water is absorbed and quinoa is cooked.

While the quinoa is cooking, pour the beans into a small saucepan and cook over low heat. Stir in the onions, lime juice, garlic, and cumin and let the flavors combine for 10 to 15 minutes.

When the quinoa is done, scoop it into individual serving bowls. Top with beans, avocado, and cilantro. Serve and enjoy!

ZUCCHINI LINGUINE WITH SPINACH LEMON PESTO

Serves 2

ONE OF the biggest challenges for me in going alkaline has been finding a substitute for pasta. I'm Italian, after all. But pasta is gluten, and it's one of the most acidic substances on earth. So when I discovered "zoodles" (or zucchini spiraled "noodles"), it changed everything. You can make them with a peeler, but I recommend investing in a spiralizer. The texture mimics pasta exactly, and it really feels like the actual thing. You can eat zoodles raw or flash sauté them

(Continues)

Zucchini Linguine with
Spinach Lemon Pesto (Continued)

for no more than four minutes, which preserves the enzymes. Add a warm sauce, and there won't be any need to sauté them. I make my zoodles myself, but more and more stores are selling them packaged in the produce section, which makes eating alkaline easier.

4 medium zucchinis

3 cups baby spinach

¼ cup basil

3 garlic cloves

¼ cup cashews

½ cup extra virgin olive oil

Juice of 1 small to medium lemon

Salt (Celtic Grey, Himalayan, or Redmond Real Salt) to taste

Pepper, to taste

½ cup cherry tomatoes sliced in half

To make the zucchini pasta: use a spiralizer to turn the zucchini into long strands. These are best raw, or they can be flash sautéed.

To make the spinach lemon pesto: in a food processor with an S blade, pulse the spinach, basil, garlic, and cashews until finely chopped.

With the food processor on, slowly add the olive oil and lemon juice. Season with sea salt and pepper.

Toss the zucchini pasta with spinach lemon pesto and serve. Garnish with cherry tomatoes.

COLLARD GREEN BANH MI

Serves 1

THIS IS a fun recipe to make. It feels like fancy restaurant food, as it's a delicate wrap with a super yummy dipping sauce. It makes an elegant presentation if you're entertaining, and it's loaded with sprouts and avocado so it's as healthy as it is enticing. It's a total crowd pleaser at a party, and it's easy to pass on trays as finger food.

Dipping Sauce

¼ cup extra virgin olive oil

1 teaspoon ginger, minced (grating it with a zester is an easy way to do this)

1 garlic clove, minced

1 green onion, sliced

(Continues)

Collard Green Banh Mi (Continued)

Banh Mi

½ cucumber, cut into matchsticks

1 carrot, cut into matchsticks

½ avocado, sliced

Small handful of mung bean sprouts (can be found in the produce section—if not available other sprouts will suffice)

2 sprigs basil, chopped

3–4 sprigs mint, chopped

Small handful of cilantro, chopped

1 large collard green with thick part of stem removed

1 endive (optional)

In a bowl, mix all the dipping sauce ingredients and set aside.

Roll the cucumber, carrot, avocado, sprouts, and herbs in the collard green like you would a burrito. (If you like, use an endive to tie the collard green). Serve with the dipping sauce.

FRIED "RICE" WITH HOT SAUCE

Serves 4

I LOVE fried rice, and this is an amazing substitute you won't recognize. A classic Asian-style dish, alkaline fried rice is a great swap for grains. I created the healthy hot sauce using Eastern flavor inspiration. Most hot sauces are loaded with artificial sugars and ingredients, but not this one. Make some extra and use it on anything—you can moderate spiciness with cayenne, too.

Dr. Daryl's Hot Sauce

¼ cup extra virgin olive oil

2 tablespoons paprika

1 teaspoon smoked paprika

¼ cup chopped white onion

1 small clove of garlic

Pinch of cayenne to taste

Pinch of salt (Celtic Grey, Himalayan, or Redmond Real Salt)

Black pepper to taste

Cauliflower Rice

1 head cauliflower

2 tablespoons coconut oil

2 tablespoons garlic, minced

½ cup purple cabbage, finely diced

¼ cup broccoli

½ medium onion, finely diced

½ cup carrots, finely diced

Salt (Celtic Grey, Himalayan, or Redmond Real Salt)

Black pepper to taste

3 tablespoons Braggs Liquid Aminos

¼ to ½ cubed avocado, for topping

(Continues)

Blend the hot sauce ingredients together in a small blender and set aside.

Cut the stem off the cauliflower head and remove any leaves. Place the cauliflower into a food processor, and pulse for 30 seconds or so (the cauliflower should look like rice, and you'll need about 2 cups worth).

In a large saucepan or wok, heat the coconut oil on medium to high heat. Add the minced garlic and vegetables, sea salt, and black pepper. Add the Braggs Liquid Aminos, mix, and sauté for about 10 to 15 minutes, until the vegetables are tender.

Top with Dr. Daryl's Hot Sauce and sliced avocado.

SPAGHETTI SQUASH WITH MARINARA

Serves 2

SPAGHETTI SQUASH is one of the coolest options for an alkaline eater. Just use your fork to pull it out of the skin, like Mother Nature's spaghetti. It's also a low-starch veggie, so you can eat it regularly and feel great about it. Add my divine marinara, sneak in extra veggies, and your kids will gobble it up with no clue how healthy it is.

Marinara

3 medium tomatoes

½ cup basil leaves (loose)

¼ cup extra virgin olive oil

¼ cup sun-dried tomatoes

¼ cup red onion, chopped

2 tablespoons fresh oregano, chopped

1 tablespoon lemon juice, freshly squeezed

1 large clove of garlic

1 teaspoon salt (Celtic Grey, Himalayan, or Redmond Real Salt)

1 teaspoon black pepper

1 tablespoon rosemary, sage, or tarragon, chopped (optional)

2 cups of spinach (optional—a great way to sneak in more greens)

Spaghetti Squash

1 medium spaghetti squash

1 large handful of spinach

2 teaspoons coconut oil

2 teaspoons garlic, minced

Salt (Celtic Grey, Himalayan, or Redmond Real Salt) to taste

Black pepper, to taste

For the marinara: for a smooth sauce, place all contents in blender and blend until desired consistency is obtained. For a chunky sauce, set aside two tomatoes and the herbs. Blend everything else until smooth and creamy. Now place the contents in a food

(Continues)

Spagehetti Squash with Marinara (Continued)

processor. Then, add the two tomatoes and herbs, pulse ingredients together, leaving the sauce a bit chunky.

For the spaghetti squash: preheat the oven to 375°F. Cut the spaghetti squash in half lengthwise. Scoop out the seeds and stringy flesh with a spoon. Rub a teaspoon of coconut oil over the inside of each half. Rub both insides with minced garlic and sprinkle with sea salt and pepper. Place the squash face down on a baking sheet and bake for 35 minutes.

Carefully, use a fork to shred the spaghetti squash into strands. Heat a saucepan over medium heat. Place the squash in the pan and cover with marinara sauce (I use about two-thirds of the sauce and save the rest). Toss to combine until warmed through. Top with fresh basil and red pepper flakes before serving.

QUINOA-STUFFED BELL PEPPERS

Serves 4

I LOVE the way all these ingredients are packaged neatly into the pepper. It's easy to make and easy to enjoy. Traditionally, this recipe from Eastern Europe is often stuffed with ground beef, cheese, and rice. You know what I think about those: acid city. My version is alkaline and equally as flavorful and satisfying. It makes a hearty meal, especially for the fall or winter seasons.

1 cup quinoa

2 cups filtered water or yeast-free vegetable broth

1 tablespoon coconut oil

½ cup yellow onion, chopped

½ cup tomatoes, chopped

1 cup canned adzuki beans (I prefer Eden Organic)

1 tablespoon cumin

¼ cup cilantro, chopped

8 red bell peppers

1½ cups vegetable broth (yeast-free)

2 sliced avocados

Salt (Celtic Grey, Himalayan, or Redmond Real Salt)

Lime juice

Black pepper to taste

For the quinoa: in a small saucepan, combine the quinoa with the water over medium heat and bring to a boil. Lower the heat, cover, and continue to cook until all of the water has evaporated and the quinoa is tender, about 15 to 20 minutes. Uncover and fluff the quinoa, and transfer it to a large bowl.

(Continues)

For the onion mixture: in a large skillet over medium heat, add the coconut oil and onions. Sauté the onions until slightly softened, about 2 minutes. Add the tomatoes and cook for another minute. Next, add in adzuki beans, cumin, and cilantro. Cook approximately another 2 minutes and remove from the heat.

Combine the quinoa and onion mixture well. Cut the tops off the bell peppers and remove the insides. Fill each pepper with the quinoa and onion mixture. Place the stuffed peppers in a large pot or Dutch oven and pour the vegetable broth into the bottom of the pot. Cover and cook over a very low flame for about 45 minutes.

When ready to serve, remove the lid and let cool for 5 to 10 minutes. Transfer the quinoa peppers to plates using a slotted spoon. Place a few slices of avocado on top, squeeze some lime juice, and season with sea salt and black pepper.

INDIAN-SPICED BOK CHOY

Serves 1 to 2

3 cups bok choy, shredded (or use spinach)

1 tablespoon coconut oil

½ cup red bell pepper, diced

2 tablespoons fresh basil, finely chopped

½ cup pine nuts

1 cup walnuts, soaked overnight

1½ tablespoons fresh lemon juice

1 tablespoon fresh ginger

1 tablespoon garam masala

½ teaspoon salt (Celtic Grey, Himalayan, or Redmond Real Salt)

1 tablespoon garlic, minced

½ tablespoon black pepper

Optional: add jalapeño or chili pepper for a kick!

Flash sauté the bok choy or spinach and diced red bell pepper with coconut oil in a pan for 5 minutes, or until the ingredients are slightly softened. Combine the bok choy, diced red bell pepper, and chopped basil in a mixing bowl and set aside.

Process the remaining ingredients in a food processor with the "S" blade until smooth. Combine this with the bok choy mixture and mix well. Let it sit for 1 to 2 hours. Serve and enjoy!

BRUSSELS SPROUTS WITH PISTACHIOS AND LEMON

Serves 4

CAULIFLOWER WASN'T the only vegetable I hated growing up; I disliked Brussels sprouts just as much! I'd like to blame my aversion for them on their potential to be bitter or sour. But truthfully, as a kid, I had an aversion to anything that was green and good for me. I would try to give them to the dog, and even the dog wouldn't eat them. Now, these powerhouse veggies are a favorite, not just of mine, but of alkaline eaters everywhere. Have you noticed how many fantastic restaurants feature roasted Brussels sprouts? They taste amazing, and they're a great source of iron, protein, vitamin C, potassium, and sulforaphane—a chemical thought to contain anti-cancer properties. Sprouts are super for anybody who's anemic, and they are antioxidant, which means they help slow premature aging. Remember never to boil them, as all that mineral goodness will cook out. Instead, sauté, roast, steam, or stir fry.

2 tablespoons coconut oil

¾ cup pistachios, shelled

Zest and juice from one lemon

16 large Brussels sprouts, leaves separated from the core. Cut the end of the sprout off and peel off leaves

Salt (Celtic Grey, Himalayan, or Redmond Real Salt) and pepper to taste

Heat coconut oil in a large wok or skillet over medium-high heat. Add pistachios and lemon zest and sauté for 1 minute. Add Brussels sprouts leaves and toss until bright green but still crisp, about 5 minutes. Squeeze lemon juice over the leaves and season with sea salt and pepper.

THE ORIGINAL
VANILLA COCONUT CHIA PUDDING

Serves 2

THIS IS my favorite dessert of all time. It takes only 10 minutes to make in the blender, but please note, you will have to let in sit overnight in the fridge. I always joke that we'd better make extra because it won't last. Chia was used for energy and strength by Mayan and Aztec civilizations, as it's 50 percent omega-3s—one of the richest sources of these fatty acids—and 20 percent protein. It's also high in fiber, which helps reduce inflammation in the gut and lowers cholesterol. It's also great for anybody who has constipation issues. A mere 2 tablespoons of chia seeds gives you 18 percent of your daily calcium, 35 percent phosphorous, 24 percent magnesium, and 50 percent manganese. For all these reasons, it's simply one of the best foods for neutralizing acid and balancing pH.

2 cups coconut water or filtered water (I prefer coconut water, it's sweeter)

½ cup raw cashews

2 tablespoons coconut oil

3 dates, pitted

⅛ teaspoon salt (Celtic Grey, Himalayan, or Redmond Real Salt)

1 tablespoon unsweetened coconut flakes

2 teaspoons vanilla (I use Medicine Flower Vanilla, 15 drops)

1 teaspoon cinnamon

6 tablespoons chia seeds

Pomegranate seeds, cinnamon, or cacao nibbs for garnish

Blend all the ingredients except the chia and pomegranate seeds in a blender until thoroughly mixed, for 40 to 60 seconds. Then, on the lowest variable speed, add the chia and blend for 1 minute to mix the chia in. If your blender does not have a low speed option, mix in the chia seeds with a spoon. Place in an airtight container, and refrigerate for at least 5 hours before serving.

Garnish with pomegranate seeds, cinnamon, or cacao nibbs.

Variation: for chocolate chia pudding, just add ¼ cup raw cacao before first blend and, optionally, 5 drops of light chocolate essential oil flavor (I like Medicine Flower).

AVOCADO CHOCOLATE MOUSSE

Serves 2

YOU'LL NEVER believe this is a healthy treat made with avocado. It's so deceptively delicious, in fact, that eating it will make you feel like you're cheating on your mindful eating. It's so thick and creamy and chocolaty, I'd say it's even *better* than the real thing.

1½ avocados

⅔ cup coconut water, ideally raw

1 tablespoon vanilla (I use Medicine Flowers Vanilla 10 drops)

2 tablespoons raw cacao

3 pitted dates (can use 5 to make a little sweeter)

1½ teaspoons sea salt (Celtic Grey, Himalayan, or Redmond Real Salt)

Blend on high in blender, enjoy! Refrigerate leftovers to make firm.

GINGER CINNAMON FRUIT WITH SWEET TAHINI DIP

Serves 2

THIS WAS one of the first recipes I put together when I was first experimenting with raw foods. I love this dessert because it uses tahini in a sweet formulation, which is rare here but common in many Israeli sweets such as halvah. It's an unexpected sesame taste, and it's great for balancing blood sugar. Plus, all the fats, cinnamon, and ginger help to neutralize the acidity of the pear and green apple.

Fruit

2 to 3 tablespoons fresh ginger, to taste

1 teaspoon cinnamon

1 teaspoon salt (Celtic Grey, Himalayan, or Redmond Real Salt)

1 pear

1 green apple

Sweet Tahini Dip

3 tablespoons tahini

3 tablespoons raw almond butter

1 tablespoon liquid coconut nectar (I use Coconut Secret Raw Coconut Nectar brand)

2 tablespoons coconut oil

2 teaspoons gluten-free tamari

¼ teaspoon cayenne (optional)

(Continues)

Ginger Cinnamon Fruit with Sweet Tahini Dip
(Continued)

Grate the ginger into a small mixing bowl. Add the sea salt and cinnamon and mix together. Dice the fruit into small cubes and add into bowl, mixing thoroughly.

In a separate bowl, mix all the dip ingredients and drizzle over the Ginger Cinnamon Fruit.

CHOPPED BERRIES WITH MINT AND COCONUT BUTTER

Serves 1

THIS IS another sweet treat where you're adding healthy fats to slow down the sugars. If you want to have fruit, this is the best way to eat it and stay alkaline. Always remember to choose your fruit based on what's organic and in season.

1 cup of mixed berries: blueberries, strawberries, and raspberries

2 tablespoons coconut butter, soft or melted

1 tablespoon chopped mint

Drizzle the coconut butter on the berries and sprinkle with mint.

DAIRY-FREE HOT CHOCOLATE

Serves 2

HOT COCOA is such a nostalgic favorite in our culture, and it would be a shame to outlaw it from a healthy eating plan. The truth is, making hot chocolate the old-fashioned way is very acidic because it combines milk, chocolate and sugar. My recipe uses almond or coconut milk and cacao so it's just as delicious but totally guilt free.

2 cups almond milk (or coconut)

¼ cup raw cacao

1 heaping teaspoon of cinnamon

Dash of cayenne pepper (optional)

Puree everything in a blender and then warm it on the stove (if you have a high-power blender like Vitamix, the mixture can heat up, so it may not need to be warmed on stove).

CHOCOLATE BANANA FRO-YO

Serves 2

YOU MIGHT think that ice cream treats are a no-no on an alkaline diet, but this dairy-free, sugar-free substitute is going to be your new best friend, especially in the summer months. With the frozen yogurt-like consistency and the chocolate-banana flavor combo, it satisfies all your dessert cravings without relying on acidic ingredients. Think of this as a great reward for eating so healthily.

2 bananas, peeled and frozen

3 tablespoons raw cacao powder

1 tablespoon raw almond butter

¼ cup unsweetened almond milk

1 tablespoon chia seeds, for topping

1 tablespoon hemp seeds, for topping

Place bananas and cacao into the blender and blend while slowly adding the almond milk until you have the consistency of frozen yogurt. You might not use all ¼ cup of almond milk. Sprinkle the chia and hemp seeds on top.

APPENDIX I

Keep a Health Cabinet

Some everyday ailments can be treated with natural foods. I always keep these on hand, and rather than calling it a medicine cabinet, I call it my health cabinet.

Activated charcoal. Activated charcoal absorbs toxins and kicks them out of the body. For any form of food poisoning, this can be a lifesaver. I always take it with me when I travel. Sometimes, moms give sick kids burnt toast because of the charcoal effect. Activated coconut charcoal is a product I like especially. It also works for hangovers and alcohol poisoning.

Baking soda. I use it in baths and on mosquito bites and bee stings. A little paste on the sting (mixed with water) is anti-inflammatory and takes the pain away. Once a week, brush your teeth with water and baking soda. It neutralizes acid and helps prevent gum and tooth disease. It's also good for removing tartar. I used to have the worst teeth in the world—I've had four root canals from all the sugar and acid I used to eat—but I haven't had a cavity since I went alkaline.

Cold-pressed coconut oil is at the top of my list because of its versatility. Every night, I put it on my skin to keep it hydrated, toned, and wrinkle free.

Elderberry syrup. This stuff not only tastes good, it's also antiviral and antibacterial. When you feel flu-like symptoms, take it three times a day. Research shows it is three times more effective than Tamiflu. I give it to kids when they're coming down with something. Get it at the natural foods store.

Epsom salt is good for stubborn splinters. Soak in warm water with baking soda and Epsom—this solution decreases inflammation and toxicity and helps push out whatever is in the skin.

Oil of oregano. This wonder stuff is antiviral, antifungal, and antibacterial. I use it anytime I feel like I'm coming down with something, I take 20 drops in 6 to 8 ounces of water. It's a very strong oil, and it almost burns. You have to dilute it and stir it, drink quickly, stir it, and drink quickly (because oil and water don't mix). And to be honest, it has a powerful taste. Grin and bear it; it's worth it. It is also great for killing bacteria that would be entering the body by breathing (put a dab under your nose before flights!).

Lavender oil is great for:

▸ Relaxation and stress relief. Add it to a bath, which aids in detoxification. Combine 8 drops of lavender oil with 2 cups of Epsom salts and 1 cup of baking soda. Add this to *very* hot water, soak for 20 minutes, then wrap yourself in a towel and jump under the covers. Do this before bed; you will sweat but will feel so relaxed and refreshed and will have one of your best night's sleep ever!

▸ Healing skin disorders and wounds: apply essential oil directly to the skin.

▸ Relieving insomnia: rub it on your neck, put a drop or two on your pillow, or diffuse it in the air.

Peppermint oil is great for:

▸ Improving concentration and energy: diffuse it into the air.

▸ Aiding digestion, including nausea and acid reflux. Take orally, using 1 drop in a glass of water (use only the highest quality oils orally).

▸ Improving breathing, especially when fighting a cold. Diffuse or apply topically to the chest.

▸ Applying topically across the forehead and on the temples effectively alleviates a tension headache (allow 30 minutes for it to take full effect)

▸ Use in a diffuser before going to sleep.

Frankincense oil is great for:

▸ Reducing inflammation. Apply to the skin or take orally (use only the highest quality oils orally).

▸ Fighting cancer. Studies have shown the oil can kill cancer cells; talk to your doctor about the best way to use frankincense oil in your treatment. Use in a diffuser at night or put it on your feet every night before going to sleep. Or place 1 drop on your thumb (along with myrrh) and rub on the roof of your mouth—effective for brain and lung cancer.

▸ Cleansing and detoxifying the body: add it to bath water.

▸ Boosting immunity: apply on the neck and behind the ears.

▸ Fighting infection: diffuse it into the air.

▸ Improving skin conditions, scars, aging effect, and acne: apply topically.

Lemon oil is great for:

▸ Detoxifying the body and lymphatic system. Take 1 drop orally a few times a day (use only the highest quality oils orally).

▸ Supporting the immune system to prevent illness: diffuse in the air.

▸ Killing bacteria: use for home cleaning or apply to hands.

▸ Lifting mood and energy levels: diffuse in the air.

Tea tree oil is great for:

▸ Killing fungus, yeast, and infections; apply directly.

▸ Improving acne. Mix it with honey and use as a face wash.

▸ Reducing and preventing dandruff. Add a few drops to shampoo.

▸ Cleaning: add a few drops to water to use in a spray bottle.

▸ Children's ear infections (always run by your pediatrician).

Silver Hydrosol. Silver has antibiotic properties. Robert Scott Bell, D.A. Hom—a good friend, colleague, and featured doctor in the docu-series *The Truth About Cancer*—offered to share his latest findings about colloidal silver.

Since the introduction of penicillin, the medical community has adopted antibiotics as the new standard of care—wonder drugs to eliminate bacterial infections. What it did not account for was the rapid and growing antibiotic resistance by the microbes they were meant to kill.

What follows is information about what I have used instead for my family and patients over the past decade: silver hydrosol, which has anti-bacterial, anti-fungal, and anti-viral properties.

How does silver work as an antimicrobial? First, silver ions rupture the outer membrane of the pathogenic cell. Then the ions attack the microbes' oxygen and energy metabolizing enzymes, suffocating the life out of the so-called bad guys. Silver is virostatic, which means it stops viral replication on contact. Unlike antibiotics, even when taken multiple times on a daily basis, silver hydrosol does not disrupt normal healthy gut flora.

Taking a reliable bioactive silver hydrosol supplement may offer advantages to anyone's daily regimen. If you're facing a medical risk, you should follow your doctor's instructions for best measures of prevention. However, since many staph infections are transmitted through the nasal passages and upper respiratory pathways, it may be wise to reinforce your defenses with a quality silver formulation via a nebulizer. Just spraying your throat with a silver hydrosol preparation every few hours gives your immune system an edge, especially before, during, and after traveling on an airplane, or whenever you are around someone who is sick or ill (especially visiting a hospital).

And when cold and flu season comes around, it's with good reason that more people are choosing to replace hand sanitizers with silver gels and sprays. They work better than benzyl alcohol and endocrine-disrupting triclosan, which are both very toxic and acidic to the human body.

Silver hydrosol is safe, nontoxic, effectively excreted, and appears to offer real advantages to help prevent or at least reduce the risk of infections. Please note I recommend only the use of *bioactive silver hydrosol* and not generic colloidal silvers, which tend to have too many compounds (salts and proteins), and inefficiently large particle sizes. I recommend the brands Sovereign Silver along with Argentyn 23 for health professionals. I have not seen a more rapidly acting intestinal-health recovery protocol.

Although I do not support the indiscriminate use of antibiotics, the only class of said drugs contraindicated with the use of silver are sulfonamides (Bactrim, Septra) due to the strong affinity that silver and sulfur have for one another.

When it comes to silver, smaller is better, and particle size is critical. Because of the purity and activity found in this quality of colloidal silver, anyone can use very safe, low concentrations to achieve the goals of pathogen burden reduction. Use these guidelines for the following health issues, but be sure to consult your health care provider first.

Adult dose: Take 1 ounce of silver with 1 ounce of aloe, swallowing directly on an empty stomach three times daily, followed by probiotic replenishment every evening for one to two weeks for mild gut dysbiosis or candida overgrowth.

Candida overgrowth or mild gut dysbiosis: Silver nanoparticles can kill antibiotic-resistant bacteria and have powerful anti-fungal properties, exhitibing powerful actions against yeast organisms, including Candida albicans (in vitro). Take 1 ounce of silver (1 to 2 tablespoons) with 1 ounce of pure aloe liquid, swallowing directly on an empty stomach three times daily, followed by a probiotic replenishment early evening for one to two weeks. Those who weigh less than 120 pounds can take half the dose.

Chronic gut inflammation: For those dealing with more serious inflammatory instetinal issues including Crohn's IBS, leaky gut, colitis, diverticulitis, and celiac, please consult your health care provider. Follow the mild gut dysbiosis protocol, but it may require four, six, or eight weeks to complete.

Maintenance: 1 teaspoon daily

Immunity-building: 3 teaspoons daily

Chronic immune support: 5 teaspoons daily

Gastrointestinal health: 1–2 tablespoons with aloe three times daily

Acute immune support: 7 teaspoons daily

APPENDIX II

The Ultimate Alkaline-Acid Food Guide

The following chart is a great quick reference guide for the most commonly consumed alkaline and acidic foods. At first look, many foods and drinks might seem to be alkaline or acidic, when, in fact, the opposite is true! Eat these alkaline foods freely! Try to incorporate 80 percent or more into your daily diet . . .

TABLE A2.1
THE ULTIMATE ALKALINE AND ACID FOOD GUIDE

ALKALINE FOODS

VEGETABLES:
HIGH ALKALINE
asparagus
barley grass
beet greens
bell pepper (capsicum)
bok choy
broccoli
burdock root
butter lettuce
celery
chards (swiss)
collard greens
cucumber
daikon radish
dandelion greens
endive
grasses
kale
kohlrabi

leaf lettuce
lettuce
lotus root
mustard greens
romaine lettuce
salad greens
spinach
sprouts
turnip greens
watercress
wheatgrass

VEGETABLES:
MODERATE ALKALINE
artichokes
beetroot
Brussels sprouts
cabbage (chinese)
cabbage (green)
cabbage (napa)

cabbage (red)
cabbage (savoy)
cabbage (white)
cauliflower
chicory
choy sum
eggplant
green beans
Jerusalem artichokes
leeks
lemongrass
okra
red onion
rutabagas
snow peas
spring onion
zucchini
zucchini noodles

(Continues)

ALKALINE FOODS (Continued)

VEGETABLES:
MILD ALKALINE
carrots
edamame
garlic
jicama
mushrooms (medicinal
   powdered)
onions
parsnips
peas
pepper (jalapeño)
pepper (shishito)
potato (new)

SEA VEGETABLES:
HIGH ALKALINE
chlorella
kelp
nori seaweed
seaweed

SEA VEGETABLES:
MODERATE ALKALINE
blue-green algae
e3live
spirulina

SEA VEGETABLES:
MILD ALKALINE
arame
dulse

FISH (WILD-CAUGHT):
MILD ALKALINE
anchovies
herring
salmon (Alaskan,
   New Zealand, Spain)
sardines
trout

NUTS, NUT-BUTTERS,
AND SEEDS (RAW):
HIGH ALKALINE
chia seeds
hemp seeds (hulled, non-
   irradiated)
hemp seed butter

NUTS, NUT-BUTTERS,
AND SEEDS (RAW):
MODERATE ALKALINE
black cumin
black seeds
cardamom seeds
cacao butter
coconut butter
cumin seeds
fennel seeds
flaxseed
flax meal
pumpkin seeds
macadamia nuts
macadamia nut butter

NUTS, NUT-BUTTERS,
AND SEEDS (RAW):
MILD ALKALINE
almond butter (in
   moderation)
almonds (in moderation)
Brazil nuts
cashews (in moderation)
cashew butter (homemade,
   in moderation)
celery seeds
chestnuts
coriander seeds
dill seeds
ghee (transitional)
grass-fed butter
   (transitional)

hazelnuts
pine nuts
pistachio nuts
psyllium seed husks
quinoa
safflower seeds
   (in moderation)
sesame seeds
sunflower seeds
   (in moderation)
tahini
walnuts

GRAINS AND CEREALS:
MILD ALKALINE
amaranth (sprouted)
buckwheat (sprouted)
buckwheat flour (sprouted)
hemp seed flour (sprouted)
kamut (sprouted)

FRUIT: HIGH ALKALINE
avocado

FRUIT:
MODERATE ALKALINE
coconuts (meat)
lemons
limes
tomato

FRUIT: MILD ALKALINE
grapefruit
olives (green)
pomegranates
watermelon (neutral)

BEVERAGES: HIGH ALKALINE

dandelion tea
essiac tea
green juice (green,
    cold-pressed, no fruit)
green smoothie (no fruit)
herbal tea
turmeric/ginger/lemon/
    black pepper tea
water (ionized)
water (H2—molecular
    hydrogen/ionized)

BEVERAGES: MODERATE ALKALINE

coconut water (raw)
ginseng tea
green smoothie
    (w/ healthy fats, and
    no more than one fruit)
hemp milk
lemon water (fresh
    squeezed)
lime water (fresh squeezed)
pomegranate juice
    (fresh, unsweetened)

BEVERAGES: MILD ALKALINE

almond milk (unsweetened)
carrot juice
chamomile tea
coconut milk (unsweetened)
grapefruit juice
    (fresh squeezed)
teecino (tea)
tomato juice (fresh)
water (filtered)

OILS AND VINEGARS: HIGH ALKALINE

avacado oil
black cumin oil
    (black seed oil)
coconut oil (cold-pressed)
fish oil (omega-3)
mct oil

OILS AND VINEGARS: MILD ALKALINE

apple cider vinegar
Bragg's liquid aminos
    (transitional b/c soy)
chia oil (fresh/consumed
    immediately)
coconut aminos
flax oil (fresh/consumed
    immediately)
hemp oil (fresh/consumed
    immediately)
macadamia nut oil
olive oil (extra virgin)
sesame oil
UDOs oil (moderation)

DAIRY AND CHEESE: (TRANSITION FOODS) MILD ALKALINE

coconut cream
coconut yogurt
ghee (clarified butter)
grass-fed butter (i.e.,
    Kerrygold)
heavy whipping cream
    (transitional)

HERBS AND SPICES: HIGH ALKALINE

arugula
cilantro
ginger
parsley
salt (Celtic Grey)
salt (Hawaiian black)
salt (Himalayan)
turmeric

HERBS AND SPICES: MODERATE ALKALINE

basil
caraway seeds
cardamom
chili powder
chives
cinnamon
coriander
cumin
curry
dill
fennel
marjoram
mint

HERBS AND SPICES: MODERATE ALKALINE

nutmeg
oregano
paprika
pepper (black)
pepper (cayenne)
sage
salt (sea unbleached)
tarragon
thyme

(Continues)

HERBS AND SPICES: MILD ALKALINE
bay leaf

BEANS AND LEGUMES: HIGH ALKALINE
sprouted beans (i.e., sprouted chickpeas)

BEANS AND LEGUMES: MODERATE ALKALINE
hummus (fresh)
lima beans

BEANS AND LEGUMES: MILD ALKALINE (ALL IN MODERATION)
adzuki beans
black-eyed peas
butter beans
cacao beans
cannellini beans
chickpeas
fava beans
kidney beans
lentils
licorice
mung beans
Navy beans
pinto beans
red clover
split peas
white haricot beans
white kidney bean

PROCESSED FOODS/ CONDIMENTS: MILD ALKALINE
beans (BPA-free can)
wasabi

BAKED GOODS/ DESSERTS: HIGH ALKALINE
baking soda

BAKED GOODS/ DESSERTS: MILD ALKALINE
sprouted breads

SWEETENERS: MILD ALKALINE
bee pollen
cacao (raw)
lo han
stevia

ACID FOODS

**Try to avoid these foods and drinks, and try to keep
to a maximum of 20 percent of your diet.**

GRAINS AND CEREALS: MILD ACIDIC
corn (fresh/non-gmo)
einkorn
emmer
farro (whole)
heirloom wheat
muesli (gluten-free)
oat bran
oat flour
oatmeal
oatmeal (gluten-free, in moderation)
oats (gluten-free, rolled, in moderation)
oats (gluten-free, steel cut, in moderation)
oats (gluten-free, whole, in moderation)
rice (white and brown)
rice cakes
rice flour
sorghum
soy flour
spelt

GRAINS AND CEREALS: MODERATE ACIDIC
barley (whole)
barley flour
bran (cereal)
farro (pearled)
granola
millet
noodles
oats (instant)
oatmeal (with gluten)
rye
wheat
wholegrain bread

GRAINS AND CEREALS: HIGH ACIDIC
corn (processed)
malt
wheat flour

BEANS: MILDLY ACIDIC
black beans
miso
soybeans (non-gmo, fermented)
tempeh
tofu (fermented)

BEANS: MODERATE ACIDIC
refried beans
shoyu (raw)
soybeans (gmo, unfermented)
tofu (unfermented)

MEAT: MODERATE ACID
chicken
duck
goat
lamb
lard
liver
rabbit
roast beef
seitan
steak
turkey
venison

MEAT: HIGH ACID
bacon
beef (hamburgers)
beef (hotdogs)
cold cuts
ham
pork
sausage
veal

FERMENTED FOODS: MILD ACIDIC
lassi
miso
natto
pickled beets
pickled cucumbers
soybeans (non-gmo)
tamari (gluten-free)
tempeh

FERMENTED FOODS: MODERATE ACIDIC
shoyu (raw)
soy sauce

FERMENTED FOODS: HIGH ACIDIC
kefir
kombucha

DAIRY AND CHEESE: MILD ACIDIC
milk (goat's, camel, sheep)
soy yogurt
whey

(Continues)

ACID FOODS (Continued)

DAIRY AND CHEESE:
MODERATE ACIDIC
butter (non grass-fed)
goat cheese
vegan cheese
yogurt

DAIRY AND CHEESE:
HIGH ACIDIC
Camembert cheese
cheddar cheese
cheese
cottage cheese
cream
cream cheese
egg (white only)
egg (whole)
gelato
gouda
ice cream
margarine
milk (cow's skim)
milk (cow's whole)
mozzarella cheese
sour cream
string cheese

VEGETABLES:
MILD ACIDIC
baked potato
potatoes (stored)
rhubarb
yams

VEGETABLES:
HIGH ACIDIC
corn
mushrooms (edible)

SEA VEGETABLES:
MILD ACIDIC
agar
hijiki
kombu
wakame

FISH: MILD ACIDIC
bass
flounder
haddock
mahi-mahi
rockfish
salmon (Atlantic)
salmon (canned)
skate
snapper
sole
white fish
whiting

FISH: MODERATE ACIDIC
blue fish
catfish
cod
mackerel
orange roughy
perch
scallops
tile fish
tuna

FISH: HIGH ACIDIC
clams
crab
grouper
lobster
marlin
mussels
oysters

sea bass
shark
shrimp
swordfish
tuna (canned)

FRUIT: MILD ACIDIC
apples (green)
berries (black)
berries (blue)
berries (raspberry)
cherries (sour)
cherries (sweet)
cranberries
dates (fresh)
dehydrated apples
guava
kiwi fruit
nectarines
olives (ripe)
papayas
persimmons
plums
raspberries
strawberries
tangerines

FRUIT: MODERATE ACIDIC
apples (other than green)
apricots
bananas
figs (fresh)
grapes
jackfruit
mandarins
mangos
mangosteen
oranges
peaches
pears

FRUIT: HIGH ACIDIC
apricots (dried)
cantaloupe
cranberries (dried)
currants
dried fruit
figs (dried)
melon
pineapples
prunes
raisins

BEVERAGES: MILD ACIDIC
decaffeinated drinks
green juice (w/fruit)
green smoothie (w/fruit)
matcha
rice milk (unsweetened)
soy milk (unsweetened)
tea (green)
water (tap)

BEVERAGES: MODERATE ACIDIC
black tea
carbonated drinks
espresso
fruit juice (fresh)
grape juice
hot cocoa
orange juice
pear juice
spirits (straight)
sports drinks
tea (black)
tea (white)
V8
water (most bottled)
wine (white)

BEVERAGES: HIGH ACIDIC
beer
cappuccino
coffee
coffee (decaf)
energy drinks
espresso (w/milk)
fruit juice (processed)
malt liquor
milk shake
pineapple juice
root beer
scotch
soda/soft drinks
spirits (w/mixer)
tequila
vodka
water (carbonated)
wine (red)

OILS AND VINEGAR: MILD ACIDIC
chia oil
    (d/t oxidation)
flaxseed oil
    (d/t oxidation)
hemp oil
    (d/t oxidationgrape
    seed oil
safflower oil
sunflower oil
walnut oil

OILS AND VINEGAR: MODERATE ACIDIC
balsamic vinegar
canola oil
cottonseed oil
grapeseed oil
soybean oil

OILS AND VINEGAR: HIGH ACIDIC
corn oil
hydrogenated vegetable oils
peanut oil
vinegar
wheat germ oil

NUTS, NUT BUTTERS, AND SEEDS: MILD ACIDIC
dry roasted nuts (i.e., almonds)
soy nut
tiger nut

NUTS, NUT BUTTERS, AND SEEDS: HIGH ACIDIC
cashew butter (store-bought)
peanuts
peanut butter

HERBS AND SPICES: MILD ACIDIC
kosher salt
sea salt (bleached)

HERBS AND SPICES: HIGH ACIDIC
salt (table)

PROCESSED FOODS AND CONDIMENTS: MILD ACIDIC
coleslaw (fresh)
mustard
popcorn

PROCESSED FOODS AND CONDIMENTS: MODERATE ACIDIC
baked beans
couscous

(Continues)

ACID FOODS (Continued)

crackers (rye)
salad dressing
soy sauce
sweet pickles
tomato paste
tomato sauce

**PROCESSED FOODS
AND CONDIMENTS:
HIGH ACIDIC**
burritos
chicken nuggets
chicken sandwich
chicken soup
corn chips
corned beef
crackers (white flour)
cranberry sauce
French fries
fruit pies
hash browns
hot dogs
jam
ketchup
lasagna
liverwurst
macaroni
mayonnaise
MSG
pancakes
pastrami
pepperoni
pickled relish
pizza
pork sausage
potato chips
preserves
puddings
spaghetti
tacos

Tabasco
tortilla
Worcestershire sauce

**BAKED GOODS
AND DESSERTS:
MODERATE ACIDIC**
nutritional yeast
pita (whole flour)
pumpernickel bread
rye bread
tapioca
whole wheat bread

**BAKED GOODS
AND DESSERTS:
HIGH ACIDIC**
apple pie
bagels
biscuits
bread sticks
brownies
carrot cake
cheese cake
cookies
croissants
danish
donuts
muffins
pastry puffs
pita (white flour)
pretzels
white bread

**SWEETENERS:
MILD ACIDIC**
chocolate (dark > 80%)
coconut nectar
coconut sugar

**SWEETENERS:
MODERATE ACIDIC**
carob
demerara sugar
honey (natural)
panela
saccharin
sugar (brown)
turbinado sugar

**SWEETENERS:
HIGH ACIDIC**
agave
artificial sweeteners
aspartame
brown rice syrup
chocolate milk
cocoa (processed)
honey (processed)
jelly
maple syrup
molasses
processed sugar
rice syrup
splenda
sucrose
sugar (white)
Sweet 'n Low

APPENDIX III

TABLE A3.1
NET CARB COUNTER

NAME OF FOOD (PER 100 GRAMS), NET CARBS (GRAMS)

Alfalfa seeds, sprouted, 0.2

Almond butter, raw, 2.8

Almonds, whole, raw, 2.9

Amanranth leaves, 4.02

Apple, Granny Smith, red delicious, 15.76

Arrowhead, 20.23

Arrowroot, 12.09

Artichokes, 5.11

Arugula, 2.05

Asparagus, 1.78

Avocado, 3.65

Balsam-pear, leafy tips, 3.29

Bamboo shoots, 3

Banana, medium, 23.85

Barley, 1 cup cooked, 39.31

Beans, butter, 6.5

Beans, chickpeas (garbanzo), 11

Beans, adzuki, 10

Beans, fava, in pod, 10.13

Beans, kidney, 35

Beans, lima, 6

Beans, navy, 13.05

Beans, pinto, 4.1

Beans, snap, green, 3.6

Beet greens, 0.63

Beets, 6.76

Blueberries, 1 cup, 17.51

Bok choy, 0.4

Brazil nuts, raw, 1.5

Bread, Ezekiel slice, 10

Bread, multigrain, 13

Bread, sprouted slice, 16

Bread, Udis slice (gluten-free), 19

Bread, white slice, 10.65

Bread, whole-wheat slice, 11.16

Broadbeans, immature seeds, 7.5

Broccoli, 4.04

Broccoli raab, 0.15

Brussels sprouts, 3

Buckwheat groats, 1 cup cooked, 29

Burdock root, 14.04

Butterbur (fuki), 3.61

Cabbage, 3.3

Cabbage, Chinese , 2.03

Cabbage, red, 5.27

Cabbage, savoy, 3

Cardoon, 2.47

Carrots, 6.78

Carrots, baby, 5.34

Cassava, 36.26

Cashews, raw, 7.9

Cauliflower, 2.97

Celeriac, 7.4

Celery, 1.37

Celtuce, 1.95

Chanterelle mushrooms, 3.06

(Continues)

NET CARB COUNTER (Continued)

Chard, Swiss, 2.14

Chayote, fruit, 2.81

Chia seeds, 1.1

Chicory greens, 0.7

Chicory, witloof, 0.9

Chives, 1.85

Cilantro (coriander), 0.87

Cranberries, 5

Coconut flakes, raw, unsweetened, 0.9

Collards, 1.42

Corn, sweet, white, 16.32

Corn, sweet, yellow, 16.7

Cowpeas (blackeyed-peas), 13.83

Cress, garden, 4.4

Cucumber, with peel, 3.13

Dandelion greens, 5.7

Date, medjool, one, 16.39

Eggplant, 2.88

Endive, 0.25

Enoki mushrooms, 5.11

Epazote, 3.64

Escarole, 0.5

Fennel, bulb, 4.2

Fiddlehead ferns, 5.54

Fireweed, leaves, 8.62

Flaxseeds, whole, raw, 0.2

Garlic (clove), 1

Ginger root, 15.77

Gourd, white-flowered (calabash), 2.89

Grape leaves, 6.31

Grapefruit, pink, red, white, 8.9

Hemp seeds, raw, 3

Honey, raw, 18.4

Hyacinth-beans, immature seeds, 5.89

Jerusalem-artichokes, 15.84

Jicama, 4

Kale, 5.15

Kiwi, whole, 8.84

Kohlrabi, 2.6

Leeks, (bulb and lower leaf-portion), 12.35

Lemon, 3.81

Lemon, juice (from one lemon), 3.86

Lemon grass (citronella), 25.31

Lentils, sprouted, 4

Lettuce, butter (includes boston and bibb types), 1.13

Lettuce, cos or romaine, 1.19

Lettuce, green leaf, 1.57

Lettuce, iceberg (includes crisphead types), 1.77

Lettuce, red leaf, 1.36

Lima beans, immature seeds, 15.27

Lime, whole, 5.16

Lime, juice (from 1 lime), 3

Lotus root, 12.33

Macadamia nuts, raw, 1.5

Mango, one whole, 31.49

Maple syrup, raw, 13.9

Milk, almond, sweetened (1 cup), 5.53

Milk, almond unsweetened (1 cup), 0.6

Milk, coconut sweetened (1 cup), 8.3

Milk, coconut unsweetened (1 cup), 1

Milk, goat raw (1 cup), 10.86

Milk, whole (1 cup), 11.03

Millet, 1 cup cooked, 38.71

Mountain yam, Hawaii, 4.27

Mung beans, mature seeds, sprouted, 2.3

Mushrooms, brown, Italian, or crimini, 13.8

Mushrooms, maitake, 4.14

Mushrooms, morel, 3.7

Mushrooms, portabella, 1.47

Mushrooms, white, 2.26

Mustard greens, 1.13

Nopales, 4.25

Oatmeal, gluten-free, 24

Oatmeal, instant, 29

Okra, 7.64

Onions, 4.74

Onions, spring or scallions (includes tops and bulb), 6.65

Onions, sweet, 3.79

Orange, 12.39

Oyster mushrooms, 24.11

Palm hearts, 13.09

Papaya, 1 small, 12.21

Parsnips, 9.35

Passion Fruit, 1 whole, 2.31

Pasta, penne, spaghetti, 1 cup, 40.45

Pasta, quinoa, 2 oz. dry, 42

Pasta, rice, 1 cup, 41

Peach, 1 small, 7.85

Pear, 1 whole, 20.56

Peas, green, 1.95

Pecans, raw, 0.5

Pepper, banana, 7.31

Peppers, green bell, 3.7

Peppers, hot chili, red, 3

Peppers, jalapeño, 2.94

Peppers, red bell, 3.93

Peppers, serrano, 5.42

Peppers, yellow bell, 18.78

Pigeonpeas, immature seeds, 2.57

Pinapple, 1 cup diced, 17.38

Pine nuts, raw, 1.9

Pistachios, hulled, raw, 5.03

Pomegranate, seeds, 1/2 cup, 13

Potatoes, red, flesh and skin, 14.2

Potatoes, russet, flesh and skin, 16.77

Potatoes, sweet, 16.9

Potatoes, white, flesh and skin, 13.31

Pumpkin, 6

Pumpkin leaves, 2.33

Pumpkin seeds, hulled, raw, 1

Purslane, 3.39

Quinoa, 1/4 cup cooked, 9

Radicchio, 3.58

Radish seeds, sprouted, 3.6

Radishes, 1.8

Raisins, 1/4 cup, 31

Raspberries, red, 6.69

Rice, brown, 1 cup cooked, 40.92

Rice, white, 1 cup cooked, 43.48

Rutabagas, 6.32

Salsify, (vegetable oyster), 15.3

Seaweed, kelp, 8.27

Seaweed, spirulina, 2.02

Seaweed, wakame, 8.64

Sesame seeds, raw, 2

Shallots, 13.6

Soybeans, green, 6.85

Soybeans, mature seeds, sprouted, 8.47

Spinach, 1.43

Squash, summer, crookneck and straightneck, 2.88

Squash, summer, scallop, 2.64

Squash, summer, zucchini, includes skin, 2.11

Squash, winter, acorn, 8.92

Squash, winter, butternut, 9.69

Squash, winter, hubbard, 4.8

Squash, winter, spaghetti, 5.41

Strawberries, 1 cup, 8.67

Succotash, corn and limas, 15.79

Sunflower seeds, hulled, raw, 2

Sweet potato leaves, 3.52

Taro, 22.36

Tomatillos, 3.94

Tomatoes, red, ripe, year round average, 2.69

Turnip greens, 3.93

Turnips, 4.63

Walnuts, raw, 1.9

Wasabi, root, 15.74

Waterchestnuts, chinese, (matai), 20.94

Watercress, 0.79

Watermelon, 1 cup, 10.88

Waxgourd, (Chinese preserving melon), 0.1

Winged bean tuber, 28.1

Yam, 23.78

Yardlong bean, 8.35

Source: Rami Abramov of Tasteaholics.com, https://www.tasteaholics.com/low-carb-vegetables/, 2017.

ACKNOWLEDGMENTS

So many have helped me along this journey, and I am humbled by their contribution.

First, my deepest thanks to my publisher, Hachette Group, and in particular my editor, Renee Sedliar. You believed in my vision and me from the first moment we met, and I'm forever grateful for giving me the opportunity to share this important information with the world. Thank you again for your endless support and for believing in me.

Thank you to my literary agent team at Stonesong, especially Ellen Scordato. This book wouldn't have been possible if it were not for you. You've shepherded me through the process, and your support was second to none. I appreciate you and what you do so much.

To my writing partner, Jamie Shaw, you took my vision and helped me turn it into a reality. Thank you for the countless hours you invested in this project, and for being as passionate and connected to it as I was. You truly are a master at what you do, and it was a privilege to work by your side.

To my other editors, Lori Hobkirk and Katie McHugh Malm, I am in awe of your skill, insight, and patience. Thank you for polishing this most extensive project, and for your meticulous time to make this book the best it can be.

To my graphic designer, Chris Cook, thank you for bringing my brand to life.

Kelly Ripa, I can't thank you enough. You are the embodiment of good health, and I am honored that you are a part of my mission to help change lives. I am forever grateful for the message you shared in the Foreword. You inspire me, and so many others with your commitment to walking the walk. You are a role model, and I know your words will bring others to better health.

Bobbi Brown, I admire you so much. You are a beauty guru, and yet you understand beauty begins with optimum health from the inside out. Thank you for not only being part of my book, but also for having me to be part of yours.

I must also thank my forefathers in health, the pioneers who led the charge in standing up to the establishment to uncover the causes of true health. Your work and collective wisdom brought me to where I am today. To D. D. Palmer, B. J. Palmer, Antoine Béchamp, Claude Bernard, Royal Raymond Rife, Günther Enderlein, and Gaston Naessens, thank you for leading the way.

There are also many professional colleagues and mentors who have inspired and informed my work. At the top of the list is Tony Robbins. You helped shaped me personally and professionally, and I would not be here today had I not been empowered with your life strategies. Endless gratitude.

Ty and Charlene Bollinger, thank you for your essential cancer research, and also for introducing me (and the world) to many cutting-edge cancer protocols that were so crucial with my father's battle. I couldn't imagine having made the journey without your help.

To my fellow health crusaders, whose methods, modalities, and messages have made my own work better, I am proud to be in league with you. Dr. Dan Murphy, your research for the chiropractic profession and nutrition for healthy aging and brain optimization was invaluable for not only this book, but also for my clinical practice. Doug Caporrino, Dr. Daniel Johnston, Richard and Mary Harvey, Ross Bridgeford, Stu Mittleman, Paulo Fernandes, Jane Goldberg, Art Jaffe, Carine Vermenot, and Leonardo Chiriboga—you are my people.

Thank you also to those who agreed to be interviewed for this book. To Paul Barattiero and Dr. Robert Scott Bell, I'm grateful for your friendship and thought leadership in such important emerging fields. Your selfless dedication to helping people is awe-inspiring. Dr. Joe Hibbeln and James Lebeau, thank you for sharing your expertise. Your work on pH testing and omega-3/omega-6 fatty acids, respectively, is at the heart of what I do.

Ernest Lupinacci, my brilliant visionary brand thinker. What can I say—you're a genius. Thank you.

To Stu Gelbard, it's thrilling to learn from someone on the cutting edge of an exciting new health frontier. Thank you for sharing your advice, knowledge, and for your never-ending support for Get Off Your Acid.

To Amy Natsoulis and my brother Tony, your legal expertise is so very appreciated. Thank you for all the complex and careful work you do on my behalf.

And alongside all the professionals who helped this book come into being were friends who held me up. Ron Tumpowsky, we go back as far as you can go—you're a true friend who has been there for me through it all. Josh Shaw, you've been one of my closest friends since childhood. I would never be where I am, personally or professionally, without your sound advice and support. You are a brilliant entrepreneur, and I am lucky to have such a trusted advisor and friend.

John Decker, Aviva Drescher, Garrett and Nicole McNamara, Tom Yates, Leslie Jacovino, Denise Werleman, and Sara Bliss—thank you for being the best ambassadors of my brand. It's beautiful to have avid believers spreading the word and helping others toward true health.

Joan Pelzer, thank you for all your help with social media, and for always being such a positive force in this world.

And, finally, my family. Sheri, George, and Rick, my Pittsburgh family, you are the best in-laws a man could ask for. Thanks for your love and endless support.

To my brothers, Tony and Brandon, and your families—you've always been there for me, by my side through all the ups and downs of life, with encouragement and as an instrumental source of inspiration to help me realize my dreams. You are my biggest supporters and advocates. I am truly blessed.

Dear Mom, your strength, resolve, and unconditional love and support has carried me through some of the hardest and most challenging moments in my life. You are the most selfless soul I've ever known, and you have always led by example. You taught me what family really means by always putting us first, and you are the most incredible role model. I love you more than I can ever express in these words.

. . . and Dad. You made me the man I am today. I can never thank you enough for how hard you worked and how much you gave up. You were a true family man, an American patriot, and you will always live in my heart. I'll do my best to carry on your legacy for our family. I will forever be touched by the battle you courageously fought as I wrote this book. You are inextricably linked to this project, and your story will inspire so many. I promise to always protect the principles you taught me and stay true to who I am. I love you, and I miss you.

Chelsea, my rock. This book would not have been possible without you. You have been there for me, through it all. You are the most incredible wife and mother, and I am so grateful for everything you do for our two beautiful children and me. You are the reason I was able to complete this challenging and enduring project during the most painful period of my life. You were by my side at every moment, to give me strength with your nurturing and caring support. I couldn't love you more.

And my babies, Brayden and Alea, you are the light of my life and bring me true joy and happiness. Having you as my children makes me want to be a better person and is what inspired me to work so hard on this book. You are our future. You represent the next generation of health for everyone I aim to serve. I am so proud to be your father—I love you both with every inch of my soul.

And finally, to the Get Off Your Acid community, you are my tribe. I am filled with joy by your curiosity, your commitment to never-ending improvement and better health, and your support for one another and me. Keep fighting the good fight and spreading the good word.

RESOURCES FOR PRODUCTS

ALKALINE SUPPLEMENTS

Alkamind
Omega-3 Acid Index Test Kit

Test your omega-3/omega-6 ratio. Use coupon code OMEGA3 at checkout to receive a special Get Off Your Acid 20 percent discount (only discounted off regular retail price).

http://www.GetOffYourAcid.com, 844-200-ALKA (2552)

Bioactive Silver Hydrosol
(Colloidal Silver)

Natural-Immunogenics Corporation, the leader in hydrosol technology. Bioactive Colloidal Silver Products, http://bit.ly/2mXIEF4.

Dehydrated Greens
Supplement

Alkamind Daily Greens. With twenty-seven of the most alkalizing raw vegetables, grasses, sprouts, and low sugar-fruits, one scoop of Daily Greens will give you five servings of organic greens to alkalize and energize your body.

http://www.GetOffYourAcid.com, 844-200-ALKA (2552)

Mineral Salt Supplement

Alkamind Daily Minerals. With the four crucial minerals—calcium citrate, magnesium glycinate, potassium bicarbonate, and sodium bicarbonate—Daily Minerals is well-balanced with the purest medical-grade mineral salts, in a light and refreshing natural lemon taste.

http://www.GetOffYourAcid.com, 844-200-ALKA (2552)

Omega-3 Fatty Acid
Supplement (Fish Oil)

Alkamind Daily Omega-3. I couldn't find the exact formula that our bodies need in regards to the EPA to DHA ratio, so I created my own. Daily Omega-3 uses a process called *molecular distillation* to organically filter and triple purify to eliminate mercury and other toxic contaminants, while at the same time concentrating the fish oil. The benefit is that instead of having to take six to eight capsules to get the recommended 3,000 mg of daily fish oil, you only have to take three—half that amount. Daily Omega-3 has the exact ratio of EPA to DHA that your body requires, which is 2:1. **We are the *only* company to have the exact ratio of 2:1 with the process of *molecular distillation*.** These two factors make

Alkamind Daily Omega-3 the world's most premier, cutting-edge fish oil.

http://www.GetOffYourAcid.com, 844-200-ALKA (2552)

Plant-Based Algae Sources for DHA (for Vegetarians)

- Deva Omega-3
- Nature's Way Neuromins DHA
- Neuromins 200 DHA
- NuTru O-Mega-Zen3
- Vitamin Shoppe Neuromins DHA

Plant-Based Protein Powder Supplement

Alkamind Organic Daily Protein. Not all protein powders are created equal. Most use whey, sugar, artificial sweeteners, and fillers, which are toxic and acidic. Organic Daily Protein is infused with the three core alkaline proteins—hemp, pea, and sachi inchi—and coconut oil, to create a delicious tasting, organic protein powder that can be used as a total meal replacement, a healthy snack, or after your workout for a quick recovery.

http://www.GetOffYourAcid.com, 844-200-ALKA (2552)

Pure MSM (Organic Sufur)

http://www.organic-sulfur.com

CLEANSE AND DETOX PROGRAMS

Alkamind 7-Day Alkaline Cleanse and 2-Day Detox Challenge

These two programs are the perfect solution to lose weight, feel great, and fight inflammation in your body. They are not deprivation based programs—in fact, the alkaline recipes are so delicious you'll feel like you're cheating!

http://www.GetOffYourAcid.com, 844-200-ALKA (2552)

EQUIPMENT
Favorite Juicer

Hurom (cold-pressed masticating juicer)

http://www.hurom.com, 800-235-2140

Favorite Blenders
NUTRIBULLET

http://www.nutribullet.com, 800-523-5993

VITAMIX

https://www.vitamix.com/us/en_us, 800-848-2649

Favorite Dehydrator

My favorite dehydrator is the Excalibur, which is just around $100. However, it can also be acquired for $30. It's a worthwhile investment if you want to start making raw, alkaline veggie treats of all kinds.

http://www.excaliburdehydrator.com, 800-875-4254

BEMER Machine (PEMF)

https://getoffyouracid.bemergroup.com/en-US, 917-572-3971

High-Altitude Training Mask

https://www.trainingmask.com, 888-407-7555

Alkaline Water Filtration System with Molecular Hydrogen

Syngery Science Echo H2 Water. There are more than 700 studies showing that molecular hydrogen has strong therapeutic benefits, with 150 of those studies done with human disease models. Hydrogen gas (H_2) is the smallest molecule in the universe, about half the size of oxygen, which gives it a higher cellular bioavailability than any other supplement, drug, or nutraceutical. Founder Paul Barattiero is the foremost authority on molecular hydrogen and has built a powerful hydration system (Echo 9 Ultra H2), which I use in my home for my family and myself.

https://www.synergyscience.com/#agent=GETOFFYOURACID, 800-337-7017

OTHER RESOURCES

All Hands and Hearts Foundation

Every year, on average, natural disasters impact the lives of 218 million people. After these disasters, aid flows into countries for basic needs, but soon after these funds dry up, leaving countless children without safe schools. The All Hands and Hearts Foundation steps in when many go home, restoring hope and rebuilding safe, resilient schools around the world.

http://www.allhandsandhearts.org

Bremmer Farms

Unpasteurized, non-irradiated organic almonds

http://www.organicalmondsraw.com/almonds, 530-893-4950

The Dr. Robert Scott Bell Show

The Robert Scott Bell Show broadcasts live Monday–Friday, 7–9 p.m. EST, and Sundays, 1–3 p.m. EST on syndicator Genesis Communications Network (GCN). It simulcasts on YouTube (RSBellMediaChannel) with rebroadcasts via UK Health Radio, iTunes, Stitcher, tunein, and SoundCloud.

Robert Scott Bell, D.A. Hom. (American Academy of Clinical Homeopathy 1994) has served on the board of the American Association of Homeopathic Pharmacists (1999–2001) and continues to provide direct support to those in need. He also works with physicians on their toughest cases. Twenty-six years ago, he personally overcame numerous chronic diseases by using homeopathy, herbal medicine, organic whole foods, minerals, essential fats, and the transformational power of belief. As a homeopath, he has dedicated his life to revealing the healing power within us all.

http://www.robertscottbell.com/

Essential Oils

My favorite brands are Young Living, Do Terra, and NOW Foods.

The Food Revolution

The Food Revolution Network is committed to healthy, sustainable, humane, and conscious food for all. Guided by John and Ocean Robbins, with more than 600,000 members and with the collaboration of many of the top food revolutionary leaders, the network aims to empower individuals, build community, and transform food systems to support healthy people and a healthy planet.

http://www.foodrevolution.org

Fresh, Wild-Caught Fish

http://www.VitalChoice.com, 800-608-4825

Hope4Cancer Institute

Founded by Dr. Antonio Jiminez, Hope4Cancer is dedicated to restoring hope and health for those diagnosed with cancer. with two clinics in Mexico, the organization offers alternative therapies to strengthen and heal patients.

http://www.hope4cancer.com, 888-544-5993

Ketone Breath Analyzer

Ketonix is the first reusable breath ketone analyzer.

http://www.ketonix.co/, 301-302-0832

Micronutrient Depletion test by SpectraCell Laboratories

http://www.spectracell.com, 800-227-5227

pH Test Strips

These are the most accurate pH strips for testing saliva and urine pH levels. The state-of-the-art dual-color test strips deliver incredible accuracy in less than fifteen seconds.

http://www.GetOffYourAcid.com, 844-200-ALKA (2552)

Raw Flavored Essential Oils (for food)

http://www.medicineflower.com /esoilpr.html, 800-787-3645

The Truth About Cancer

This is a website aimed at taking cancer into our own hands. There are many articles from doctors, researchers, experts, and survivors about the education and prevention of cancer.

http://www.thetruthaboutcancer.com

REFERENCES

"2013 Milliman Medical Index," Milliman, 2013.

ABC News. "The Big Business of Falling Asleep." December 9, 2004. Retrieved from http://abcnews.go.com/GMA/story?id=343792&page=1.

"Abdominal Fat and What to Do About It." *Harvard Family Health Guide,* October 9, 2015.

Adebamowo, C. A., D. Spiegelman, C. S. Berkey, et al. "Milk Consumption and Acne in Adolescent Girls." *Dermatology Online Journal* 12 (2006): 1.

Albert, B. B. "Higher Omega-3 Index Is Associated with Increased Insulin Sensitivity and More Favourable Metabolic Profile in Middle-Aged Overweight Men." *Scientific Reports* 4.6697 (2014).

Ali, Sadia, Sachin K. Garg, Beth E. Cohen, Prashant Bhave, William S. Harris, and Mary A. Whooleya. "Association between Omega-3 Fatty Acids and Depressive Symptoms among Patients with Established Coronary Artery Disease: Data from the Heart and Soul Study." US National Library of Medicine, National Institutes of Health, Feb 18, 2009.

Altered States. "Monitoring Your Body's pH Levels." 2013. Retrieved from http://altered-states.net/barry/update178/.

Alzheimer's Association. 2016. "Facts and Figures." Retrieved from http://www.alz.org/facts/

Alzheimer's Research UK. "Dementia Deaths Set to Quadruple by 2040." May 18, 2017.

American Cancer Society. "Cancer Facts & Figures." 2017. Retrieved from https://www.cancer.org/research/cancer-facts-statistics/all-cancer-facts-figures/cancer-facts-figures-2017.html.

Anand, Preetha, et al. "Cancer Is a Preventable Disease that Requires Major Lifestyle Changes." *Pharmaceutical Research* 25.9 (Sept 2008).

Anxiety and Depression Association of America. "Facts & Statistics." 2017. Retrieved from https://adaa.org/about-adaa/press-room/facts-statistics.

Aubrey, Allison. "The Average American Ate (Literally) a Ton This Year." NPR, December 31, 2011. Retrieved from http://www.npr.org/sections/thesalt/2011/12/31/144478009/the-average-american-ate-literally-a-ton-this-year.

Ballantyne, Coco. "Fact or Fiction? Vitamin Supplements Improve Your Health." *Scientific American*, May 17, 2007. Retrieved from https://www.scientificamerican.com/article/fact-or-fiction-vitamin-supplements-improve-health/.

Barefoot, Robert R., and Carl M. Reich. *The Calcium Factor: The Scientific Secret of Health and Youth.* Wickenburg, AZ: Bokar Consultants, 2002.

Barnard, Neal. "Got Truth? The Dairy Industry's Junk Science." *Naked Food Magazine*, 2012. Retrieved from http://nakedfoodmagazine.com/got-truth/.

Barron, Jon. *Lessons from the Miracle Doctors: A Step-by-Step Guide to Optimum Health and Relief from Catastrophic Illness.* Laguna Beach, CA: Basic Health Publications, 2008, 77–80 and 111–114.

Bartels, Elmer C., Marios C. Balodimos, and Lester R. Corn. "The Association of Gout and Diabetes Mellitus." *Medical Clinics of North America* 44.2 (March 1960): 433–438.

Berger, T. J., et al. "Antifungal Properties of Electrically Generated Metallic Ions." *Antimicrobial Oligodynamic Agents and Chemotherapy* 10.5 (1976): 856–860.

Bernstein, A. M., and W. C. Willett. "Trends in 24-Hour Urinary Sodium Excretion in the United States, 1957–2003: A Systematic Review." *American Journal of Clinical Nutrition* 92.5 (Nov 2010): 1172–1180.

Better Health Foundation. "State of the Plate Report." 2011. Retrieved from http://www .pbhfoundation.org/pdfs/about/res/pbh _res/stateplate.pdf.

Bittman, Mark. "Is Junk Food Really Cheaper?" *New York Times*, Sept. 24, 2011.

Blaylock, Russell. *Natural Strategies for Cancer Patients.* New York: Kensington Publishing, 2003.

Blumenthal, Robin Goldwyn. "Drink Up!" *Barron's*, July 23, 2012. Retrieved from http: //www.barrons.com/articles/SB50001424053 111904346504577531063244598398.

Bollinger, Ty. *Cancer: Step Outside the Box*, 6th edition. Infinity 510^2 Partners, 2014.

Boswell, Mark, and B. Eliot Cole, eds. *American Academy of Pain Management, Weiner's Pain Management: A Practical Guide for Clinicians*, 7th edition. Boca Raton, FL: CRC Press, 2006, 584–585.

Boutenko, Victoria. "Oxalic Acid in Spinach." Raw Family Newsletter, July 11, 2014. Retrieved from http://www.rawfamily.com /oxalic-acid-in-spinach.

Breau, Anne. "The Mathematics of Middle-age Spread: Getting Older, Losing Muscle." Indiana Public Media, February 3, 2012. Retrieved from http://indianapublicmedia .org/amomentofscience/the-mathematics -of-middle-age-spread/.

Brewer, George J., and Sukhvir Kaur. "Zinc Deficiency and Zinc Therapy Efficacy with Reduction of Serum Free Copper in Alzheimer's Disease." *International Journal of Alzheimer's Disease* (Oct. 10, 2013).

Brogan, Kelly. "Taming the Monkey Mind: How Meditation Affects Your Health and Wellbeing." Mercola.com, February 20, 2014. Retrieved from http://articles.mercola.com /sites/articles/archive/2014/02/20 /meditation-relaxation-response.aspx.

Brown, M. D., C. A. Hart, E. Gazi, S. Bagley, and N. W. Clarke. "Promotion of Prostatic Metastatic Migration Toward Human Bone Marrow Stoma by Omega 6 and Its Inhibition by Omega 3 PUFAs." *British Journal of Cancer* 94 (2006): 842–853.

Burdge, G. C., and P. C. Calder. "Conversion of A-Linolenic Acid to Longer-Chain Polyunsaturated Fatty Acids in Human Adults." *Reproductive Nutrition and Development* 45 (2005): 581–597.

Burdge, G. C., and S. A. Wootton. "Conversion of A-Linolenic Acid to Eicosapentaenoic, Docosapentaenoic and Docosahexaenoic Acids in Young Women." *British Journal of Nutrition* 88 (2002): 411–420.

Burdge, G. C., et al. "Eicosapentaenoic and Docosahexaenoic Acids Are the Principal Products of Alpha-Linolenic Acid Metabolism in Young Men." *British Journal of Nutrition* 88 (2002): 355–363.

Burris, J., W. Rietkerk, and K. Woolf. "Acne: The Role of Medical Nutrition Therapy," *Journal of the Academy of Nutrition and Diet* 113.2 (2013): 416–430; doi: 10.1016/j.jand.2012.11.016.

Burrows, T., et al. "Omega-3 Index, Obesity and Insulin Resistance in Children." *International Journal of Pediatric Obesity* 6.2–2 (June 2011): e532–539.

Campbell, T. Colin. *The China Study*. Dallas, TX: BenBella Books, 2006.

"Cancer Overtakes Heart Disease as the Main Cause of Death in 12 European Countries." *ScienceDaily*, August 14, 2016.

CDC (Centers for Disease Control and Prevention). "Behavioral Risk Factor Surveillance System." 2017. Retrieved from https://www.cdc.gov/brfss/index.html.

CDC. "Childhood Obesity Facts." 2013. Retrieved from https://www.cdc.gov/healthyschools/obesity/facts.htm.

CDC. "Health: United States." 2016. Retrieved from https://www.cdc.gov/nchs/hus/index.htm.

CDC. "Heart Disease Risk Factors." 2012. Retrieved from https://www.cdc.gov/heartdisease/risk_factors.htm.

CDC. "Inflammatory Bowel Disease." 2017. Retrieved from https://www.cdc.gov/ibd/index.htm.

CDC. "Insufficient Sleep Is a Public Health Epidemic." 2015. Retrieved from https://www.cdc.gov/features/dssleep/index.html.

CDC. "Long-Term Trends in Diagnosed Diabetes." April 2017. Retrieved from https://www.cdc.gov/diabetes/statistics/slides/long_term_trends.pdf.

CDC. "National Diabetes Statistics Report." 2017. Retrieved from https://www.cdc.gov/diabetes/pdfs/data/statistics/national-diabetes-statistics-report.pdf.

CDC. "Nearly 1 in 10 US Adults Report Depression." 2010. Retrieved from http://thechart.blogs.cnn.com/2010/10/01/cdc-nearly-1-in-10-u-s-adults-depressed/.

CDC. "Types of Fungal Diseases." 2017. Retrieved from https://www.cdc.gov/fungal/diseases/index.html.

Chan, J. K., et al. "Effects of Dietary Alpha-Linolenic Acid and Its Ratio to Linoleic Acid on Platelet and Plasma Fatty Acids and Thrombogenesis." *Lipids* 28 (1993): 811–817.

Chen, X., and H. J. Schluesener. "Nanosilver: A Nanoproduct in Medical Application." *Toxicology Letters* 176 (2008): 1–12.

Chestnut, James. *The Wellness Prevention Paradigm*. Singapore: TWP Press, 2011.

"Chlorophyll and Chlorophyll in Chlorophyllin Is Effective in Limiting Aflatoxin Absorption in Humans." *News Medical Life Sciences*, December 30, 2009.

Cleland, et al. "A High Omega-3 Index May Provide Effective Pain Relief for People with Chronic Musculoskeletal Pain." *Nutrition & Dietetics* 66 (2009): 4–6.

Colliver, Victoria. "Medi-Cal Costs Soar as Alzheimer's Takes a Huge Financial Toll in State." *San Francisco Chronicle*, November 4, 2015.

Consumer Search. "Best Juicers—Top 5 Juicer Reviews." 2012.

Council for Agricultural Science and Technology. *Mycotoxins: Economic and Health Risks*. Task Force Report Number 116. Ames, IA, Nov. 1989.

Critser, Greg. *Fat Land: How Americans Became the Fattest People in the World*. Boston, MA: Houghton Mifflin Harcourt, 2004.

Crohns and Colitis Foundation of America. "IBS and IBD: Two Very Different Disorders." June 1, 2012. Retrieved from http://www.crohnscolitisfoundation.org/resources/ibs-and-ibd-two-very.html?print=t.

Cryer, B., and M. Feldman. "Effects of Very Low Doses of Daily, Long-Term Aspirin Therapy on Gastric, Duodenal and Rectal Prostaglandins on Mucosal Injury in Healthy Humans." *Gastroenterology* (1999): 117.

Cryer, Byron. "NSAID-Associated Deaths: The Rise and Fall of NSAID-Associated GI Mortality." *American Journal of*

Gastroenterology 100 (2005): 1694–1695. doi: 10.1111/j.1572-0241.2005.50565.

Cytokine Research Laboratory, Dept of Experimental Therapeutics, University of Texas M. D. Anderson Cancer Center, Houston TX.

David, A. Rosalie, and Michael R. Zimmerman. "Cancer: An Old Disease, a New Disease, or Something In Between?" *Nature Reviews Cancer* 10 (Oct 2010): 728–733.

Davis, D. R. "Declining Fruit and Vegetable Nutrient Composition: What Is the Evidence?" *Horticultural Science* 44.1 (Feb 2009): 15–19.

De Mello, V. D., A. T. Erkkila, U. S. Schwab, et al. "The Effect of Fatty or Lean Fish Intake on Inflammatory Gene Expression in Peripheral Blood Mononuclear Cells of Patients with Coronary Heart Disease." *European Journal of Nutrition* 48.8 (Dec 2009): 447–455.

de Nadai, T. R., et al. "Metabolic Acidosis Treatment as Part of a Strategy to Curb Inflammation." *International Journal of Inflammation* (2013).

"Deadly NSAIDS." American Nutrition Association, *Nutrition Digest* 38.2. Retrieved from http://americannutritionassociation. org/newsletter/deadly-nsaids.

Dean, Carolyn. *The Magnesium Miracle.* New York: Ballantine Books, 2014.

Deangela, Emma. "Hormones in Milk." The Alkaline Diet, March 2013. Retrieved from http://thealkalinediet.org/blog/hormones -in-milk.

Deardorff, Julie. "A Nutrition Gap in Modern Medicine," *Chicago Tribune*, March 26, 2013.

Dhingra, R., L. Sullivan, and P. F. Jacques, et al. "Soft Drink Consumption and Risk of Developing Cardiometabolic Risk Factors and the Metabolic Syndrome in Middle-Aged Adults in the Community." *Circulation* 116 (2007): 480–488.

Diamond, D. M., and U. Ravnskov. "How Statistical Deception Created the Appearance That Statins Are Safe and Effective in Primary and Secondary Prevention of Cardiovascular Disease." *Expert Review of Clinical Pharmacology* 8.2 (March 2015): 201–210.

Didymus, John Thomas. "Study: High Fructose Corn Syrup Is as Addictive as Cocaine." *Digital Journal,* June 8, 2013. Retrieved from http:// www.digitaljournal.com/article/351810.

"Dirt Poor: Have Fruits and Vegetables Become Less Nutritious?" *Scientific American*, 2011.

Dorfman, Kelly. "Do You Have One of the Most Common Nutritional Deficiencies?" *Huffington Post*, August 29, 2012. Retrieved from http://www.huffingtonpost.com/kelly -dorfman/vitamin-deficiency_b_1633446 .html.

Doyle, Kathryn. "Drinking Diet Soda Linked to a Widening Waistline with Age: People Over Age 65 Who Drink Diet Soda Daily Tend to Expand Their Waistlines by Much More Than Peers Who Prefer Other Beverages, Possibly Contributing to Chronic Illnesses That Go Along with Excess Belly Fat." *Reuters*, March 18, 2015. Retrieved from http://www.reuters .com/article/us-health-aging-soda-belly- idUSKBN0ME2MH20150318.

Earth Policy Institute, US Dept of Agriculture. "U.S. Meat Consumption Per Person, 1902– 2012," 2013. Retrieved from www.earth-policy. org/datacenter/xls/highlights25_1.xls.

Eating Well. "What Is a Serving of Vegetables?" 2017. Retrieved from http://www.eatingwell .com/article/17573/what-is-a-serving-of -vegetables/.

Emken, E. A., et al. "Dietary Linolenic Acid Influences Desaturation and Acylation of Deuterium-Labeled Linoleic and Linolenic Acids in Young Adult Males." *Biochimica et Biophysica Acta* 1213 (1994): 277–288.

Environmental Working Group. "Body Burden: The Pollution in Newborns." A Benchmark Investigation of Industrial Chemicals, Pollutants, and Pesticides in Umbilical Cord Blood." July 14, 2005.

Epel, Elissa S., Elizabeth H. Blackburn, Jue Lin, Firdaus S. Dhabhar, Nancy E. Adler, Jason D. Morrow, and Richard M. Cawthon. "Accelerated Telomere Shortening in Response to Life Stress." *Proceedings of the National Academy of Sciences of the United States of America* 101.49 (December 7, 2004): 17312–17315.

Ergas, D. E. Eilat, S. Mendlovic, and Z. M. Sthoeger. "N-3 Fatty Acids and the Immune System in Autoimmunity." *Israel Medical Association Journal* 4.1 (Jan 2002): 34–38.

Fairfield, Hannah. "Metrics: Factory Food." *New York Times*, April 3, 2010.

Feskanich, D., W. C. Willett, and G. A. Colditz. "Calcium, Vitamin D, Milk Consumption, and Hip Fractures: A Prospective Study Among Postmenopausal Women." *American Journal of Clinical Nutrition* 77 (2003): 504–511.

Fife, Bruce. *Oil Pulling Therapy, Detoxifying and Healing the Body Through Oral Cleansing.* Colorado Springs, CO: Piccadilly Books, 2008.

Fisher, M. C., D. A. Henk, and C. J. Briggs, et al. "Emerging Fungal Threats to Animal, Plant and Ecosystem Health." *Nature* 484 (2012): 186–219. doi: 10.1038/nature10947.

Food and Nutrition Board, Institute of Medicine. "Dietary Reference Intakes for Energy, Carbohydrate, Fiber, Fat, Fatty Acids, Cholesterol, Protein, and Amino Acids (Macronutrients): A Report of the Panel on Macronutrients, Subcommittees on Upper Reference Levels of Nutrients and Interpretation and Uses of Dietary Reference Intakes, and the Standing Committee on the Scientific Evaluation of Dietary Reference Intakes." National Academy Press, Washington, DC, 2002.

Fowler, Sharon P. G., Ken Williams, and Helen P. Hazuda. "Diet Soda Intake Is Associated with Long-Term Increases in Waist Circumference in a Biethnic Cohort of Older Adults: The San Antonio Longitudinal Study of Aging." *Journal of American Geriatrics Society*, March17, 2015.

Francois, C. A., et al. "Supplementing Lactating Women with Flaxseed Oil Does Not Increase Docosahexaenoic Acid in Their Milk." *American Journal of Clinical Nutrition* 77 (2003): 226–233.

Freuman, Tamara Duker. "Why Juice Cleanses Don't Deliver." *U.S. News & World Report*, December 26, 2012. Retrieved from http://health.usnews.com/health-news/blogs/eat-run/2012/12/26/why-juice-cleanses-dont-deliver.

Friedman, Lindsay. "Americans More Proactive in Personal Healthcare," *USA Today*, August 1, 2013.

Fryar, Cheryl D., Margaret D. Carroll, and Cynthia L. Ogden. "Prevalence of Overweight, Obesity, and Extreme Obesity Among Adults." Centers for Disease Control and Prevention, 2012. Retrieved from https://www.cdc.gov/nchs/data/hestat/obesity_adult_11_12/obesity_adult_11_12.htm.

Fung, Jason, and Jimmy Moore. *The Complete Guide to Fasting.* Las Vegas, NV: Victory Belt Publishing, 2016, 199–208.

Gan, X., T. Liu, J. Zhong, X. Liu, and G. Li. "Effect of Silver Nanoparticles on the Electron Transfer Reactivity and the Catalytic Activity of Myoglobin." *ChemBioChem* 5.12 (Dec 3, 2004): 1686–1691.

Garber, C. E., et al. "Quantity and Quality of Exercise for Developing and Maintaining Cardiorespiratory, Musculoskeletal, and

Neuromotor Fitness in Apparently Healthy Adults: Guidance for Prescribing Exercise." *Medical Science Sports Exercise* 43.7 (July 2011): 1334–1359. doi: 10.1249 /MSS.0b013e318213fefb.

Gedgaudas, Nora. *Primal Fat Burner: Live Longer, Slow Aging, Super-Power Your Brain, and Save Your Life with a High-Fat, Low-Carb Paleo Diet.* Atria Books, 2017, 80, 161, 199.

Gerster, H. "Can Adults Adequately Convert A-Linolenic Acid (18:3n-3) to Eicosapentaenoic Acid (20:5n-3) and Docosahexaenoic Acid (22:6n-3)?" *International Journal of Vitamin and Nutrition Research* 68 (1998): 159–173.

Goldberg, Jane G. "Almonds: Raw or Rocket Fuel?" 2015. Retrieved from http:// drjanegoldberg.com/almonds-raw-or -rocket-fuel/.

Golubovich, V. N., et al. "Binding of Silver Ions by Candida Utilis Cells." *Mikrobiolgiia* 15.1 (1976): 119–122.

Gu, Q., C. F. Dillon, and V. L. Burt. "Prescription Drug Use Continues to Increase." *NCHS Data Brief* 42 (Sept 2010): 1–8.

Gu, Qiuping, Ryne Paulose-Ram, Vicki L. Burt, and Brian K. Kit. "Prescription Cholesterol-Lowering Medication Use in Adults Aged 40 and Over." Centers for Disease Control and Prevention, December 2014. Retrieved from https://www.cdc.gov/nchs/products /databriefs/db177.htm.

Gunnars, Kris. "44 Healthy Low-Carb Foods that Taste Incredible." *Authority Nutrition*, August 18, 2016.

Hageman, William. "Living Healthier at Higher Elevations: The Benefits Are Seen in Lifespan and Disease, Obesity Rates." *Journal of Epidemiology and Community Health*, Sept. 7, 2011.

Halldorsson, Thorhallur I., Marin Strøm, Sesilje B. Petersen, and Sjurdur F. Olsen. "Intake of Artificially Sweetened Soft Drinks and Risk of Preterm Delivery: A Prospective Cohort Study in 59,334 Danish Pregnant Women." *American Journal of Clinical Nutrition*, 2010.

Harvard Health Publications. "Cutting Red Meat for a Longer Life." Harvard Men's Health Watch, June 2012.

Harvard School of Public Health. "Food Pyramids and Plates: What Should You Really Eat?" 2013. Retrieved from https://www.hsph .harvard.edu/nutritionsource/healthy-eating -plate/.

Harvard Women's Health Watch. "Anxiety and Physical Illness." June 2017. Retrieved from https://www.health.harvard.edu/staying -healthy/anxiety_and_physical_illness.

He, F. J., C. A. Nowson, and G. A. MacGregor. "Fruit and Vegetable Consumption and Stroke: Meta-Analysis of Cohort Studies." *Lancet* 367.9507 (2006): 320–326.

He, F. J., et al. "Increased Consumption of Fruit and Vegetables Is Related to a Reduced Risk of Coronary Heart Disease: Meta-Analysis of Cohort Studies." *Journal of Human Hypertension* 21.9 (2007): 717–728.

Hendry, G. A., and O. T. Jones. "Haems and Chlorophylls: Comparison of Function and Formation." *Journal of Medical Genetics* 17.1 (Feb 1980): 1–14. PMCID: PMC1048480.

Hess, B. "Pathophysiology, Diagnosis, and Conservative Therapy in Calcium Kidney Calculi." *Therapeutische Umschau* (Feb. 2003), Medizinische Klinik, Spital Zimmerberg, Wädenswil, Switzerland.

Holmes, R., and D. Assimos. "The Impact of Dietary Oxalate on Kidney Stone Formation." Urological Research, Oct. 2004, Department of Urology, Wake Forest University Medical School, Winston-Salem, NC.

Hung, H. C., et al. "Fruit and Vegetable Intake and Risk of Major Chronic Disease." *National Cancer Institute* 96.21 (2004): 1577–1584.

Hussein, N., et al. "Long-Chain Conversion of [13C]Linoleic Acid and A-Linolenic Acid in Response to Marked Changes in the Dietary Intake in Men." *Journal of Lipid Research* 46: 269–280, 2005.

Inflammatory Bowel Disease Center at Baylor College of Medicine. "Crohns Disease." 2013.

Jansson, G., and M. Harms-Ringdahl. "Stimulating Effects of Mercuric and Silver Ions on the Superoxide Anion Production in Human Polymorphonuclear Leukocytes." *Free Radical Research Communications* 18.2 (1993): 87–98.

Kaluza, J., A. Wolk, and S. C. Larsson. "Red Meat Consumption and Risk of Stroke: A Meta-analysis of Prospective Studies." *Stroke* 43.10 (October 2012): 2556–2560.

Kaplan, Karen. "Stress, Anxiety and Pain Disturb Americans' Sleep, Survey Finds." *Los Angeles Times*, June 3, 2013. Retrieved from http://articles.latimes.com/2013/jun/03/science/la-sci-sn-sleep-problems-survey-20130603.

Kimball, Molly. "30 Days of Daily Juicing." *Times-Picayune*, May 6, 2013.

Kimopoulos, Artemis, ed. "Prevention of Coronary Heart Disease: From the Cholesterol Hypothesis to O6/O3 Balance." *World Review of Nutrition and Dietetics*. Basel, Switzerland: Karger Publishers, 2007.

King, V. R., W. L. Huang, S. C. Dyall, O. E. Curran, J. V. Priestley, and A. T. Michael-Titus. "Omega-3 Fatty Acids Improve Recovery, Whereas Omega-6 Fatty Acids Worsen Outcome, After Spinal Cord Injury in the Adult Rat." *Journal of Neuroscience* 26.17 (2006): 4672–4680.

Klein, S., and R. R. Wolfe. "Carbohydrate Restriction Regulates the Adaptive Response to Fasting." *American Journal of Physiology, Endocrinology, and Metabolism* 262.5 (May 1, 1992): E631–E636.

Knapton, Sarah. "High-Protein Diet 'as Bad for Health as Smoking.' Research Finds that People Who Eat Diet Rich in Animal Protein Carry Similar Cancer Risk to Those Who Smoke 20 Cigarettes Each Day." *The Telegraph*, March 4, 2014.

Kok, Dirk J., et al. "The Effects of Dietary Excesses in Animal Protein and in Sodium on the Composition and the Crystallization Kinetics of Calcium Oxalate Monohydrate in Urines of Healthy Men." *Journal of Clinical Endocrinology and Metabolism*, Oct. 1990, Department of Endocrinology, University Hospital, Leiden, the Netherlands.

Krumholz, Harlan M., Teresa E. Seeman, and Susan S. Merrill. "Lack of Association Between Cholesterol and Coronary Heart Disease Mortality and Morbidity and All-Cause Mortality in Persons Older Than 70 Years." *Journal of the American Medical Association* 272.17 (1994): 1335–1340. doi: 10.1001/jama.1994.03520170045034.

Lamptey, M. S., and B. L. Walker. "A Possible Essential Role for Dietary Linolenic Acid in the Development of the Young Rat." *Journal of Nutrition* 106.1 (1976): 86–93.

Landa, Jennifer. "More Than 24,500 Chemicals Found in Bottled Water." FoxNews.com, Jan. 13, 2014.

Lanou, A. J., S. E. Berkow, and N. D. Barnard. "Calcium, Dairy Products, and Bone Health in Children and Young Adults: A Reevaluation of the Evidence." *Pediatrics* 115 (2005): 736–743.

Lardner, Anne. "The Effects of Extracellular pH on Immune Function." *Journal of Leukocyte Biology* 69 (April 2001).

LeBeau, James. *Balance Your pH*. Thiensville, WI: The Perfect Health Foundation, 1995.

Lembke, et al. "Higher Omega-3 Levels Could Reduce the Incidence of Neck and Back Pain and Reduce the Need for Medication." *Journal of Sports Science Medicine* 13.1 (Jan 2014): 151–156.

Lenoir, M., F. Serre, L. Cantin, and S. H. Ahmed. "Intense Sweetness Surpasses Cocaine Reward." *PLoS ONE* 2.8 (2007): e698.

Leung, Cindy W., Barbara A. Laraia, Belinda L. Needham, David H. Rehkopf, Nancy E. Adler, Jue Lin, Elizabeth H. Blackburn, and Elissa S. Epel. "Soda and Cell Aging: Associations Between Sugar-Sweetened Beverage Consumption and Leukocyte Telomere Length in Healthy Adults From the National Health and Nutrition Examination Surveys." *American Journal of Public Health* (October 16, 2014).

Levine, Morgan E., et al. "Low Protein Intake Is Associated with a Major Reduction in IGF-1, Cancer, and Overall Mortality in the 65 and Younger but Not Older Population." *Cell Metabolism* 19.3 (March 4, 2014): 407–417.

Lindeberg, Staffan. "Paleolithic Diets as a Model for Prevention and Treatment of Western Disease." *American Journal of Human Biology* 24.2 (March/April 2012): 110–115.

Loyola University Health System. "New Evidence for Link Between Depression and Heart Disease." ScienceDaily, February 19, 2013. Retrieved from https://www.sciencedaily.com/releases/2013/02/130219121604.htm.

Ludwig, David S., and Walter C. Willett. "Three Daily Servings of Reduced-Fat Milk: An Evidence-Based Recommendation?" *Journal of the American Medical Association, Pediatrics* 167.9 (September 2013): 788–789.

Lustig, Robert H. *Fat Chance: Beating the Odds Against Sugar, Processed Food, Obesity, and Disease.* New York: Avery, 2013, 119.

Lutsey, P. L., L. M. Steffen, and J. Stevens. "Dietary Intake and the Development of the Metabolic Syndrome: The Atherosclerosis Risk in Communities Study." *Circulation* 117 (2008): 754–761.

Mangels, Reed. "Protein in the Vegan Diet." Vegetarian Resource Group, 2017. Retrieved from http://www.vrg.org/nutrition/protein.php.

Marieb, Elaine N., and Katja N. Hoehn. *Human Anatomy and Physiology*, 3rd edition. New York: Pearson, 2005.

Marler, John B., and Jeanne R. Wallin. "Human Health: The Nutritional Quality of Harvested Food and Sustainable Farming Systems." Nutrition Security Institute, 2010. Retrieved from http://www.nutritionsecurity.org/PDF/NSI_White%20Paper_Web.pdf.

Mayer, Mark. *Calcification: The Phosphate Factor in Aging and Disease.* Create Space Independent Publishing, 2014.

Mayo Clinic. "Stress: Constant Stress Puts Your Health at Risk." 2017. Retrieved from http://www.mayoclinic.org/healthy-lifestyle/stress-management/in-depth/stress/art-20046037.

Mayo Clinic. "Water: How Much Should You Drink Every Day?" 2013. Retrieved from http://www.mayoclinic.org/healthy-lifestyle/nutrition-and-healthy-eating/in-depth/water/art-20044256.

Mazza, A., et al. "Predictors of Cancer Mortality in Elderly Subjects." *European Journal of Epidemiology* 15.5 (June 1999): 421–427.

Meier, Barry. "More Emergency Room Visits Linked to Energy Drinks." *New York Times*, January 11, 2013.

Mensah, G. "Global and Domestic Health Priorities: Spotlight on Chronic Disease." National Business Group on Health Webinar, May 23, 2006.

Mercola, Joseph, et al. *Total Health Program*, 2005. Ebook available at http://www.mercola.com/ebook/total-health-book.aspx.

Mercola, Joseph. "Artificial Sweeteners Gaining Increasingly Bad Press—And For Good Reason." Mercola.com, October 2013. Retrieved from http://articles.mercola.com/sites/articles/archive/2013/10/23/aspartame-artificial-sweeteners.aspx.

Mercola, Joseph. *Fat for Fuel.* Carlsbad, CA: Hay House Publishing, 2017, 36.

Mercola.com. "Alkaline Water: If You Fall for This 'Water Fad' You Could Do Some Damage." September 11, 2010. Retrieved from http://articles.mercola.com/sites/articles/archive/2010/09/11/alkaline-water-interview.aspx.

Mercola.com. "The Truth About Soy Foods: Can Soy Damage Your Health?" September 18, 2010. Retrieved from http://articles.mercola.com/sites/articles/archive/2010/09/18/soy-can-damage-your-health.aspx.

Moschos, S. J., and C. S. Mantzoros. "The Role of the IGF System in Cancer: From Basic to Clinical Studies and Clinical Applications." *Oncology* 63.4 (2002): 317–332.

Murthy, G. K., and U. Rhea. "Cadmium and Silver Content of Market Milk." Food Protection Research, National Center for Urban and Industrial Health, US Public Health Service. *Journal of Dairy Science* 51.4 (1968): 610–613.

Mychaskiw, Marianne. "Women Spend an Average of $15,000 on Makeup in Their Lifetimes." *InStyle*, April 17, 2013. Retrieved from http://www.instyle.com/beauty/15-under-15-best-bargain-beauty-products.

Nafar, F., and K. M. Mearow. "Coconut Oil Attenuates the Effects of Amyloid-! on Cortical Neurons In Vitro." *Journal of Alzheimer's Disease* 39.2 (Jan. 1, 2014): 233–237. doi: 10.3233/JAD-131436.

Naish, John. "The Rotten Truth: Why Fruit Sugar Is One of the Most Damaging Ingredients in Our Food." *Daily Mail*, October 3, 2011. Retrieved from http://www.dailymail.co.uk/health/article-2044880/The-rotten-truth-Why-fruit-sugar-damaging-ingredients-food.html.

Nakayama, T. "Studies on Acetic Acid-Bacteria I. Biochemical Studies on Ethanol Oxidation." *Journal of Biochemistry* 46.9 (1959): 1217–1225.

Natural Resources Defense Council. "Select the Right Filter." 2011. Retrieved from http://www.laondaverde.org/living/waterair/select-right-filter.asp.

Newport, Mary. *Alzheimer's Disease: What If There Was a Cure?* Nashville, TN: Basic Health, 2011.

Novelli B. "Health Care Reform Hinges on Private-Sector Collaboration." *Preventing Chronic Disease* 6.2 (2009).

Offit, Paul. "The Vitamin Myth: Why We Think We Need Supplements." *The Atlantic*, July 19, 2013. Retrieved from https://www.theatlantic.com/health/archive/2013/07/the-vitamin-myth-why-we-think-we-need-supplements/277947/.

Okuyama, H., et al. "Statins Stimulate Atherosclerosis and Heart Failure: Pharmacological Mechanisms." *Expert Review of Clinical Pharmacology* 8.2 (March 2015): 189–199.

Olmsted, Larry. *Real Food, Fake Food: Why You Don't Know What You're Eating & What You Can DO About It.* Chapel Hill, NC: Algonquin Books, 2016, 80–85.

Ophardt, Charles E. "pH Scale." Elmhurst College Chemistry Department, 2003. Retrieved fro. http://chemistry.elmhurst.edu/vchembook/184ph.html.

Organisation for Economic Co-operation and Development (OECD). "How Does the United States Compare," 2014. Retrieved from http://www.oecd.org/unitedstates/Briefing-Note-UNITED-STATES-2014.pdf.

Osterud, Bjarne, and Edel O. Elvevoll. "Dietary Omega-3 Fatty Acids and Risk of Type-2 Diabetes: Lack of Antioxidants?" *American Journal of Clinical Nutrition* 94.2 (August 2011): 618–619.

Padova, James N., and Gordon Bendersky. "Hyperuricemia in Diabetic Ketoacidosis." *New England Journal of Medicine* 267 (Sept 13, 1962): 530–534. doi: 10.1056/NEJM1962 0913267110.

Pai, Sunil. *An Inflammation Nation: The Definitive 10-Step Guide to Preventing and Treating All Diseases Through Diet, Lifestyle, and the Use of Natural Anti-Inflammatories.* San Francisco, CA: RocDoc Publications, 2014, 138–139, 142–143.

Pan, A., Q. Sun, A. M. Bernstein, J. E. Manson, W. C. Willett, and F. B. Hu. "Changes in Red Meat Consumption and Subsequent Risk of Type 2 Diabetes Mellitus," *Journal of the American Medical Association, Internal Medicine* 173.14 (July 22, 2013): 1328–1335.

Park, Alice. "A Thin Gene Is Linked to Heart Disease and Diabetes Risk Factors," *Time,* June 27, 2011.

Park, H. J. "Silver-Ion-Mediated Reactive Oxygen Species Generation Affecting Bactericidal Activity." *Water Research* 43 (2009): 1027–1032.

Parletta, N., T. Niyonsenga, J. Duff. "Omega-3 and Omega-6 Polyunsaturated Fatty Acid Levels and Correlations with Symptoms in Children with Attention Deficit Hyperactivity Disorder, Autistic Spectrum Disorder and Typically Developing Controls." *PLoS ONE* 11.5 (2016): e0156432. https://doi.org /10.1371/journal.pone.0156432.

Patek, Arthur J., Jr. "Chlorophyll and Blood Regeneration." *Journal of the American Medical Association* 106.11 (March 4, 1936): 925.

Pawlosky, R. J., et al. "Physiological Compartmental Analysis of Alpha-Linolenic Acid Metabolism in Adult Humans." *Journal of Lipid Research* 42.8 (2001): 1257–1265.

Penna, Dean Della. "Testimony on Nutrition; Vitamins: The Bottom Line." Harvard School of Public Health, 2013.

Phelan, et al. "Hormonal and Metabolic Effects of Polyunsaturated Fatty Acids in Young Women with Polycystic Ovary Syndrome: Results from a Cross-Sectional Analysis and a Randomized, Placebo-Controlled Crossover Trial." *American Journal of Clinical Nutrition* 93 (March 2011): 652–662.

PHuel. "How to Measure Your pH with pH Test Strips." 2015. Retrieved from http:// www.phuelup.com/portfolio/how-to-test -your-ph/.

Physicians Committee for Responsible Medicine. "Survey Finds Americans Lack Basic Nutrition Information." 2012. Retrieved from http:// www.pcrm.org/health/reports/survey -americans-lack-basic-nutrition-info.

Physicians Committee for Responsible Medicine. "The Power Plate" 2017. Retrieved from http://www.pcrm.org/health/diets/pplate /power-plate.

Physicians Committee for Responsible Medicine. "The Protein Myth." 2016. Retrieved from http://www.pcrm.org/health/diets/vsk /vegetarian-starter-kit-protein.

Pizzorno, Joseph. "What We Have Learned About Vitamin D Dosing?" *Integrative Medicine* 9.1 (Feb/Mar 2010).

PR Daily. "Most Employed Americans Work More Than 40 Hours Per Week." July 12, 2012. Retrieved from http://m.prdaily.com /Main/Articles/Most_employed_Americans _work_more_than_40_hours_pe_12123.aspx.

Price, Maria Z. "What Is Superfood?" LiveStrong, 2011. Retrieved from http://www.livestrong .com/article/45305-superfood/.

Puusa, Seppo. "Research Shows Inflammation Causes Acne." *Natural News,* March 7, 2011.

Retrieved from http://www.naturalnews.com/031605_inflammation_acne.html.

Ramsden, Christopher E., Daisy Zamora, Sharon Majchrzak-Hong, Keturah R. Faurot, Steven K. Broste, Robert P. Frantz, John M. Davis, Amit Ringel, Chirayath M. Suchindran, and Joseph R. Hibbeln. "Re-Evaluation of the Traditional Diet-Heart Hypothesis: Analysis of Recovered Data from Minnesota Coronary Experiment (1968–1973)." *British Medical Journal* 353 (April 2016): 1246.

Ravn, Karen. "Don't Just Sit There. Really." *Los Angeles Times*, May 25, 2013. Retrieved from http://articles.latimes.com/2013/may/25/health/la-he-dont-sit-20130525.

RayStrand.com. "My Concept of Nutritional Medicine." 2017. Retrieved from http://www.raystrand.com/nutritional-medicine.asp.

Rentz, E. J. "Viral Pathogens and Severe Acute Respiratory Syndrome: Oligodynamic Ag+ for Direct Immune Intervention." *Journal of Nutritional and Environmental Medicine* 13.2 (June 2003): 109–118.

"Retirement & Survivors Benefits: Life Expectancy Calculator," Social Security Administration, 2013.

Ridgeway, Leslie. "High Fructose Corn Syrup Linked to Diabetes." *USC News*, November 28, 2012.

Riell, Howard. "Bursting With Energy." Convenience Store Decisions, July 17, 2013. Retrieved from http://www.cstoredecisions.com/2012/12/10/bursting-with-energy-3/.

Robbins, Anthony. *Unleash the Power Within: Personal Coaching from Anthony Robbins That Will Transform Your Life.* New York: Simon and Schuster Audio, 2012.

Rosen, Meghan. "All Bodies Don't Act Their Age." *Science News* (December 26, 2015): 20.

Roth, Stephen M. "Why Does Lactic Acid Build Up in Muscles? And Why Does It Cause Soreness?" *Scientific American*, Jan 23, 2006.

Retrieved from https://www.scientificamerican.com/article/why-does-lactic-acid-buil/.

Rubenstein, Grace. "New Health Rankings: Of 17 Nations, U.S. Is Dead Last." *The Atlantic*, January 10, 2013. Retrieved from https://www.theatlantic.com/health/archive/2013/01/new-health-rankings-of-17-nations-us-is-dead-last/267045/.

Runtuwene, Joshua, Haruka Amitani, Marie Amitani, Akihiro Asakawa, Kai-Chun Cheng and Akio Inui. "Hydrogen-Water Enhances 5-Fluorouracil-Induced Inhibition of Colon Cancer." Department of Psychosomatic Internal Medicine, Kagoshima University Graduate School of Medical and Dental Sciences, Kagoshima, Japan. *Peer Journal*, April 7, 2015.

Saey, Tina Hesman. "Age Is More Than Just a Number." *Science News* (August 2015): 10.

Samuni, A., et al. "On the Cytotoxicity of Vitamin C and Metal Ions. *European Journal of Biochemistry* 99 (1983): 562.

Schaefer, et al. "Higher Level of Certain Fatty Acid Associated with Lower Dementia Risk." *JAMA Neurology* 63 (2006): 1527–1528.

Schaefer, et al. "Individuals with High Blood Cell DHA Had a 47% Lower Risk of Developing Dementia Than Those with Low DHA." *Journal of the American Medical Association, Neurology* 63 (2006): 1527–1528.

Schatz, Irwin J., et al. "Cholesterol and All-Cause Mortality in Elderly People from the Honolulu Heart Program: A Cohort Study." *The Lancet* 358.9279: 351–355.

Schmid, Ron. *Primal Nutrition: Paleolithic and Ancestral Diets for Optimal Health.* Golden, CO: Healing Arts, 2015.

Schulze, M. B., J. E. Manson, and D. S. Ludwig, et al. "Sugar-Sweetened Beverages, Weight Gain, and Incidence of Type 2 Diabetes in Young and Middle-Aged Women." *Journal of* the *American Medical Association* 292 (2004): 927–934.

Schwalfenberg, Gerry K. "The Alkaline Diet: Is There Evidence That an Alkaline pH Diet Benefits Health?" *Journal of Environmental and Public Health* (Oct 2012).

Sears, Barry. *The Anti-Inflammation Zone: Reversing the Silent Epidemic That's Destroying Our Health.* New York: ReganBooks, 2005, 217–218.

Short, Matthew W., and Jason E. Domagalski. "Iron Deficiency Anemia." *American Family Physician* 87.2 (Jan 15 2007): 98–104.

Sidhu, H., R. P. Holmes, M. J. Allison, and A. B. Peck. "Direct Quantification of the Enteric Bacterium Oxalobacter formigenes in Human Fecal Samples by Quantitative Competitive-Template PCR." *Journal of Clinical Microbiology* 37.5 (May 1999): 1503–1509. PMCID: PMC84815.

Simonetti, N., et al. "Electrochemical Oligodynamic Ag+ for Preservative Use." *Applied and Environmental Microbiology* 58.12 (1992): 3834–3836.

Simopoulos, A. P. "Omega-3 Fatty Acids in Health and Disease and in Growth and Development." *American Journal of Clinical Nutrition* 54.3 (Sept 1991): 438–463.

Simopoulos, A. P. "Omega-3 Fatty Acids in Inflammation and Autoimmune Diseases." *Journal of the American College of Nutrition* 21.6 (Dec 2002): 495–505.

Simopoulos, A. P. "The Importance of the Omega-6/Omega-3 Fatty Acid Ratio in Cardiovascular Disease and Other Chronic Diseases." *Experimental Biology and Medicine* 233.6 (June 2008): 674–688, diuL 10,3181.0711-MR-311.

Simopoulos, A. P. "The Omega-6/Omega-3 Fatty Acid Ratio, Genetic Ariation, and Cardiovascular Disease." *Asia Pacific Journal of Clinical Nutrition* 17.1 (2008): 131–134.

Simopoulos, A. P. "An Increase in the Omega-6/Omega-3 Fatty Acid Ratio Increases the Risk for Obesity." *Nutrients* 8.3 (March 2, 2016): 128. doi: 10.3390/nu8030128.

Simopoulos, A. P., ed. *International Conference on the Return of Omega-3 Fatty Acids into the Food Supply I. Land-Based Animal Food Products and Their Health Effects.* The Center for Genetics, Nutrition, and Health, Washington, DC, 1998.

Simopoulos, A. P., et al. "Dietary Omega-3 Fatty Acid Deficiency and High Fructose Intake in the Development of Metabolic Syndrome, Brain Metabolic Abnormalities, and Non-Alcoholic Fatty Liver Disease." *Nutrients* 5.8 (Aug 2013): 2901–2923.

Singh, M, et al. "Nanotechnology in Medicine and Antibacterial Effect of Silver Nanoparticles." *Digest Journal of Nanomaterials and Biostructures* 3.3 (September 2008): 115–122.

Sircus, Mark. *Anti-Inflammatory Oxygen Therapy: Your Complete Guide to Understanding and Using Natural Oxygen Therapy.* New Hyde Park, NY: Square One Publishers, 2015.

Sircus, Mark. *Sodium Bicarbonate: Nature's Unique First Aid Remedy.* New Hyde Park, NY: Square One Publishers, 2014.

Sisson, Mark. *The Primal Blueprint.* Malibu, CA: Primal Nutrition Inc., 2009.

SnyderHealth. "Food 'Ash' pH Chart." 2003. Retrieved from https://www.snyderhealth.com/documents/FoodAshPHChart.pdf.

Soedamah-Muthu, S. S., and E. L. Ding EL, et al. "Milk and Dairy Consumption and Incidence of Cardiovascular Diseases and All-Cause Mortality." *American Journal of Clinical Nutrition* 93.1 (2011): 158–171.

Soscia, S. J., J. E. Kirby, and K. J. Washicosky, et al. "The Alzheimer's Disease-Associated Amyloid Beta-Protein Is an Antimicrobial Peptide." *PLoS One* 5.3 (2010): e9505.

Squitti, R., I. Simonelli, M. Ventriglia, M. Siotto, P. Pasqualetti, A. Rembach, J. Doecke, and A. I. Bush. "Meta-Analysis of Serum Non-Ceruloplasmin Copper in Alzheimer's Disease." *Journal of Alzheimer's Disease* 38.4 (Jan. 1, 2014): 809–822. doi: 10.3233/JAD-131247.

Stewart, C. S., S. H. Duncan, and D. R. Cave. "Oxalobacter Formigenes and Its Role in Oxalate Metabolism in the Human Gut." *FEMS Microbiology Letters* 230.1 (Jan 15, 2004): 1–7.

Stock, Robert, John D. Currence, and Elizabeth Swanson. "The Uric Acid and Glutathione Content of Blood in Diabetes Mellitus." *Journal of Clinical Endocrinology Metabolism* 10.3 (1950): 313–317.

Stoll, Andrew. *The Omega-3 Connection: The Groundbreaking Omega-3 Anti-Depression Diet and Brain Program.* New York: Simon & Schuster, 2001, 208.

Taubes, Gary. *Good Calories Bad Calories: Fats, Carbs, and the Controversial Science of Diet and Health.* New York: Anchor, 2008.

Taylor, Eric N., and Gary C. Curhan. "Oxalate Intake and the Risk for Nephrolithiasis." *Journal of the American Society of Nephrology* (May 30, 2007).

The Dr. Oz Show. "The Healing Properties of Juicing: Why Juice Cleanses Don't Deliver," *U.S. News & World Report,* 2012.

Thompson, Chuck. "You're Breathing All Wrong." *Men's Journal,* 2013. Retrieved from http://www.mensjournal.com/magazine/you-re-breathing-all-wrong-20130227#ixzz3IaHG9phN.

Tribole, Evelyn. *The Ultimate Omega-3 Diet.* New York: McGraw Hill, 2007, 32, 73, 99, 130, 163–165, 174, 182.

University of New Hampshire. "College Students Face Obesity, High Blood Pressure, Metabolic Syndrome." *ScienceDaily.* June 18, 2007.

Retrieved from https://www.sciencedaily.com/releases/2007/06/070614113310.htm.

US Census Bureau. "Demographic Trends in the 20th Century." 2002.

Vanderhaeghe, Lorna, and Karlene Kasrst. *Healthy Fats For Life: Preventing and Treating Common Health Problems with Essential Fatty Acids.* Hoboken, NJ: Wiley, 2004.

Velasquez-Manoff, Moises. "Are Happy Gut Bacteria Key to Weight Loss?" *Mother Jones,* April 22, 2013.

Wahls, Terry. *The Wahls Protocol.* New York: Avery, 2014, 117.

Wannamethee, Goya, A. Gerald Shaper, Peter H. Whincup, and Mary Walker. "Low Serum Total Cholesterol Concentrations and Mortality in Middle Aged British Men." *British Medical Journal* 311 (1995): 409.

Wilson, Jacque. "Eat More 'Superfoods' to Lose Weight," *CNN,* April 10, 2012. Retrieved from http://www.cnn.com/2012/04/10/health/superfoods-weight-loss-diet/index.html.

Winter, Michael. "Study Links 180,000 Global Deaths to Sugary Drinks." March 19, 2013.

World Health Organization (WHO). "Silver in Drinking Water." Background Document for Development of WHO Guidelines for Drinking-Water Quality. Geneva, Switzerland, 2003.

Wright, Jonathan V., and Lane Lenard. Why Stomach Acid Is Good for You: Natural Relief from Heartburn, Indigestion, Reflux and GERD. Lanham, MD: M. Evans & Co., 2001.

Xu, Qun, and Christine G. "Multivitamin Use and Telomere Length in Women." *American Journal of Clinical Nutrition* 89.6 (June 2009): 1857–1863

Yale Rudd Center. "Added Sugars Fact Sheet." August 2012. Retrieved from http://www.uconnruddcenter.org/files/Pdfs/SSB_AddedSugars.pdf.

Yarrow, Kit. "Paying For a Good Night's Sleep." *Psychology Today*, January 29, 2013. Retrieved from https://www.psychologytoday.com/blog/the-why-behind-the-buy/201301/paying-good-nights-sleep

Zhou, Y., Z. Ning, Y. Lee, B. D. Hambly, and C. S. McLachlan. "Shortened Leukocyte Telomere Length in Type 2 Diabetes Mellitus: Genetic Polymorphisms in Mitochondrial Uncoupling Proteins and Telomeric Pathways." *Clinical and Translational Medicine* 1 (Dec 5, 2016): 8. doi: 10.1186/s40169-016-0089-2.

INDEX

stress management, 165–166
  chiropractic care for,
    168–169
  and emotional acids, 176
  meditation for, 167–168
  and moving more, 169
success, 65
sucralose, 72
sugar(s)
  as acidic food, 67–70
  acids created by, 6
  and Alzheimer's disease, 48
  author's addiction to,
    xii–xiii
  and cancer, 46–47
  cravings for, 74–77, 101
  and exercise, 161–162
  fat burner versus sugar
    burner quiz, 99–100
  fifteen-minute crash, 97
  and obesity in children,
    58–59
  quitting, 114
  as trigger food, 11
sulfur, 125
sulfuric acid, 3, 79
sulfur-rich vegetables, 125
Summer Gazpacho, 216
Summer Greens, Ultimate
  Chilled, 217
sunflower seeds
  Apple Cabbage Salad with
    Beetroot, 211–212
  Green Spring Salad with
    Jalapeño Mint Dressing,
    209
  Raw Chopped Salad
    with Lemon Tarragon
    Dressing, 210–211
supplements, 147–150
sushi
  cravings for, 110–111
  Zucchini Sushi, 205

swap outs, 183
sweet potatoes
  Boneless Broth, 213–214
Sweet Tahini Dip, 228–229
swimming, 161

table salt, 92
tahini
  Carrot Ginger Avocado
    Salad, 212
  Garlic Hummus, 200
  Ginger Cinnamon Fruit
    with Sweet Tahini Dip,
    228–229
  Green Tahini Kale Salad,
    207
  in hummus, 133
  Spiced Cold Tomato
    Ginger Soup, 218
  Tahini Dressing, 207
  Thai Quinoa Salad, 208
Tahini Dressing, 207
tamari
  Carrot Ginger Avocado
    Salad, 212
  Ginger Cinnamon Fruit
    with Sweet Tahini Dip,
    228–229
  Green Tahini Kale Salad,
    207
  Thai Quinoa Salad, 208
tarragon
  Raw Chopped Salad
    with Lemon Tarragon
    Dressing, 210–211
  Spaghetti Squash with
    Marinara, 223–224
teas, 6, 153–154
tea tree oil, 233
telomeres, 36–38
Thai Dressing, 208
Thai Quinoa Salad, 208
thyroid health, 129

Toasted Curry Kale Chips,
  200–201
tomatoes
  Avocado, Tomato, and Red
    Onion Salad, 208–209
  Bloody Mary Smoothie, 195
  Carrot Ginger Avocado
    Salad, 212
  Dr. Daryl's Favorite
    Marinated Kale Salad
    and Dressing, 206
  Green Tahini Kale Salad,
    207
  Quinoa-Stuffed Bell
    Peppers, 224–225
  Savory Avocado Wraps,
    203
  Spaghetti Squash with
    Marinara, 223–224
  Spiced Cold Tomato
    Ginger Soup, 218
  storing, 181
  Summer Gazpacho, 216
  Thai Quinoa Salad, 208
  Zucchini Linguine with
    Spinach Lemon Pesto,
    220–221
toxicity. See also
    environmental acids
  of almonds, 82
  and cancer, 45–46
  daily detox, 151–157
  reducing, 5
trans fats, 83
trigger foods, 11
triglycerides, 42–43
Truth About Cancer, The,
  47–48
Truvia, 73
turmeric, 128, 153–154
turnip and turnip greens
  Boneless Broth, 213–214
type 2 diabetes, 50–52